Biomarkers of Renal Diseases

Biomarkers of Renal Diseases

Editors

Joaquín García-Estañ
Felix Vargas

MDPI • Basel • Beijing • Wuhan • Barcelona • Belgrade • Manchester • Tokyo • Cluj • Tianjin

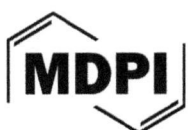

Editors
Joaquín García-Estañ
Universidad de Murcia
Spain

Felix Vargas
Universidad de Granada
Spain

Editorial Office
MDPI
St. Alban-Anlage 66
4052 Basel, Switzerland

This is a reprint of articles from the Special Issue published online in the open access journal *International Journal of Molecular Sciences* (ISSN 1422-0067) (available at: https://www.mdpi.com/si/ijms/Biomarkers_Renal_Diseases).

For citation purposes, cite each article independently as indicated on the article page online and as indicated below:

LastName, A.A.; LastName, B.B.; LastName, C.C. Article Title. *Journal Name* **Year**, *Volume Number*, Page Range.

ISBN 978-3-03943-911-9 (Hbk)
ISBN 978-3-03943-912-6 (PDF)

© 2020 by the authors. Articles in this book are Open Access and distributed under the Creative Commons Attribution (CC BY) license, which allows users to download, copy and build upon published articles, as long as the author and publisher are properly credited, which ensures maximum dissemination and a wider impact of our publications.

The book as a whole is distributed by MDPI under the terms and conditions of the Creative Commons license CC BY-NC-ND.

Contents

About the Editors vii

Preface to "Biomarkers of Renal Diseases" ix

Joaquín García-Estañ and Felix Vargas
Editorial for Special Issue—Biomarkers of Renal Disease
Reprinted from: *Int. J. Mol. Sci.* **2020**, *21*, 8077, doi:10.3390/ijms21218077 1

Koen E. Groeneweg, Jacques M.G.J. Duijs, Barend W. Florijn, Cees van Kooten,
Johan W. de Fijter, Anton Jan van Zonneveld, Marlies E.J. Reinders and Roel Bijkerk
Circulating Long Noncoding RNA LNC-EPHA6 Associates with Acute Rejection after
Kidney Transplantation
Reprinted from: *Int. J. Mol. Sci.* **2020**, *21*, 5616, doi:10.3390/ijms21165616 5

Špela Borštnar, Željka Večerić-Haler, Emanuela Boštjančič, Živa Pipan Tkalec,
Damjan Kovač, Jelka Lindič and Nika Kojc
Uromodulin and microRNAs in Kidney Transplantation—Association with Kidney
Graft Function
Reprinted from: *Int. J. Mol. Sci.* **2020**, *21*, 5592, doi:10.3390/ijms21165592 15

Francesco Guzzi, Luigi Cirillo, Elisa Buti, Francesca Becherucci, Carmela Errichiello,
Rosa Maria Roperto, James P. Hunter and Paola Romagnani
Urinary Biomarkers for Diagnosis and Prediction of Acute Kidney Allograft Rejection:
A Systematic Review
Reprinted from: *Int. J. Mol. Sci.* **2020**, *21*, 6889, doi:10.3390/ijms21186889 27

Marco Quaglia, Guido Merlotti, Gabriele Guglielmetti, Giuseppe Castellano and
Vincenzo Cantaluppi
Recent Advances on Biomarkers of Early and Late Kidney Graft Dysfunction
Reprinted from: *Int. J. Mol. Sci.* **2020**, *21*, 5404, doi:10.3390/ijms21155404 49

Yury E. Glazyrin, Dmitry V. Veprintsev, Irina A. Ler, Maria L. Rossovskaya,
Svetlana A. Varygina, Sofia L. Glizer, Tatiana N. Zamay, Marina M. Petrova,
Zoran Minic, Maxim V. Berezovski and Anna S. Kichkailo
Proteomics-Based Machine Learning Approach as an Alternative to Conventional Biomarkers
for Differential Diagnosis of Chronic Kidney Diseases
Reprinted from: *Int. J. Mol. Sci.* **2020**, *21*, 4802, doi:10.3390/ijms21134802 85

Hee-Sung Ahn, Jong Ho Kim, Hwangkyo Jeong, Jiyoung Yu, Jeonghun Yeom,
Sang Heon Song, Sang Soo Kim, In Joo Kim and Kyunggon Kim
Differential Urinary Proteome Analysis for Predicting Prognosis in Type 2 Diabetes Patients
with and without Renal Dysfunction
Reprinted from: *Int. J. Mol. Sci.* **2020**, *21*, 4236, doi:10.3390/ijms21124236 97

Wei-Cheng Tseng, Ming-Tsun Tsai, Nien-Jung Chen and Der-Cherng Tarng
Trichostatin A Alleviates Renal Interstitial Fibrosis Through Modulation of the M2
Macrophage Subpopulation
Reprinted from: *Int. J. Mol. Sci.* **2020**, *21*, 5966, doi:10.3390/ijms21175966 117

Michele Provenzano, Salvatore Rotundo, Paolo Chiodini, Ida Gagliardi, Ashour Michael, Elvira Angotti, Silvio Borrelli, Raffaele Serra, Daniela Foti, Giovambattista De Sarro and Michele Andreucci
Contribution of Predictive and Prognostic Biomarkers to Clinical Research on Chronic Kidney Disease
Reprinted from: *Int. J. Mol. Sci.* **2020**, *21*, 5846, doi:10.3390/ijms21165846 133

Nadezda Petejova, Arnost Martinek, Josef Zadrazil, Marcela Kanova, Viktor Klementa, Radka Sigutova, Ivana Kacirova, Vladimir Hrabovsky, Zdenek Svagera and David Stejskal
Acute Kidney Injury in Septic Patients Treated by Selected Nephrotoxic Antibiotic Agents—Pathophysiology and Biomarkers—A Review
Reprinted from: *Int. J. Mol. Sci.* **2020**, *21*, 7115, doi:10.3390/ijms21197115 159

Satoshi Washino, Keiko Hosohata and Tomoaki Miyagawa
Roles Played by Biomarkers of Kidney Injury in Patients with Upper Urinary Tract Obstruction
Reprinted from: *Int. J. Mol. Sci.* **2020**, *21*, 5490, doi:10.3390/ijms21155490 175

Félix Vargas, Rosemary Wangesteen, Isabel Rodríguez-Gómez and Joaquín García-Estañ
Aminopeptidases in Cardiovascular and Renal Function. Role as Predictive Renal Injury Biomarkers
Reprinted from: *Int. J. Mol. Sci.* **2020**, *21*, 5615, doi:10.3390/ijms21165615 193

Wojciech Wołyniec, Wojciech Ratkowski, Joanna Renke and Marcin Renke
Changes in Novel AKI Biomarkers after Exercise. A Systematic Review
Reprinted from: *Int. J. Mol. Sci.* **2020**, *21*, 5673, doi:10.3390/ijms21165673 213

Laura Martinez Valenzuela, Juliana Draibe, Xavier Fulladosa and Juan Torras
New Biomarkers in Acute Tubulointerstitial Nephritis: A Novel Approach to a Classic Condition
Reprinted from: *Int. J. Mol. Sci.* **2020**, *21*, 4690, doi:10.3390/ijms21134690 233

Armando Coca, Carmen Aller, Jimmy Reinaldo Sánchez, Ana Lucía Valencia, Elena Bustamante-Munguira and Juan Bustamante-Munguira
Role of the Furosemide Stress Test in Renal Injury Prognosis
Reprinted from: *Int. J. Mol. Sci.* **2020**, *21*, 3086, doi:10.3390/ijms21093086 243

Takahiro Uchida and Takashi Oda
Glomerular Deposition of Nephritis-Associated Plasmin Receptor (NAPlr) and Related Plasmin Activity: Key Diagnostic Biomarkers of Bacterial Infection-related Glomerulonephritis
Reprinted from: *Int. J. Mol. Sci.* **2020**, *21*, 2595, doi:10.3390/ijms21072595 255

About the Editors

Joaquín García-Estañ studied medicine at the University of Murcia in 1974–1980 and began his academic activity in 1982 in the Department of Physiology of the Faculty of Medicine of the University of Murcia. He earned his medical degree in 1986 at the University of Murcia. He completed a postdoctoral stay at the Medical College of Wisconsin (Milwaukee, USA) in 1987 and 1988, under the guidance of Dr. Richard J. Roman. He became Associate Professor of Physiology at the University of Murcia in 1987 and became Full Professor in 2002. Since 1989, he has been Principal Investigator in the Research Group of Physiopathology of the Liver Cirrhosis and Arterial Hypertension. He has been Principal Investigator in 10 research projects funded by the National Plan of Biomedicine, Carlos III Health Institute, and Seneca Foundation since 1989. He has authored or co-authored almost 130 articles and book chapters, many of them in international journals with medium–high impact. He has been the director of nine doctoral theses, four of them receiving the Extraordinary Doctorate Award. He has held the positions of Vice-Dean of the Faculty of Medicine of the University of Murcia (1992–1995), Coordinator of International Relations for the Health Sciences (1992–1999), Coordinator of Curriculum Planning of the Vice-Rectorate of Studies and Postgraduate Studies of the University of Murcia (from July 2002 to March 2006), Dean of the Faculty of Medicine of the University of Murcia (2006–2014), and President of the National Conference of Deans of Spanish Medical Schools (2008–2012). He is the founder (2014) and current secretary of the Center of Studies on Medical Education.

Felix Vargas studied medicine at the University of Granada in 1973–1979 and began his academic activity in 1980 in the Department of Physiology of the Faculty of Medicine of the University of Granada. He earned his doctoral degree in 1984 at the University of Granada. He completed a postdoctoral stay in the Blood Pressure Unit (Glasgow, UK) in 1986, under the guidance of Dr. A. F. Lever. He completed another scientific stay at Paris INSERM Unite 400, directed by Dr. R. P. Garay. He became Associate Professor of Physiology at the University of Granada in 1984 and became Full Professor in 2000. Since 1990, he has been Principal Investigator in the Research Group of Physiopathology of the Thyroid Disorders and Arterial Hypertension. He has completed studies and obtained a patent on the aminopeptidases as early renal biomarkers of renal diseases. He has been Principal Investigator in 10 research projects funded by the National Plan of Biomedicine, Carlos III Health Institute, and the Department of Innovation and Science since 1990. He is a member of the National Group of Investigation of Renal Diseases (REDinREN). He has authored or co-authored almost 135 articles and reviews, many of them in international journals with medium–high impact. He has been the director of 23 doctoral theses, 10 of them receiving the Extraordinary Doctorate Award. He is the coordinator of teaching activities at the Department of Physiology of the University of Granada (2008–2020).

Preface to "Biomarkers of Renal Diseases"

The National Institutes of Health (NIH) Biomarkers Definitions Group has defined a biomarker as "A characteristic that is objectively measured and evaluated as an indicator of normal biologic processes, pathogenic processes, or pharmacologic responses to a therapeutic intervention." For acute or chronic kidney diseases, the ideal biomarker should, among others, show rapid and reliable changes with the progression of the disease and be highly sensitive and specific, be able to detect injury to the different segments of the nephron, and be rapidly and easily measurable. Creatinine, for instance, is not a good renal marker since acute injuries would not show changes in filtration rate until the progression of the disease allows its accumulation. Similarly, in chronic renal disease, the elevation in serum creatinine is a late indicator of the reduction in glomerular filtration. Other conventional biomarkers such as proteinuria, cell cylinders, and fractional excretion of sodium have shown a lack of sensitivity and specificity for the early recognition of acute kidney injury, leading to the need for and the enormous interest surrounding the possibility of using other biomarkers with the ability to perform early detection, differential diagnosis, prognostic assessment, response to treatment, and functional recovery. In this Special Issue, we have published reviews and experimental papers showing significant advances in the field of renal biomarkers.

Joaquín García-Estañ, Felix Vargas
Editors

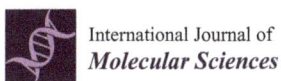

Editorial

Editorial for Special Issue—Biomarkers of Renal Disease

Joaquín García-Estañ [1,*] and Felix Vargas [2,*]

1. Departamento de Fisiologia, Facultad de Medicina, IMIB, Universidad de Murcia, 30120 Murcia, Spain
2. Departamento de Fisiologia, Facultad de Medicina, Universidad de Granada, 18071 Granada, Spain
* Correspondence: jgestan@um.es (J.G.-E.); fvargas@ugr.es (F.V.)

Received: 21 October 2020; Accepted: 27 October 2020; Published: 29 October 2020

The National Institutes of Health (NIH) Biomarkers Definitions Group has defined a biomarker as "A characteristic that is objectively measured and evaluated as an indicator of normal biologic processes, pathogenic processes, or pharmacologic responses to a therapeutic intervention." For acute or chronic kidney diseases, the ideal biomarker should, among others, show rapid and reliable changes with the progression of the disease and be highly sensitive and specific, be able to detect injury to the different segments of the nephron, and be rapidly and easily measurable. Creatinine, for instance, is not a good renal marker since acute injuries would not show changes in filtration rate until the progression of the disease allows its accumulation. Similarly, in chronic renal disease, the elevation in serum creatinine is a late indicator of the reduction in glomerular filtration. Other conventional biomarkers such as proteinuria, cell cylinders, and fractional excretion of sodium have shown lack of sensitivity and specificity for the early recognition of acute kidney injury; hence, leading to the need and the enormous interest surrounding the possibility of using other biomarkers with the ability to perform early detection, differential diagnosis, assessment prognostic, response to treatment, and functional recovery. In this Special Issue [1], we have published reviews or experimental papers showing significant advances in the field of renal biomarkers.

Regarding research articles, we have an interesting contribution by Groeneweg et al. [2] to the topic of rejection of a kidney graft. These authors demonstrate that the use of circulating long noncoding RNAs (lncRNAs) may be a suitable marker for vascular injury in that setting, specially LNC-EPHA6, a substance that has been found to relate to diabetic nephropathy. An additional paper [3] by Borštnar et al., working with microRNAs (miRNAs), concluded that six selected miRNAs (miR-29c, miR-126, miR-146a, miR-150, miR-155, and miR-223) were shown to be independent of kidney graft function, indicating their potential as biomarkers of associated kidney graft disease processes, but using serum uromodulin levels, which were also analyzed, depended entirely on kidney graft function and thus reflected functioning tubules rather than any specific kidney graft injury. In line with these studies, a good review by Guzzi et al. [4] followed the Preferred Reporting Items for Systematic Reviews and Meta-Analysis (PRISMA) guidelines to conclude that urinary C-X-C motif chemokine ligands were the most promising and frequently studied biomarkers for diagnosis and prediction of acute kidney allograft rejection. In the same field, the review by Quaglia and colleagues [5] explores new biomarkers of early and late graft dysfunction, which are very much needed in renal transplants to improve the management of complications and prolong graft survival. Thus, OMIC technology (all technologies aimed at detection of genes (genomics), mRNA (transriptomics), proteins (proteomics) and metabolites (metabolomics)) has allowed the identification of many candidate biomarkers, providing diagnostic and prognostic information at very early stages of pathological processes. Donor-derived cell-free DNA and extracellular vesicles are further promising tools. However, most of these biomarkers still need to be validated in multiple independent cohorts and standardized, and prospective studies are needed to assess whether introduction of these new sets of biomarkers into clinical practice could actually reduce the need for renal biopsy, integrate traditional tools, and ultimately improve graft survival compared to current management.

In an interesting study [6], Glazyrin and coworkers examined several machine learning algorithms linked to a full-proteomic approach, which were examined for the differential diagnosis of chronic kidney disease (CKD) of three origins, diabetic nephropathy, hypertension, and glomerulonephritis—three of the most common causes of CKD. While the group of hypertensive nephropathy could not be reliably separated according to plasma data, this group of hypertensive nephropathy was reliably separated from all other renal patients by urine proteome data. However, the analysis of the entire proteomics data of urine did not allow differentiating between the three diseases. Thus, it seems that the urine proteome, compared with the plasma proteome, is of much less importance. Clearly, this is an area of interest that will benefit from the incorporation of data technicians and proteomic analysts to these hospital services. Additional information came with the results shown in the article by Ahn et al. [7]. They used proteome analysis for the prediction of type 2 diabetic patients with or without renal dysfunction. In the results of these authors, it looks that several proteins (ACP2, CTSA, GM2A, MUC1, and SPARCL1) performed better than mucin-1 or albumin as predictors of direct kidney function in these diabetic patients with kidney impairment.

Tseng et al. [8], in the field of renal fibrosis, showed that histone deacetylase inhibition by trichostatin A significantly attenuated renal fibrosis through promoting an M1(proinflammatory) to M2 (anti-inflammatory) macrophage transition in obstructed kidneys, therefore alleviating the renal fibrosis in obstructed kidneys. However, it is first necessary to establish the role of M2 macrophages regarding its profibrotic or antifibrotic roles.

An important review by Provenzano and coworkers [9] has reported a framework for implementing biomarkers in observational and intervention studies. To that end, biomarkers are classified as either prognostic or predictive, the first type is used to identify the likelihood of a patient to develop an endpoint regardless of treatment, whereas the second type is used to determine whether the patient is likely to benefit from a specific treatment. Thus, the authors revise current biomarkers useful for chronic kidney patients, not only kidney biomarkers but also markers of oxidative stress, tissue remodeling, metabolism, and cardiac biomarkers, together with some important paragraphs on the role, either prognostic or predictive, of proteomics, metabolomics, and genomics. A final page on biomarkers in intervention studies should be of interest to clinical studies and those in the experimental phase of drug development.

The contribution by Petejova et al. [10] covered the pathophysiology of vancomycin and gentamicin nephrotoxicity. In particular, septic acute kidney injury (AKI) and the microRNAs involved in the pathophysiology of both syndromes and also the pathophysiology and potential biomarkers of septic and toxic acute kidney injury in septic patients was studied. In addition, five miRNAs (miR-15a-5p, miR-192-5p, miR-155-5p, miR-486-5p and miR-423-5p) specific to septic and toxic acute kidney injury in septic patients, treated by nephrotoxic antibiotic agents (vancomycin and gentamicin), were identified.

Partial or complete obstruction of the urinary tract is a common and challenging urological condition caused by a variety of conditions, eventually impairing renal function. Washino and coworkers [11] report that biomarkers of acute kidney injury are useful for the early detection and monitoring of kidney injury induced by upper urinary tract obstruction, including levels of neutrophil gelatinase-associated lipocalin (NGAL), monocyte chemotactic protein-1, kidney injury molecule 1, N-acetyl-b-D-glucosaminidase, and vanin-1 in the urine and serum NGAL and cystatin C concentrations.

In a review by the group of Vargas et al. [12], they focused on the role of four aminopeptidases in the control of blood pressure (BP) and renal function and their association with different cardiovascular and renal diseases. Beyond their role as therapeutic tools for BP control and renal diseases, they also explored their role as urinary biomarkers of renal injury in both acute and chronic renal nephropathies, including those induced by nephrotoxic agents, obesity, hypertension, or diabetes.

The review by Wołyniec et al. [13] has identified and analyzed several studies that have studied these markers after physical exercise, concluding that there is evidence that cystatin C is a better indicator of glomerular filtration rate (GFR) in athletes after exercise than creatinine. Additionally, serum and plasma NGAL are increased after prolonged exercise, but the level also depends on inflammation and hypoxia; therefore, it seems that in physical exercise, it is too sensitive for AKI diagnosis. It may, however, help to diagnose subclinical kidney injury, e.g., in rhabdomyolysis. Although urinary biomarkers are increased after many types of exercise, such as NGAL, KIM-1, cystatin-C, L-FABP and interleukin 18, their levels decrease rapidly after exercise; thus, the importance of this short-term increase in AKI biomarkers after exercise lacks a physiological explanation and it merits further studies that show their relation to kidney injury.

In the search for biomarkers of acute tubulointerstitial nephritis, Martinez-Valenzuela and coworkers [14] have summarized the available evidence on this topic, with a special focus on urinary cytokines and chemokines that may reflect kidney local inflammation. However, they conclude that to date, there is a lack of reliable non-invasive diagnostic and follow-up markers and that the gold standard for diagnosis is still kidney biopsy, which shows a pattern of tubulointerstitial leukocyte infiltrate.

Coca et al. have revised the [15] furosemide stress test as a low-cost, fast, safe, and easy-to-perform test to assess tubular integrity, to allow for risk stratification and accurate patient prognosis in the management of patients with kidney disease. However, the findings published so far regarding its clinical use provide insufficient evidence to recommend the generalized application of the test in daily clinical routine, and they recommend the need for standardization in the application of the test in order to facilitate the comparison of results.

Finally, Uchida et al. [16] write about the glomerulonephritis that often develops after the curing of an infection, such as the glomerulonephritis (GN) in children following streptococcal infections (poststreptococcal acute glomerulonephritis, PSAGN). Nephritis-associated plasmin receptor (NAPlr), isolated from the cytoplasmic fraction of group A streptococcus, has been shown to trap plasmin and maintain its activity and was originally considered as a nephritogenic protein for PSAGN. Indeed, NAPlr deposition and related plasmin activity have been observed to have an almost identical distribution in the glomeruli of early phase PSAGN patients at a high frequency. The authors conclude that the interactions among NAPlr, plasmin activity, and the streptococcal cysteine proteinase SpeB, and the association between these elements and complements or immune complexes, both in vitro and in vivo, should be investigated in future studies.

Author Contributions: Both authors have contributed equally. All authors have read and agreed to the published version of the manuscript.

Funding: This research received no external funding.

Conflicts of Interest: The authors declare no conflict of interest.

References

1. Biomarkers of Renal Disease. Special Issue. Available online: https://www.mdpi.com/journal/ijms/special_issues/Biomarkers_Renal_Diseases#published (accessed on 15 October 2020).
2. Groeneweg, K.E.; Duijs, J.M.; Florijn, B.W.; van Kooten, C.; de Fijter, J.W.; van Zonneveld, A.J.; Reinders, M.E.; Bijkerk, R. Circulating Long Noncoding RNA LNC-EPHA6 Associates with Acute Rejection after Kidney Transplantation. *Int. J. Mol. Sci.* **2020**, *21*, 5616. [CrossRef] [PubMed]
3. Borštnar, Š.; Večerić-Haler, Ž.; Boštjančič, E.; Pipan Tkalec, Ž.; Kovač, D.; Lindič, J.; Kojc, N. Uromodulin and microRNAs in Kidney Transplantation—Association with Kidney Graft Function. *Int. J. Mol. Sci.* **2020**, *21*, 5592. [CrossRef] [PubMed]
4. Guzzi, F.; Cirillo, L.; Buti, E.; Becherucci, F.; Errichiello, C.; Roperto, R.M.; Hunter, J.P.; Romagnani, P. Urinary Biomarkers for Diagnosis and Prediction of Acute Kidney Allograft Rejection: A Systematic Review. *Int. J. Mol. Sci.* **2020**, *21*, 6889. [CrossRef] [PubMed]
5. Quaglia, M.; Merlotti, G.; Guglielmetti, G.; Castellano, G.; Cantaluppi, V. Recent Advances on Biomarkers of Early and Late Kidney Graft Dysfunction. *Int. J. Mol. Sci.* **2020**, *21*, 5404. [CrossRef] [PubMed]

6. Glazyrin, Y.E.; Veprintsev, D.V.; Ler, I.A.; Rossovskaya, M.L.; Varygina, S.A.; Glizer, S.L.; Zamay, T.N.; Petrova, M.M.; Minic, Z.; Berezovski, M.V.; et al. Proteomics-Based Machine Learning Approach as an Alternative to Conventional Biomarkers for Differential Diagnosis of Chronic Kidney Diseases. *Int. J. Mol. Sci.* **2020**, *21*, 4802. [CrossRef] [PubMed]
7. Ahn, H.-S.; Kim, J.H.; Jeong, H.; Yu, J.; Yeom, J.; Song, S.H.; Kim, S.S.; Kim, I.J.; Kim, K. Differential Urinary Proteome Analysis for Predicting Prognosis in Type 2 Diabetes Patients with and without Renal Dysfunction. *Int. J. Mol. Sci.* **2020**, *21*, 4236. [CrossRef] [PubMed]
8. Tseng, W.-C.; Tsai, M.-T.; Chen, N.-J.; Tarng, D.-C. Trichostatin A Alleviates Renal Interstitial Fibrosis through Modulation of the M2 Macrophage Subpopulation. *Int. J. Mol. Sci.* **2020**, *21*, 5966. [CrossRef] [PubMed]
9. Provenzano, M.; Rotundo, S.; Chiodini, P.; Gagliardi, I.; Michael, A.; Angotti, E.; Borrelli, S.; Serra, R.; Foti, D.; De Sarro, G.; et al. Contribution of Predictive and Prognostic Biomarkers to Clinical Research on Chronic Kidney Disease. *Int. J. Mol. Sci.* **2020**, *21*, 5846. [CrossRef] [PubMed]
10. Petejova, N.; Martinek, A.; Zadrazil, J.; Kanova, M.; Klementa, V.; Sigutova, R.; Kacirova, I.; Hrabovsky, V.; Svagera, Z.; Stejskal, D. Acute Kidney Injury in Septic Patients Treated by Selected Nephrotoxic Antibiotic Agents—Pathophysiology and Biomarkers—A Review. *Int. J. Mol. Sci.* **2020**, *21*, 7115. [CrossRef] [PubMed]
11. Washino, S.; Hosohata, K.; Miyagawa, T. Roles Played by Biomarkers of Kidney Injury in Patients with Upper Urinary Tract Obstruction. *Int. J. Mol. Sci.* **2020**, *21*, 5490. [CrossRef] [PubMed]
12. Vargas, F.; Wangesteen, R.; Rodríguez-Gómez, I.; García-Estañ, J. Aminopeptidases in Cardiovascular and Renal Function. Role as Predictive Renal Injury Biomarkers. *Int. J. Mol. Sci.* **2020**, *21*, 5615. [CrossRef] [PubMed]
13. Wołyniec, W.; Ratkowski, W.; Renke, J.; Renke, M. Changes in Novel AKI Biomarkers after Exercise. A Systematic Review. *Int. J. Mol. Sci.* **2020**, *21*, 5673.
14. Martinez Valenzuela, L.; Draibe, J.; Fulladosa, X.; Torras, J. New Biomarkers in Acute Tubulointerstitial Nephritis: A Novel Approach to a Classic Condition. *Int. J. Mol. Sci.* **2020**, *21*, 4690. [CrossRef] [PubMed]
15. Coca, A.; Aller, C.; Reinaldo Sánchez, J.; Valencia, A.L.; Bustamante-Munguira, E.; Bustamante-Munguira, J. Role of the Furosemide Stress Test in Renal Injury Prognosis. *Int. J. Mol. Sci.* **2020**, *21*, 3086. [CrossRef] [PubMed]
16. Uchida, T.; Oda, T. Glomerular Deposition of Nephritis-Associated Plasmin Receptor (NAPlr) and Related Plasmin Activity: Key Diagnostic Biomarkers of Bacterial Infection-related Glomerulonephritis. *Int. J. Mol. Sci.* **2020**, *21*, 2595. [CrossRef] [PubMed]

Publisher's Note: MDPI stays neutral with regard to jurisdictional claims in published maps and institutional affiliations.

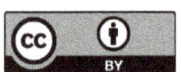

© 2020 by the authors. Licensee MDPI, Basel, Switzerland. This article is an open access article distributed under the terms and conditions of the Creative Commons Attribution (CC BY) license (http://creativecommons.org/licenses/by/4.0/).

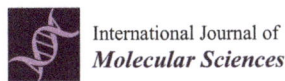

Article

Circulating Long Noncoding RNA LNC-EPHA6 Associates with Acute Rejection after Kidney Transplantation

Koen E. Groeneweg, Jacques M.G.J. Duijs, Barend W. Florijn, Cees van Kooten, Johan W. de Fijter, Anton Jan van Zonneveld, Marlies E.J. Reinders and Roel Bijkerk *

Department of Internal Medicine (Nephrology) and the Einthoven Laboratory for Vascular and Regenerative Medicine, Leiden University Medical Center, Albinusdreef 2, 2333 ZA Leiden, Zuid Holland, The Netherlands; k.e.groeneweg@lumc.nl (K.E.G.); J.M.G.J.Duijs@lumc.nl (J.M.G.J.D.); b.w.florijn@lumc.nl (B.W.F.); C.van_Kooten@lumc.nl (C.v.K.); J.W.de_Fijter@lumc.nl (J.W.d.F.); A.J.van_Zonneveld@lumc.nl (A.J.v.Z.); M.E.J.Reinders@lumc.nl (M.E.J.R.)
* Correspondence: R.Bijkerk@lumc.nl

Received: 29 June 2020; Accepted: 3 August 2020; Published: 5 August 2020

Abstract: Acute rejection (AR) of a kidney graft in renal transplant recipients is associated with microvascular injury in graft dysfunction and, ultimately, graft failure. Circulating long noncoding RNAs (lncRNAs) may be suitable markers for vascular injury in the context of AR. Here, we first investigated the effect of AR after kidney transplantation on local vascular integrity and demonstrated that the capillary density markedly decreased in AR kidney biopsies compared to pre-transplant biopsies. Subsequently, we assessed the circulating levels of four lncRNAs (LNC-RPS24, LNC-EPHA6, MALAT1, and LIPCAR), that were previously demonstrated to associate with vascular injury in a cohort of kidney recipients with a stable kidney transplant function ($n = 32$) and recipients with AR ($n = 15$). The latter were followed longitudinally six and 12 months after rejection. We found higher levels of circulating LNC-EPHA6 during rejection, compared with renal recipients with a stable kidney function ($p = 0.017$), that normalized one year after AR. In addition, LNC-RPS24, LNC-EPHA6, and LIPCAR levels correlated significantly with the vascular injury marker soluble thrombomodulin. We conclude that AR and microvascular injury are associated with higher levels of circulating LNC-EPHA6, which emphasizes the potential role of lncRNAs as biomarker in the context of AR.

Keywords: long noncoding RNA; kidney transplantation; rejection; microvascular injury

1. Introduction

Acute rejection (AR) is considered to be a prominent cause of graft failure in the first year after transplantation in kidney transplant recipients [1,2], although the long-term consequences of AR remain a subject of discussion. Despite better screening and improved immune suppressive therapies, rejection is still suspected to cause a significant proportion of death censored graft failure after kidney transplantation [3,4]. Previous research showed a prolonged effect on kidney function deterioration as well as graft survival after a rejection episode [2]. Microvascular endothelial cells (ECs) are very susceptible to injury, that can result from episodes of AR. Following the alloimmune response, cytokines and growth factors are produced that can lead to EC activation and microvascular destabilization [5–10]. These rejection-associated events can result in perpetual EC damage and promotion of (aberrant) angiogenesis within the allograft [5,7,9]. Together, these insults can lead to the loss of the microvasculature, chronic ischemia and cell death [11,12], and ultimately, to the development of interstitial fibrosis/tubular atrophy and graft dysfunction [5,6,9]. Therefore, monitoring the course of microvascular injury after rejection could be beneficial in deciding on the best treatment strategies. Previously, we found the vascular injury markers soluble thrombomodulin (sTM) and Angiopoietin-2 (Ang-2) to increase upon AR. sTM normalized in the first year after AR, while Ang-2 remained elevated [13]. Noncoding RNA, such as micro RNAs (miRNA) and long noncoding RNAs (lncRNA)are increasingly recognized to play an important role in vascular injury [14]. The functions of lncRNAs appear to be very diverse as they can bind DNA, proteins, and other RNAs. E.g. lncRNAs have been demonstrated to serve as a scaffold for transcription factors or can assist chromatin-modifying enzymes, thereby regulating gene expression [15]. LncRNAs were also found to be important for miRNA processing, (alternative) splicing, translation and post-transcriptional regulation, for instance via sponging miRNAs [16,17]. In addition, lncRNAs can be promising biomarkers in a variety of vascular diseases and kidney injury [14,16]. Furthermore, lncRNAs have previously been associated with AR [18], but their dynamics after rejection have not been studied before. Earlier, we described that specific lncRNAs (MALAT1, LNC-RPS24, LNC-EPHA6, and LIPCAR) associate with microvascular damage and angiogenic factors in patients with diabetic nephropathy that received simultaneous kidney-pancreas transplantation [19], but their relation with AR and associated vascular damage is unclear. As such, in this study we first explored the relation of AR with local microvascular injury. Then, in a cross-sectional study of patients with T cell mediated AR, we analyzed selected vascular injury related lncRNAs as potential biomarkers for vascular damage in the context of kidney transplant rejection and assess the dynamics in these lncRNAs after rejection.

2. Results

2.1. Decreased Capillary Density in Acute Rejection Biopsies

To assess the impact of AR on the local capillary density in the kidney, we quantified the number of endothelial cells (EC) and pericytes in archival acute rejection biopsies by immunohistochemical staining of the EC for CD34 antigen and the pericytes for the CD73 marker (resp. $n = 102$ and $n = 29$). Subsequently, we compared these parameters to the available pre-transplant biopsies (resp. $n = 78$ and $n = 66$) of these patients [20]. Patient characteristics can be found in Supplementary Table S1. As shown in Figure 1, we observed a strong decrease in both the number of endothelial cells (~2.5-fold, mboxemphp < 0.0001) as well as pericytes (~6-fold, $p < 0.0001$) in AR, indicating loss of the peritubular capillary network in AR.

2.2. Patient Characteristics of Cross Sectional and Longitudinal AR Study Population

Next, we sought to investigate the relation of circulating lncRNAs with AR. To that end, we included plasma samples of a different cross-sectional study cohort that included patients with acute T cell mediated rejection and a control group of patients with stable kidney transplant function after transplantation (hereafter mentioned as 'stable'). In addition, AR patients were studied longitudinally at 6 and 12 months after rejection to determine the dynamics after AR. The baseline characteristics of the transplant recipients in this cohort are described in Table 1. Most common causes of initial kidney failure before transplantation were autosomal dominant polycystic kidney disease (23%), focal segmental glomerulosclerosis (17%) and IgA nephropathy (13%). The mean time after transplantation (12 months) was comparable. Immunosuppressive regimen did not differ significantly. eGFR was lower and proteinuria higher in patients with AR, compared with stable patients (resp. $p < 0.001$ and $p = 0.003$). Factors that can influence the amount of vascular injury next to rejection, such as donor age, dialysis before transplantation, and months since transplantation, did not differ significantly. Incidence of active smokers was 7% in AR patients and 13% in stable patients. Panel reactive antibodies (PRA), mismatch, immunosuppressive regimen and the presence of previous transplantations did not differ between stable patients and patients with AR. Patients with AR had interstitial rejection, with or without involvement of the vasculature, and were treated with methylprednisolone (67%), ATG alone (13%), or a combination of methylprednisolone and ATG (13%) or alemtuzumab (13%).

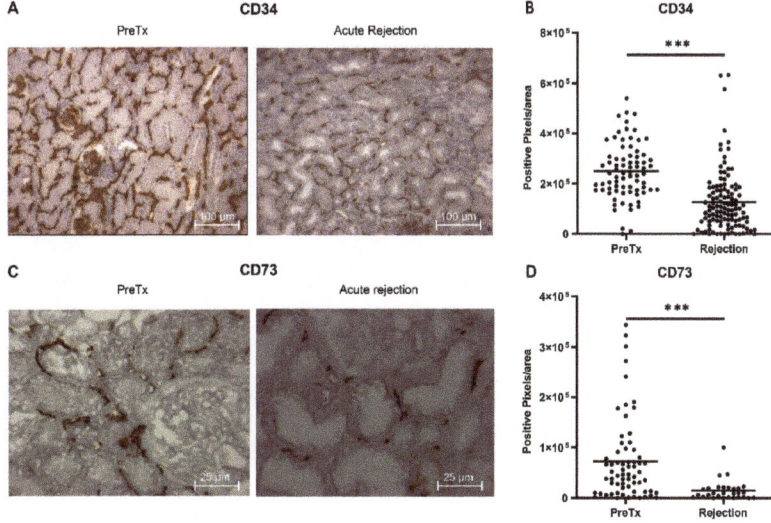

Figure 1. Decreased capillary density after acute rejection. (**A**) Representative images of CD34 staining for pre-transplantation and acute rejection (AR) biopsies. (**B**) Quantification of CD34 staining (PreTx, $n = 78$; AR, $n = 102$). (**C**) Representative images of CD73 staining for pre-transplantation and acute rejection (AR) biopsies. (**D**) Quantification of CD73 staining (PreTx, $n = 66$, AR, $n = 29$). *** p-value < 0.001.

Table 1. Cross-sectional study patient characteristics of patients with a stable kidney transplant function (stable) and patients with acute rejection (AR).

	Stable ($n = 32$)	AR ($n = 15$)	p-Value
Sex, Male, n (%)	21 (66%)	10 (67%)	1.00 [1]
Age, Years ± SD	51 ± 14	54 ± 12	0.35 [2]
BMI (kg/m^2)	26.4 ± 4.6	24.4 ± 3.5	0.15 [1]
Preemptive, n (%)	16 (50%)	5 (33%)	0.36 [1]
Months Since KTx, Median (IQR)	12 ± 1	12 ± 15	0.97 [2]
PRA >5%, n (%)	6 (19%)	1 (7%)	0.40 [1]
Previous Transplantations, n (%) Mismatch A/B/DR, Mean	2 (6%) 1.0/1.2/0.8	3 (20%) 0.9/1.3/1.0	0.31 [1] 0.76/0.81/0.63 [1]
Donor Characteristics Sex, male, n (%) Age, years ± SD	 11 (34%) 50 ± 17	 7 (47%) 47 ± 12	 0.52 [1] 0.64 [2]
Induction Therapy, n (%) Alemtuzumab IL-2 receptor inhibitor	 3 (9%) 29 (91%)	 0 15 (100%)	0.54 [1]
Immunosuppressive Drugs, n (%) Tacrolimus Cyclosporine Prednisone Mycophenolate mofetil Everolimus	 22 (69%) 5 (16%) 32 (100%) 25 (78%) 6 (19%)	 8 (53%) 3 (20%) 14 (93%) 8 (53%) 1 (7%)	 0.20 [1] 1.00 [1] 0.32 [1] 0.07 [1] 0.40 [1]

Table 1. *Cont.*

	Stable ($n = 32$)	AR ($n = 15$)	p-Value
Acute Rejection Therapy, n (%)			
ATG		2 (13%)	
methylprednisolone	-	10 (67%)	
methylprednisolone + ATG	-	2 (13%)	
methylprednisolone + alemtuzumab	-	1 (7%)	
eGFR (mL/min/1.73 m^2)	54 ± 12	34 ± 14	<0.001 [2]
Proteinuria (g/24 h), Median *(IQR)*	0.17 (0.13–0.25)	0.36 (0.23–1.19)	0.003 [3]

[1] Fisher's exact test, [2] unpaired t-test, [3] Mann-Whitney U test, KTx = kidney transplantation, PRA = panel reactive antibody.

2.3. Circulating LNC-EPHA6 Levels Directly Correlate with Acute Rejection

In order to assess the relationship between AR and vascular injury related lncRNAs LNC-RPS24, MALAT1, LNC-EPHA6, and LIPCAR, circulating levels of these lncRNAs were measured in stable patients and AR patients. In this cohort, MALAT1 levels were only detectable in less than 30% of patients and therefore not included in further analyses. Relative expression of circulating LNC-EPHA6 was significantly higher in patients with AR, compared with stable patients ($p = 0.017$; Figure 2). LNC-RPS24 and LIPCAR showed a similar trend, although these differences did not reach statistical significance (resp. $p = 0.11$ and $p = 0.16$).

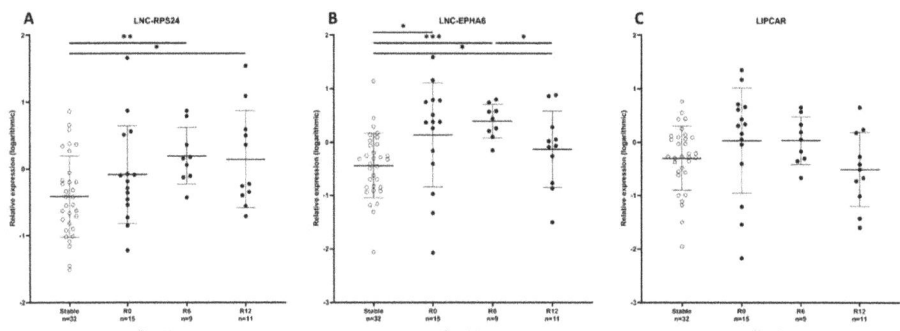

Figure 2. Circulating lncRNA levels are effected by acute rejection. Relative expression of LNC-RPS24 (**A**), LNC-EPHA6 (**B**), and LIPCAR (**C**) in the cross-sectional cohort; kidney recipients with a stable kidney function (Stable; $n = 32$), kidney recipients with acute rejection at the time of rejection (R0), and 6 and 12 months after rejection (R6 and R12). Data are presented as mean ± SD, * p-value < 0.05, ** p-value < 0.01, *** p-value < 0.001.

2.4. Circulating LNC-EPHA6 Decreases in the First Year After Acute Rejection

Since vascular damage persists after a rejection episode, patients with AR were followed longitudinally to study the dynamics of lncRNAs in the first year after AR. Elevated levels of circulating LNC-EPHA6 persisted until six months after AR ($p < 0.001$) and decreased significantly one year after rejection, although LNC-EPHA6 levels at one year after rejection remained slightly higher levels than in stable patients ($p = 0.03$; Figure 2). LIPCAR showed a similar pattern without reaching significance ($p = 0.16$), while LNC-RPS24 increased one year after transplantation (Figure 2). eGFR did not change significantly the year after AR.

2.5. LNC-RPS24, LNC-EPHA6 and LIPCAR Correlate with Soluble Thrombomodulin

In order to analyze the association of lncRNAs with vascular injury due to AR, we studied the correlation of LNC-RPS24, LNC-EPHA6, and LIPCAR with vascular injury markers sTM and Ang-2 that were previously assessed [13]. There, we showed a significant increase of sTM levels in patients with acute rejection, followed by a subsequent normalization one year after transplantation, while the ratio between Ang-2 and Ang-1 (mainly determined by Ang-2) significantly increased during AR without significant changes afterwards. Here, no significant associations were found between LNC-RPS24, LNC-EPHA6, and LIPCAR with Ang-2. However, interestingly, LNC-RPS24, LNC-EPHA6, and LIPCAR correlated positively with sTM (Table 2).

Table 2. Correlation of lncRNAs with vascular injury markers sTM, Ang-2. Values represent correlation coefficient and p-value.

	LNC-RPS24	LNC-EPHA6	LIPCAR
Vascular injury markers			
sTM	0.331 ($p = 0.035$)	0.383 ($p = 0.013$)	0.321 ($p = 0.041$)
Ang-2	ns	ns	ns

sTM = soluble thrombomodulin, Ang-2 = Angiopoietin-2.

3. Discussion

Our study shows that levels of circulating LNC-EPHA6 are significantly higher in patients with T cell-mediated AR after renal transplantation, compared with kidney transplant recipients with a stable allograft function. LNC-EPHA6 remains elevated after AR, followed by a decrease one year after rejection. LIPCAR shows a similar pattern, but did not reach statistical significance. In addition, LNC-EPHA6, LIPCAR, and LNC-RPS24 correlate with the vascular injury marker sTM. This suggests that, in particular, LNC-EPHA6 may be related to microvascular damage, of which we confirmed its relation to AR by demonstrating a significantly lower presence of endothelial cells and pericytes in our renal biopsy study.

LNC-EPHA6 was earlier found to relate to diabetic nephropathy [19], but was not studied in the context of AR before. Our finding of higher LNC-EPHA6 levels in patients with AR compared with patients without AR provided proof of principle of the biomarker potential of lncRNAs in AR. However, here we analyzed four pre-selected lncRNAs, thus analyses of other lncRNAs in AR may yield additional associations and may potentially be important for prediction of (vascular injury after) AR. This is in line with two other studies that showed an association between lncRNAs and AR that suggested their value for diagnosis of AR in kidney transplantation [21,22]. Moreover, in a rat study, the lncRNA PRINS was shown to be significantly up-regulated in kidneys of rats with cold ischemia-elicited allograft rejection, compared with rats without rejection [23]. In addition, lncRNAs may also be of value in predicting the development of chronic damage after kidney transplantation [24].

Interestingly, levels of circulating LNC-EPHA6 decrease after AR, while eGFR remains stable. This substantiates that changes in LNC-EPHA6 are likely not to be related to changes in kidney function, but other factors in the pathogenesis of AR, such as persisting microvascular injury. This suggestion is supported by the strong correlation with sTM. However, although significant differences between immunosuppressive drug regimen were not observed, we cannot exclude that differences in rejection treatment altered levels of circulating lncRNAs. Furthermore, an association with the function of the EPHA6 gene might be possible, since lncRNAs are frequently co-regulated and co-expressed with their neighboring genes [25]. The EPHA6 gene is part of a EPH receptor tyrosine kinases family, and thereby interacts with ephrins which subsequently regulates several cellular processes including angiogenesis [26,27].

LIPCAR showed a similar trend after rejection as LNC-EPHA6. This could suggest a similar association as LNC-EPHA6 with rejection. However, changes in LIPCAR did not reach statistical significance due to a large variation. Analysis of LIPCAR in a larger cohort of patients with AR may confirm the link with vascular injury in rejection, since the size of our groups limits the interpretation of LIPCAR in our study. Circulating LNC-RPS24 was only marginally higher in rejection, but increased six months after year after rejection and remained higher. Although speculative, this may be the result of persistent vascular injury after AR or a consequence of the rejection treatment. Lastly, we found LncRNA MALAT1 to be only detectable in less than 30% of the patients in our cohort. Previously, MALAT1 was however detectable in most diabetes mellitus patients [19], suggesting that diabetes mellitus may increase circulating Malat1 levels. However, next to the previously mentioned limited group size, a relatively large spread of lncRNA levels within groups limits the possibility of drawing robust conclusions. The interpretation of subtle changes (e.g., correlation of lncRNAs with the specific Banff classification score for tubulitis, interstitial inflammation, and intimal arteritis) is difficult and larger groups are necessary for the identification of a specific lncRNA as a novel biomarker. However, differences in lncRNAs levels point out the interesting possible added value of lncRNAs in the context of acute cellular rejection. Identification of lncRNAs in the context of antibody-mediated rejection would be interesting as well, since this rare condition also has major implications for the amount of vascular injury.

In conclusion, LNC-EPHA6 is higher in kidney transplant recipients with rejection, compared with those without. This is the first study that shows changes in vascular injury related lncRNAs the first year after rejection. The results suggest that lncRNAs may reflect (micro)vascular damage in the context of rejection and emphasizes the potential role of lncRNAs as biomarkers to monitor vascular injury in kidney transplant rejection.

4. Materials and Methods

4.1. Renal Biopsy Study

Renal biopsies were selected from patients that had a biopsy proven acute renal allograft rejection, as previously described [20]. Patient and transplantation characteristics are summarized in Supplementary Table S1. Frozen biopsy tissue sections (4 μm) were fixed in acetone, endogenous peroxidase was blocked with H2O2, and slides were blocked with 1% bovine serum albumin and 5% normal human serum in PBS. Sections were then incubated with specific antibodies directed against CD34 (BD Biosciences, Breda, The Netherlands) and CD73 (BD Biosciences, Breda, The Netherlands) followed by appropriate secondary antibodies that were HRP-conjugated (Jackson Immunoresearch, Westgrove, PA, USA). Stainings were visualized using Nova RED (Vector Labs, Peterborough, UK). Quantification of immunohistological staining results was performed using image J software.

4.2. Patient Study Cohort

A total of 47 patients were enrolled in a cross-sectional, observational, single center study. All patients were transplanted between 2006 and 2012 in the Leiden University Medical Center (LUMC) in Leiden, The Netherlands. The cohort consisted of 2 groups, namely renal transplant recipients with AR ($n = 15$) and a control group consisting of renal recipients 12 months after transplantation without rejection and with a stable kidney transplant function ($n = 32$). In addition, recipients from the rejection group were followed longitudinally. Plasma samples were obtained at 6 and 12 months after rejection.

The cohort has been described earlier where analysis of circulating Ang-2 and sTM in plasma was performed [13].

All subjects gave their informed consent for inclusion before they participated in the study. The study was conducted in accordance with the Declaration of Helsinki, and the protocol was approved by the Ethics Committee of The Leiden University Medical Center (P09.141).

4.3. Immunosuppressive Drugs, Rejection and Rejection Treatment

All patients received immunosuppressive drug therapy according to the standard of care at the time of transplantation. IL-2 receptor inhibitor as induction therapy was the standard of care and alemtuzumab was administered in case the treating physician expected a higher risk of rejection. The presence and type of rejection was assessed using the Banff classification. The choice for a specific rejection treatment was made according to the standard of care at the time of rejection [13].

4.4. RNA Isolation

The RNeasy Micro Kit (Qiagen, Venlo, The Netherlands) was used with an adapted protocol, to isolate total RNA from 200 µL plasma. In summary, using 800 trizol µL reagent (Invitrogen, Breda, The Netherlands), the plasma/Trizol sample was centrifuged for 15 min (15,000× g) after the addition of 160 µL chloroform. Then, 100% ethanol (1.5 volume) was added to the aqueous phase and transferred to a MinElute Spin column (Qiagen) followed by centrifugation for 15 s (18,000× g). Subsequently, 700 µL RWT buffer and twice 500 µL RPE buffer was used to wash the column. The column was centrifuged (18,000× g) for 15 s after the first two washing steps and 2 min (18,000× g) after the third washing step. 15 µL RNase-free water was added for elution of the RNA.

4.5. RT-qPCR

To quantify circulating lncRNA levels we performed RT-qPCR. Isolated RNA was reverse transcribed using Iscript (Biorad) according to the protocol of the manufacturer. RT-qPCR of target genes was done using SYBR Green Master Mix (Applied Biosystems, Waltham, MA, USA). The primer sequences of target lncRNAs are given in Supplementary Table S2.

4.6. Statistical Analyses

Categorical data are described as total count and percentages, parametric data as mean ±standard deviation (SD), and non-parametric data as median and interquartile range (IQR). Testing for differences of baseline characteristics was performed by using Fishers exact test for categorical data and the unpaired t test and Mann–Whitney U test for parametric and non-parametric data.

Circulating lncRNA levels were normalized by the double delta CT method to miR-16 and subsequently transformed logarithmically (with base 10). The logarithmic relative expression of all three lncRNAs was normally distributed. In the longitudinal study the data was analyzed by using a linear mixed model analysis. Analysis of correlations between the lncRNAs and vascular markers was performed using Spearman rank correlation.

A p-value < 0.05 was considered to be statistically significant. SPSS version 23.0 (SPSS, Inc., Chicago, IL, USA) was used for the data analysis and Graphpad Prism version 8.0 (Graphpad Prism Software, Inc., San Diego, CA, USA).

Supplementary Materials: Supplementary Materials can be found at http://www.mdpi.com/1422-0067/21/16/5616/s1. Supplementary Table S1: Patient and transplantation characteristics of patients in the renal biopsy study. Supplementary Table S2: Used primer sequences of target lncRNAs.

Author Contributions: Conceptualization, R.B. and A.J.v.Z.; Methodology, R.B.; Software, K.E.G.; Validation K.E.G., R.B. and J.M.G.J.D.; Formal Analysis, K.E.G.; Investigation J.M.G.J.D. and B.W.F.; Resources M.E.J.R.; Data Curation K.E.G.; Writing–Original Draft Preparation K.E.G. and R.B.; Writing–Review & Editing, J.M.G.J.D., B.W.F., C.v.K., J.W.d.F., A.J.v.Z., M.E.J.R. and R.B.; Visualization K.E.G.; Supervision, A.J.v.Z., M.E.J.R. and R.B.; Project Administration K.E.G. and R.B.; Funding Acquisition, A.J.v.Z. and R.B. All authors have read and agreed to the published version of the manuscript.

Funding: This research was supported by a grant from the Dutch Kidney Foundation (grant number 16OKG16). R.B. and A.J.v.Z. are supported by a grant from the European Foundation for the Study of Diabetes (EFSD).

Conflicts of Interest: The authors declare no conflict of interest, besides the funding described above. The Dutch Kidney Foundation and European Foundation for the Study of Diabetes had no role in the design, execution, interpretation, or writing of the study.

References

1. Chand, S.; Atkinson, D.; Collins, C.; Briggs, D.; Ball, S.; Sharif, A.; Skordilis, K.; Vydianath, B.; Neil, D.; Borrows, R. The Spectrum of Renal Allograft Failure. *PLoS ONE* **2016**, *11*, e0162278. [CrossRef]
2. Clayton, P.A.; McDonald, S.P.; Russ, G.R.; Chadban, S.J. Long-Term Outcomes after Acute Rejection in Kidney Transplant Recipients: An ANZDATA Analysis. *J. Am. Soc. Nephrol.* **2019**, *30*, 1697–1707. [CrossRef]
3. El-Zoghby, Z.M.; Stegall, M.D.; Lager, D.J.; Kremers, W.K.; Amer, H.; Gloor, J.M.; Cosio, F.G. Identifying specific causes of kidney allograft loss. *Am. J. Transpl.* **2009**, *9*, 527–535. [CrossRef]
4. Park, W.Y.; Paek, J.H.; Jin, K.; Park, S.B.; Choe, M.; Han, S. Differences in Pathologic Features and Graft Outcomes of Rejection on Kidney Transplant. *Transpl. Proc.* **2019**, *51*, 2655–2659. [CrossRef]
5. Bruneau, S.; Woda, C.B.; Daly, K.P.; Boneschansker, L.; Jain, N.G.; Kochupurakkal, N.; Contreras, A.G.; Seto, T.; Briscoe, D.M. Key Features of the Intragraft Microenvironment that Determine Long-Term Survival Following Transplantation. *Front Immunol.* **2012**, *3*, 54. [CrossRef]
6. Contreras, A.G.; Briscoe, D.M. Every allograft needs a silver lining. *J. Clin. Investig.* **2007**, *117*, 3645–3648. [CrossRef]
7. Denton, M.D.; Davis, S.F.; Baum, M.A.; Melter, M.; Reinders, M.E.; Exeni, A.; Samsonov, D.V.; Fang, J.; Ganz, P.; Briscoe, D.M. The role of the graft endothelium in transplant rejection: Evidence that endothelial activation may serve as a clinical marker for the development of chronic rejection. *Pediatr. Transpl.* **2000**, *4*, 252–260. [CrossRef]
8. Reinders, M.E.; Fang, J.C.; Wong, W.; Ganz, P.; Briscoe, D.M. Expression patterns of vascular endothelial growth factor in human cardiac allografts: Association with rejection. *Transplantation* **2003**, *76*, 224–230. [CrossRef]
9. Reinders, M.E.; Rabelink, T.J.; Briscoe, D.M. Angiogenesis and endothelial cell repair in renal disease and allograft rejection. *J. Am. Soc. Nephrol.* **2006**, *17*, 932–942. [CrossRef]
10. Reinders, M.E.; Sho, M.; Izawa, A.; Wang, P.; Mukhopadhyay, D.; Koss, K.E.; Geehan, C.S.; Luster, A.D.; Sayegh, M.H.; Briscoe, D.M. Proinflammatory functions of vascular endothelial growth factor in alloimmunity. *J. Clin. Investig.* **2003**, *112*, 1655–1665. [CrossRef]
11. Bishop, G.A.; Waugh, J.A.; Landers, D.V.; Krensky, A.M.; Hall, B.M. Microvascular destruction in renal transplant rejection. *Transplantation* **1989**, *48*, 408–414. [CrossRef]
12. Long, D.A.; Norman, J.T.; Fine, L.G. Restoring the renal microvasculature to treat chronic kidney disease. *Nat. Rev. Nephrol.* **2012**, *8*, 244–250. [CrossRef] [PubMed]
13. Bijkerk, R.; Florijn, B.W.; Khairoun, M.; Duijs, J.; Ocak, G.; de Vries, A.P.J.; Schaapherder, A.F.; Mallat, M.J.; de Fijter, J.W.; Rabelink, T.J.; et al. Acute Rejection After Kidney Transplantation Associates With Circulating MicroRNAs and Vascular Injury. *Transpl. Direct.* **2017**, *3*, e174. [CrossRef] [PubMed]
14. Lorenzen, J.M.; Thum, T. Long noncoding RNAs in kidney and cardiovascular diseases. *Nat. Rev. Nephrol.* **2016**, *12*, 360–373. [CrossRef]
15. Vierbuchen, T.; Fitzgerald, K.A. Long non-coding RNAs in antiviral immunity. In *Seminars in Cell and Developmental Biology*; Elsevier: London, England, 2020; E4977.
16. Ignarski, M.; Islam, R.; Müller, R.U. Long Non-Coding RNAs in Kidney Disease. *Int. J. Mol. Sci.* **2019**, *20*, 3276. [CrossRef]
17. Geisler, S.; Coller, J. RNA in unexpected places: Long non-coding RNA functions in diverse cellular contexts. *Nat. Rev. Mol. Cell. Biol.* **2013**, *14*, 699–712. [CrossRef] [PubMed]
18. Nafar, M.; Kalantari, S.; Ghaderian, S.M.H.; Omrani, M.D.; Fallah, H.; Arsang-Jang, S.; Abbasi, T.; Samavat, S.; Dalili, N.; Taheri, M.; et al. Expression Levels of lncRNAs in the Patients with the Renal Transplant Rejection. *Urol. J.* **2019**, *16*, 572–577.
19. Groeneweg, K.E.; Au, Y.W.; Duijs, J.M.; Florijn, B.W.; van Kooten, C.; de Fijter, J.W.; Reinders, M.E.; van Zonneveld, A.J.; Bijkerk, R. Diabetic nephropathy alters circulating long noncoding RNA Levels that normalize following simultaneous pancreas-kidney transplantation. *Am. J. Transpl.* **2020**. [CrossRef]
20. Zuidwijk, K.; de Fijter, J.W.; Mallat, M.J.; Eikmans, M.; van Groningen, M.C.; Goemaere, N.N.; Bajema, I.M.; Van Kooten, C. Increased influx of myeloid dendritic cells during acute rejection is associated with interstitial fibrosis and tubular atrophy and predicts poor outcome. *Kidney Int.* **2012**, *81*, 64–75. [CrossRef]

21. Ge, Y.Z.; Xu, T.; Cao, W.J.; Wu, R.; Yao, W.T.; Zhou, C.C.; Wang, M.; Xu, L.W.; Lu, T.Z.; Zhao, Y.C.; et al. A Molecular Signature of Two Long Non-Coding RNAs in Peripheral Blood Predicts Acute Renal Allograft Rejection. *Cell. Physiol. Biochem.* **2017**, *44*, 1213–1223. [CrossRef]
22. Zou, Y.; Zhang, W.; Zhou, H.H.; Liu, R. Analysis of long noncoding RNAs for acute rejection and graft outcome in kidney transplant biopsies. *Biomark Med.* **2019**, *13*, 185–195. [CrossRef] [PubMed]
23. Zou, X.F.; Song, B.; Duan, J.H.; Hu, Z.D.; Cui, Z.L.; Yang, T. PRINS Long Noncoding RNA Involved in IP-10-Mediated Allograft Rejection in Rat Kidney Transplant. *Transpl. Proc.* **2018**, *50*, 1558–1565. [CrossRef] [PubMed]
24. Xu, J.; Hu, J.; Xu, H.; Zhou, H.; Liu, Z.; Zhou, Y.; Liu, R.; Zhang, W. Long Non-coding RNA Expression Profiling in Biopsy to Identify Renal Allograft at Risk of Chronic Damage and Future Graft Loss. *Appl. Biochem. Biotechnol.* **2020**, *190*, 660–673. [CrossRef]
25. Cabili, M.N.; Trapnell, C.; Goff, L.; Koziol, M.; Tazon-Vega, B.; Regev, A.; Rinn, J.L. Integrative annotation of human large intergenic noncoding RNAs reveals global properties and specific subclasses. *Genes Dev.* **2011**, *25*, 1915–1927. [CrossRef]
26. Das, G.; Yu, Q.; Hui, R.; Reuhl, K.; Gale, N.W.; Zhou, R. EphA5 and EphA6: Regulation of neuronal and spine morphology. *Cell Biosci.* **2016**, *6*, 48. [CrossRef]
27. Li, S.; Ma, Y.; Xie, C.; Wu, Z.; Kang, Z.; Fang, Z.; Su, B.; Guan, M. EphA6 promotes angiogenesis and prostate cancer metastasis and is associated with human prostate cancer progression. *Oncotarget* **2015**, *6*, 22587–22597. [CrossRef] [PubMed]

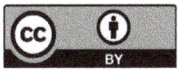

© 2020 by the authors. Licensee MDPI, Basel, Switzerland. This article is an open access article distributed under the terms and conditions of the Creative Commons Attribution (CC BY) license (http://creativecommons.org/licenses/by/4.0/).

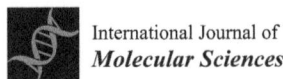 International Journal of
Molecular Sciences

Article

Uromodulin and microRNAs in Kidney Transplantation—Association with Kidney Graft Function

Špela Borštnar [1,2], Željka Večerić-Haler [1,2], Emanuela Boštjančič [3], Živa Pipan Tkalec [3], Damjan Kovač [1,2], Jelka Lindič [1,2] and Nika Kojc [3,*]

[1] Department of Nephrology, University Medical Centre Ljubljana, Zaloška 7, 1000 Ljubljana, Slovenia; spela.borstnar@kclj.si (Š.B.); zeljka.veceric@gmail.com (Ž.V.-H.); damjan.kovac@kclj.si (D.K.); jelka.lindic@kclj.si (J.L.)
[2] Faculty of Medicine, University of Ljubljana, Vrazov trg 2, 1000 Ljubljana, Slovenia
[3] Institute of Pathology, Faculty of Medicine, University of Ljubljana, Korytkova 2, 1000 Ljubljana, Slovenia; emanuela.bostjancic@mf.uni-lj.si (E.B.); ziva.pipan-tkalec@mf.uni-lj.si (Ž.P.T.)
* Correspondence: nika.kojc@mf.uni-lj.si; Tel.: +386-1-543-7125

Received: 30 June 2020; Accepted: 30 July 2020; Published: 5 August 2020

Abstract: Uromodulin and microRNAs (miRNAs) have recently been investigated as potential biomarkers for kidney graft associated pathology and outcome, with a special focus on biomarkers indicating specific disease processes and kidney graft survival. The study's aim was to determine whether expression of serum uromodulin concentration and selected miRNAs might be related to renal function in kidney transplant recipients (KTRs). The uromodulin concentration and expression of six selected miRNAs (*miR-29c*, *miR-126*, *miR-146a*, *miR-150*, *miR-155*, and *miR-223*) were determined in the serum of 100 KTRs with stable graft function and chronic kidney disease of all five stages. Kidney graft function was estimated with routine parameters (creatinine, urea, cystatin C, and Chronic Kidney Disease Epidemiology Collaboration study equations) and precisely measured using chromium-51 labelled ethylenediaminetetraacetic-acid clearance. The selected miRNAs were shown to be independent of kidney graft function, indicating their potential as biomarkers of associated kidney graft disease processes. In contrast, the serum uromodulin level depended entirely on kidney graft function and thus reflected functioning tubules rather than any specific kidney graft injury. However, decreased concentrations of serum uromodulin can be observed in the early course of tubulointerstitial injury, thereby suggesting its useful role as an accurate, noninvasive biomarker of early (subclinical) kidney graft injury.

Keywords: microRNA; uromodulin; kidney graft function; biomarker; kidney transplantation

1. Introduction

Serum creatinine, urea, cystatin C, and estimation of glomerular filtration rate (GFR) via different equations are currently routinely used biomarkers of kidney graft function in clinical transplantation. Although they are characterized by low cost and rapid accessibility of results, these biomarkers are significantly less sensitive and specific than the aggressive and time-consuming gold standard, i.e., the measurement of GFR by an exogenous marker, such as chromium-51-ethylenediaminetetraacetic acid (^{51}CrEDTA). Many new candidate biomarkers in kidney transplantation have been proposed and tested in recent years, which address specific pathologic processes and not merely glomerular, tubular, or overall kidney graft function. Uromodulin (also known as Tamm–Horsfall's protein) is a urinary mucoprotein that is synthesized only in the thick ascending limb of Henle's loop and early distal convoluted tubules of the kidneys [1]. In addition to this classical tubular secretion, to a minor degree uromodulin also sorts to the basolateral pole of tubular epithelial cells, as shown by its presence in circulation [2]. The reduced number of tubular cells seen in chronic kidney disease (CKD) due to interstitial fibrosis/tubular atrophy (IF/TA) is paralleled by the reduced urinary and serum concentrations of uromodulin [3–5]. The potential utility of serum [4,6,7] and urine [8] uromodulin measurement in kidney transplant recipients (KTRs) has been studied, showing an association of lower serum uromodulin levels with progression to end-stage renal disease and graft failure. Although normative ranges for serum/plasma uromodulin concentration were established over 30 years ago, its characteristics have not yet been sufficiently identified as a priority in certain instances, resulting in a failure to fully implement uromodulin in clinical practice.

MicroRNAs (miRNAs) are short, endogenous non-coding ribonucleic acids (RNAs) involved in the modulation of gene expression, mainly by inhibition of messenger RNA translation [9,10]. Recent studies have indicated an association of miRNAs with pathological processes following kidney transplantation, such as T-cell or antibody-mediated rejection, delayed graft function, and IF/TA [9–11]. The diagnostic accuracy of such molecules as biomarkers is still questionable, since many of them emerge on the vascular side of the glomerular filtration barrier and can therefore reflect glomerular filtration rather than a specific disease process. We have focused on searching for miRNAs that were among the most studied in the context of fibrosis (anti-fibrotic *miR-29c*) [12], endothelial dysfunction (*miR-126*) [13–15], and immune response (*miR-146a*) [16,17], or might even be involved in more than one physiological and/or pathogenetic process, e.g., *miR-150* [18,19], *miR-155* [16,17], and *miR-223* [20–22]. Moreover, our previous pilot research on miRNA association with certain most common kidney graft pathologies, such as kidney graft rejection and the recurrence of primary glomerular disease, offered interesting insights into a possible connection of selected miRNAs with underlying kidney graft pathology. For details, see also Supplementary Table S1 and Figure S1.

In this study, we investigated the association of serum uromodulin concentration (s-Uromodulin) (which emerges on the urinary side of the filtration barrier) and selected miRNAs (which emerge on the vascular side of the glomerular filtration barrier) with standard biomarkers of kidney graft function, including measurement of ^{51}CrEDTA clearance. The study's aim was firstly to investigate whether any of the proposed biomarkers are associated with the glomerular filtration and renal function in KTRs. Based on these results, the proposed biomarkers could or could not be a reliable indicator of kidney graft associated disease processes. The possible association of reliable biomarker(s) with the course of the associated disease process and kidney graft outcome is a long-term aim of this study protocol.

2. Results

2.1. Characteristics of the Study Population

The study included 100 KTRs, all Caucasian, 55 men and 45 women. The mean age was 55 ± 11 years (range 19 to 79 years). The average time from transplantation was 10 ± 7 years (range 2 to 28 years). The cohort included in the analysis had chronic kidney disease of transplanted kidney (CKD-T) of all five stages, including patients just before starting renal replacement therapy. The data presenting parameters of GFR are shown in Figure 1.

For investigation of uromodulin, the study included also 15 patients with non-kidney diseases, all Caucasian, 7 men and 8 women. The mean age was 43 ± 13 years (range 20 to 58 years).

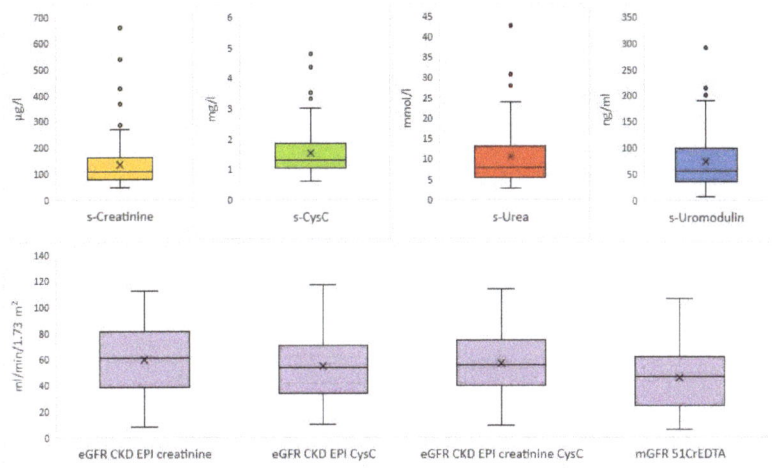

Figure 1. Boxplots for each parameter of glomerular filtration rate. Boxplots for serum creatinine concentration (s-Creatinine), serum cystatin C concentration (s-CysC), serum urea concentration (s-Urea), serum uromodulin concentration (s-Uromodulin), estimated glomerular filtration rate with Chronic Kidney Disease Epidemiology Collaboration study formula with s-Creatinine (eGFR CKD EPI creatinine), estimated glomerular filtration rate with Chronic Kidney Disease Epidemiology Collaboration study formula with s-CyC (eGFR CKD EPI CysC), estimated glomerular filtration rate with Chronic Kidney Disease Epidemiology Collaboration study formula with s-Creatinine and s-CysC (eGFR CKD EPI creatinine CysC), and measured glomerular filtration rate with Chromium-51-ethylenediaminetetraacetic acid clearance (mGFR ^{51}CrEDTA).

2.2. Relation between Kidney Function Parameters and s-Uromodulin

In the control group, the mean level of s-Uromodulin was 291 ± 71 ng/mL. S-Uromodulin levels decreased significantly in the group of KTRs ($p < 0.001$), in which the mean s-Uromodulin was 74 ± 53 ng/mL. We further analyzed s-Uromodulin in different stages of CKD-T (1–5, based on measured GFR with ^{51}CrEDTA (mGFR ^{51}CrEDTA)), in relation to the s-Uromodulin in the control group. We found that already in stage 1 of CKD-T, the s-Uromodulin significantly dropped compared to the control group ($p = 0.013$). In the other four stages (2–4), the significance of reduced s-Uromodulin compared to that in the control group was even lower ($p < 0.001$). Between CKD-T stage 1 and 2, the drop of s-Uromodulin showed borderline significance ($p = 0.067$), while s-Uromodulin was significantly lower in CKD-T stage 2 compared to CKD-T stage 3 ($p < 0.05$) and in CKD-T stage 3 compared to CKD-T stage 4 ($p < 0.05$). There were no significant differences between stages CKD-T 4 and 5 (Figure 2A).

According to receiver operating characteristics (ROC), the area under the curve (AUC) represents the probability that a randomly selected patient will have a lower or higher test result than a randomly selected control. The ROC curve of s-Uromodulin in KTRs demonstrated an AUC of 0.991 (SE-0.007) (95% CI 0.977–1.00, $p < 0.001$) at an optimal cut-off of 191.5 ng/mL with 97% sensitivity and 100% specificity (Figure 2B).

Analyzing bivariate correlations using Spearman's correlation coefficient, s-Uromodulin was significantly associated with all parameters of kidney graft function. The highest correlation coefficient was noted for estimated glomerular filtration rate (eGFR) with Chronic Kidney Disease Epidemiology Collaboration study formula with serum creatinine concentration (s-Creatinine) and serum cystatin C concentration (s-CysC) (eGFR CKD EPI creatinine CysC) (Rho = 0.758, $p < 0.001$), followed by serum urea concentration (s-Urea) (Rho = −0.740, $p < 0.001$), eGFR with Chronic Kidney Disease Epidemiology

Collaboration study formula with s-Creatinine (eGFR CKD EPI creatinine) (Rho = −0.736, $p < 0.001$), s-CysC (Rho = −0.720, $p < 0.001$), eGFR with Chronic Kidney Disease Epidemiology Collaboration study formula with s-CysC (eGFR CKD EPI CysC) (Rho = 0.718, $p < 0.001$), s-Creatinine (Rho = −0.698, $p < 0.001$), and mGFR ^{51}CrEDTA (Rho = 0.669, $p < 0.001$) (Table 1).

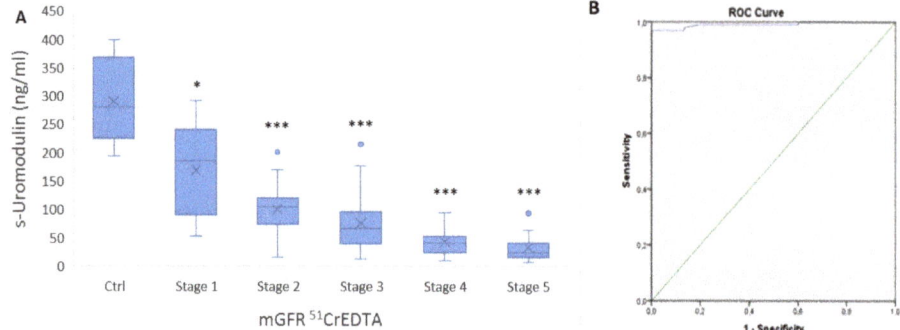

Figure 2. Uromodulin concentration in serum. (**A**) The boxplots for serum uromodulin concentration (s-Uromodulin) in chronic kidney disease of transplanted kidney (CKD-T) stages 1–5 based on measured GFR with ^{51}CrEDTA (mGFR ^{51}CrEDTA) (stage 1, $n = 5$; stage 2, $n = 21$; stage 3, $n = 43$; stage 4, $n = 17$; and stage 5, $n = 11$, with mGFR ^{51}CrEDTA not possible to perform for 3 patients) in comparison to the control group (Ctrl); (**B**) ROC curve and AUC distinguishing CKD-T from the control group without any renal diseases. Legend: * $p < 0.05$, *** $p < 0.001$ (Ctrl versus Stage 1–5).

Table 1. Bivariate correlations between serum uromodulin concentration (s-Uromodulin) and parameters of kidney graft function: serum creatinine concentration (s-Creatinine), serum cystatin C concentration (s-CysC), serum urea concentration (s-Urea), estimated glomerular filtration rate with Chronic Kidney Disease Epidemiology Collaboration study formula with s-Creatinine (eGFR CKD EPI creatinine), estimated glomerular filtration rate with Chronic Kidney Disease Epidemiology Collaboration study formula with s-CysC (eGFR CKD EPI CysC), estimated glomerular filtration rate with Chronic Kidney Disease Epidemiology Collaboration study formula with s-Creatinine and s-CysC (eGFR CKD EPI creatinine CysC) and measured GFR with Chromium-51-ethylenediaminetetraacetic acid (mGFR ^{51}CrEDTA).

Parameters of Kidney Graft Function	Spearman Correlation to s-Uromodulin	p
s-Creatinine	−0.698	<0.001
s-CysC	−0.720	<0.001
s-Urea	−0.740	<0.001
eGFR CKD EPI creatinine	0.736	<0.001
eGFR CKD EPI CysC	0.718	<0.001
eGFR CKD EPI creatinine CysC	0.758	<0.001
mGFR ^{51}CrEDTA	0.669	<0.001

2.3. Relation between Kidney Function Parameters and Expression of Selected miRNAs

While *miR-126*, *miR-146a*, and *miR-150* were expressed in all 100 samples of serum, *miR-29c*, *miR-155*, and *miR-223* were not expressed in 12, 8, and 8 serum samples, respectively. Using the Pearson correlation coefficient, none of the six analyzed miRNAs significantly correlated with the parameters of kidney graft function (Figure 3).

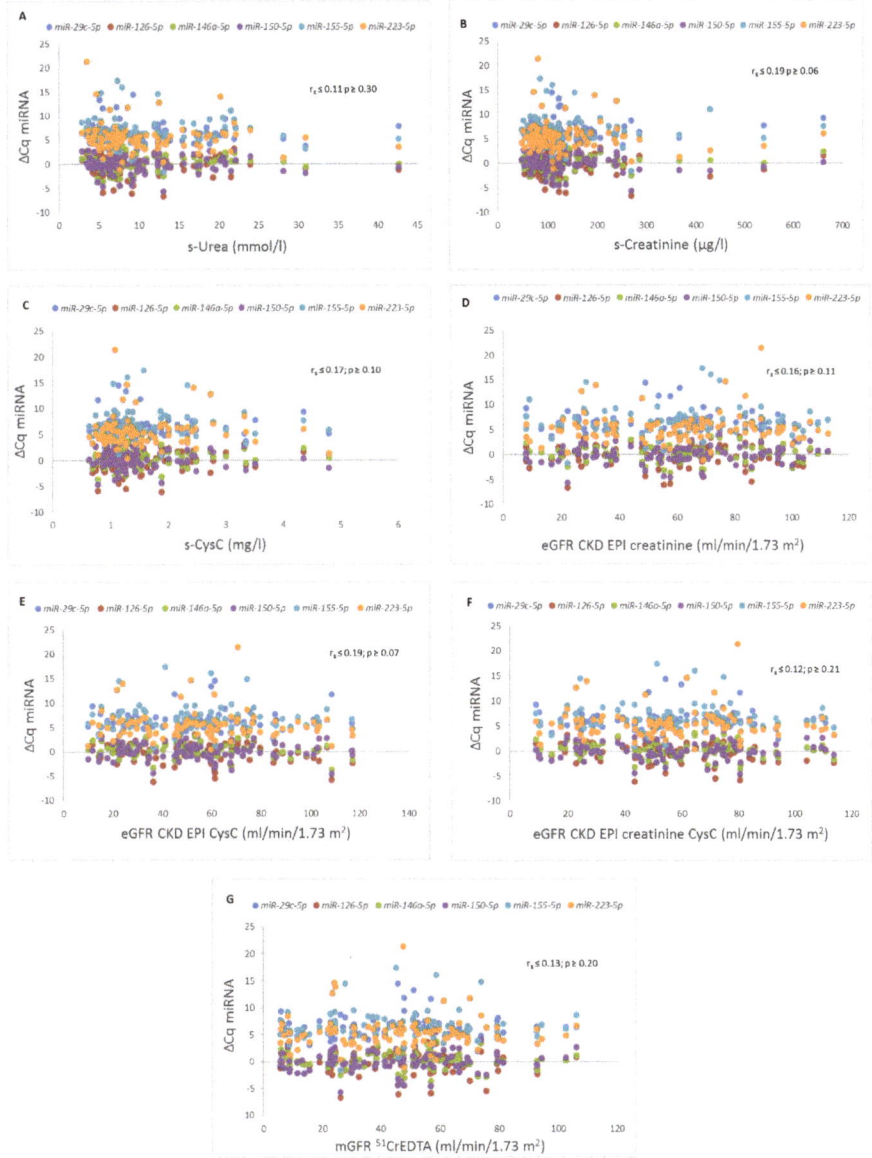

Figure 3. Correlations between different microRNAs (miRNAs) and parameters of kidney graft function. Correlation between different miRNAs and (**A**) serum urea concentration (s-Urea), (**B**) serum creatinine concentration (s-Creatinine), (**C**) serum cystatin C concentration (s-CysC), (**D**) estimated glomerular filtration rate with Chronic Kidney Disease Epidemiology Collaboration study formula with s-Creatinine (eGFR CKD EPI creatinine), (**E**) estimated glomerular filtration rate with Chronic Kidney Disease Epidemiology Collaboration study formula with s-CysC (eGFR CKD EPI CysC), (**F**) estimated glomerular filtration rate with Chronic Kidney Disease Epidemiology Collaboration study formula with s-Creatinine and s-CysC (eGFR CKD EPI creatinine CysC), (**G**) measured glomerular filtration rate with Chromium-51-ethylenediaminetetraacetic acid clearance (mGFR ^{51}CrEDTA).

3. Discussion

Although extensive scientific effort has been focused on developing biomarkers to detect kidney allograft disease processes such as rejection or IF/TA, few assays have moved from the research arena to clinical routine. The obstacle to the successful initiation of their clinical use is the still insufficiently validated specificity for renal pathology. Similar to other molecules and proteins, these biomarkers are also subject to glomerular filtration, tubular secretion, and reabsorption. Many of them, depending on the site of their production and paths of elimination, probably reflect merely kidney function and not disease. The identification of sensitive biomarkers able to reflect the subclinical steps of a pathologic process, such as rejection, is therefore of the utmost relevance to recipients of kidney transplants [23–25].

Our research confirmed previous reports showing significantly higher s-Uromodulin in healthy controls (patients without kidney disease) compared to KTRs, who in general belong to the group of CKD patients [4,5,26]. In line with the findings of other similar research in patients with kidney transplants [6], s-Uromodulin levels in our KTRs decreased stepwise from those with almost preserved graft function to the lowest values in KTRs with pre-dialysis CKD-T. We also showed in this study that s-Uromodulin correlates with all parameters of kidney graft function, the strongest association being observed for eGFR CKD EPI creatinine CysC, followed by the serum level of urea, eGFR CKD EPI creatinine, serum level of CysC, eGFR CKD EPI CysC, serum level of creatinine, and ^{51}CrEDTA. Decreased s-Uromodulin was observed in the earliest stages of CKD-T when other markers, such as serum creatinine and even the precise method of GFR determination with ^{51}CrEDTA, had still not crossed the reference range. This indicates that reabsorption of uromodulin, which is exclusively a product of tubules, is probably compromised from the earliest stages of tubulo-interstitial injury. Reduced s-Uromodulin may therefore be a more sensitive indicator of early kidney graft dysfunction not detected by serum glomerular filtration markers. In view of the simple routine of s-Uromodulin measurement and its low costs, monitoring the dynamics of s-Uromodulin concentration may serve as an accurate, noninvasive predictive biomarker of kidney graft injury and outcome.

Given that the concentration of uromodulin strongly reflects renal function, one would assume that it would never be able to act as a reliable parameter of specific kidney graft pathology. However, exceptions have already been found in the field of specificity for certain pathologies of native kidneys, such as gout [27] or Balkan nephropathy [2]. Accordingly, in the case of kidney transplantation, s-Uromodulin could be especially useful to clinicians aware of the advantages of biomarkers reflecting subclinical tubular injury. Regular s-Uromodulin checkups in KTRs could, in our opinion, become a useful tool for early detection of subclinical processes involving tubules and interstitium (such as acute tubulointerstitial rejection), or timely surveillance of IF/TA. This assumption, however, needs further exploration.

The miRNAs investigated in the present study have so far been extensively related to various physiological and pathological states of kidney graft pathology (see also Supplementary Table S1). We did not observe any association between the circulating levels of selected miRNAs (*miR-29c*, *miR-126*, *miR-146a*, *miR-150*, *miR-155*, and *miR-223*) and kidney graft function (estimated and measured by the reference method at the same time point of miRNA analysis). Previously published studies have shown that the expression of some miRNAs, such as *miR-126* or *miR-223*, is associated with renal function in an up- or downregulated manner [11,15,28]. However, many of those studies were performed with patients with CKD without kidney transplants [15] and/or focused on the functionally unstable period of delayed graft function immediately after transplantation [11,17]. The essential advantage of our analysis is that we used the reference method for GFR measurement (^{51}CrEDTA) and not only routinely used noninvasive biomarkers and/or GFR equations, but the patient cohort in this study was also larger than in most of the so far published research in the field of biomarkers in kidney transplantation [10,11,17,28].

Since selected miRNAs are independent of kidney graft function, they can be reliably used as biomarkers of various pathological processes in KTRs without adjustments to kidney function. In line with previous findings, the results of our pilot study performed on a subgroup of patients with indications of kidney graft biopsy showed a significant association with the miRNAs selected here, with histologically proven antibody-mediated kidney graft rejection and recurrence of primary glomerulonephritis. In this regard, *miR-29c* expression especially has shown potential for differentiating between these two pathologies (see also Supplementary Figure S1). Unfortunately, the sample examined was too small for reliable inference, but nevertheless pointed to the feasibility of conducting further prospective analysis with systematic serum sampling for miRNA determination and planned implementation of kidney graft biopsy, which is the long term aim of this study.

4. Materials and Methods

A prospective clinical study (NCT04413916) was conducted at the Department of Nephrology, University Medical Centre Ljubljana, Slovenia and the Institute of Pathology, Faculty of Medicine, University of Ljubljana. The study was approved by the National Medical Ethics Committee of the Republic of Slovenia (permit number 24k/06/12 approved on 15/06/2012 and 0120-625/2017/4 on 18/12/2017 (revised version number 0120-625/2017/11 on 12/12/2019)) and conducted in accordance with the Declaration of Helsinki. All patients signed informed consent.

4.1. Study Population Inclusion and Exclusion Criteria

The study included 100 kidney transplant recipients from the Slovenian Center for Kidney Transplantation. Inclusion criteria were stable graft function for more than 3 months (changes in creatinine concentration < 20%) and a time of transplantation at least two years before the study entry, since we wanted to study the expression of miRNAs in stable conditions and eliminate the influence of recent transplantation, replacement therapy, and rapid changes in renal function. The subsequent data analysis revealed unstable graft function in only one patient. Exclusion criteria were an age less than 18 years, symptomatic heart failure, malignancy, pregnancy or lactation, newly introduced drugs that may affect the function of the graft, and treatment with trimethoprim-sulfamethoxazole or cimetidine. As a control group, 15 patients with non-kidney diseases were included (nonspecific skin lesions $n = 13$, erosive stomatitis $n = 1$, and paraneoplastic dermatitis $n = 1$).

4.2. Measurement of Serum Creatinine, Serum Urea, and Cystatin C Concentration

Blood sampling was performed on the same day as the measurement of GFR ^{51}CrEDTA clearance, but before the injection of ^{51}CrEDTA. S-Creatinine was measured with the kinetic colorimetric compensated Jaffe assay (Siemens Healthcare Diagnostics Inc., Tarrytown, NY, USA) and with a calibrator traceable to primary reference material with values assigned by isotope dilution mass spectrometry [29]. S-CysC was measured using the particle-enhanced immunonephelometric method (Siemens Healthcare Diagnostics, Marburg, Germany) [30]. S-urea was determined by a Roch-Ramel enzyme reaction with urease and glutamate dehydrogenase (Siemens Healthcare Diagnostics Inc., Tarrytown, NY, USA).

4.3. eGFR

eGFR was calculated using Chronic Kidney Disease Epidemiology Collaboration study formulae with s-Creatinine (eGFR CKD EPI creatinine) and s-CysC (eGFR CKD EPI CysC) or with both s-Creatinine and s-CysC (eGFR CKD EPI creatinine CysC) [31].

4.4. Measurement of ^{51}CrEDTA Clearance

mGFR ^{51}CrEDTA was determined from a single ^{51}CrEDTA injection (activity 3 MBq) and four blood samples taken 120, 180, 240, and 300 min after intravenous application of the marker according to British Nuclear Medicine Society guidelines, using the By weight method. Samples were measured using a gamma counter (Hidex, Turku, Finland); mGFR ^{51}CrEDTA was calculated and then adjusted to the patient's body surface area (Haycock formula) and specified as mL/min/1.73 m^2 [32].

4.5. Measurement of s-Uromodulin

S-Uromodulin was assessed in 20 controls and in 100 KTRs. All serum samples were stored at −80 °C before measurements were performed. Measurements of s-Uromodulin were performed using commercial ELISA (Euroimmun, Medizinische Labordiagnostika AG, Lübeck, Germany), as described previously, based on the manufacturer's instructions [5]. Characteristics of the ELISA were as follows, given by the manufacturer: detection limit for plasma samples 2 ng/mL; mean linearity recovery 97% (83–107% at 59–397 ng/mL); intra-assay precision 1.8–3.2% (at 30–214 ng/mL); inter-assay precision 6.6–7.8% (at 35–228 ng/mL); and inter-lot precision 7.2–10.1% (at 37–227 ng/mL). Data analysis was performed using the program Analysis Software Gen5 (Gen5 2.09, BioTek).

4.6. miRNA Quantification

Total RNA isolation was performed using 200 μL of serum and a miRNeasy serum/plasma advanced kit (Qiagen, Hilden, Germany) according to the manufacturer's protocol. Elution was performed using 20 μL of RNAse-free water. The successful isolation procedure was confirmed by adding spike-ins and subsequent quantification of these spike-ins.

miRNAs *miR-29c*, *miR-126*, *miR-146a*, *miR-150*, *miR-155*, and *miR-223* were analyzed using the miRCURY LNA miRNA PCR system (Qiagen, Hilden, Germany). As the reference genes, *miR-103a-3p*, *miR-191*, and *miR-423* were used according to the manufacturer's instruction. The possibility of hemolysis was excluded by quantifying *miR-23a* and *miR-451a*. All the reagents were from Qiagen, except where otherwise indicated. qPCR was carried out using Rotor Gene Q.

For reverse transcription, a miRCURY LNA RT Kit was used in a 10 μL reaction master mix containing 2 μL of total RNA, according to the manufacturer's instructions. The resulting reverse transcription was diluted 20-fold and 3 μL was used in a 10 μL reaction master mix, according to the manufacturer's instructions. All the qPCR reactions were performed in duplicate. Prior to qPCR, RNA samples were pooled, followed by RT and qPCR as described above. Efficiency was tested for each analyzed miRNA using 10-fold dilutions and qPCR was performed in triplicate. The signal was collected at the endpoint of every cycle. Following amplification, melting curve analysis of PCR products was performed to verify the specificity and identity. Melting curves were acquired on the SYBR channel using a ramping rate of 0.7 °C/60 s for 60–95 °C.

4.7. Statistical Analysis

Correlations were analyzed using Spearman's rank correlation coefficient (Spearman's rho) or the Pearson correlation coefficient. To present relative gene expression, ΔCq was calculated for miRNA expression [33]. The *t*-test was used to calculate the difference between the expression of uromodulin between the control group and the kidney transplant group. For all statistical analyses, SPSS analytical software (IBM SPSS statistics, version 24.0, Armonk, NY, USA) was used with a cut-off point at $p < 0.05$.

5. Conclusions

In the present study, we evaluated six selected miRNAs (*miR-29c*, *miR-126*, *miR-146a*, *miR-150*, *miR-155*, and *miR-223*) and s-Uromodulin as biomarkers of kidney function in KTRs. The selected miRNAs and s-Uromodulin were compared not only with conventional GFR biomarkers (creatinine, cystatin, and estimated GFR), but also, as a novelty, with the radioisotope method, providing significant reinforcement to the credibility of the findings. To the best of our knowledge, this is the first study to compare these markers with the clinical gold standard of GFR (i.e., ^{51}CrEDTA clearance) in KTRs.

In brief, the selected miRNAs are independent of kidney graft function, indicating their potential as biomarkers of associated etiopathogenesis of kidney graft disease processes. In contrast, s-Uromodulin is dependent on all observed parameters of kidney graft function. However, s-Uromodulin reliably reflects the early stages of kidney graft disfunction, in which conventional GFR-related biomarkers, including ^{51}Cr EDTA, are still within normal limits. Since uromodulin is synthetized exclusively within tubules, though it is not a disease-specific marker, it can point to a predominantly tubular injury. Further research is needed to explore the timely expression of uromodulin and miRNAs associated with transplant pathology patterns, in order to detect kidney allograft pathology on a subclinical level, tailor response to therapy, and predict graft outcome.

Supplementary Materials: Supplementary materials can be found at http://www.mdpi.com/1422-0067/21/16/5592/s1, Table S1: Association of selected miRNAs with kidney graft disorder and relevant gene target(s), Figure S1: Association of miRNAs (*miR-29c, miR-126, miR-146a, miR-150, miR-155, miR-223*) with kidney graft disease in patients with performed kidney graft biopsy due to indication after miRNA measurement.

Author Contributions: Conceptualization, Ž.V.-H., N.K.; methodology, Š.B., E.B., Ž.P.T., D.K.; software, Š.B., E.B., Ž.P.T.; formal analysis, Š.B., Ž.V.-H., E.B., Ž.P.T., J.L., D.K., N.K.; investigation, Š.B., Ž.V.-H., E.B., Ž.P.T., J.L., D.K., N.K.; data curation, Š.B., Ž.V.-H., E.B., Ž.P.T., J.L., D.K., N.K.; writing—original draft preparation, Š.B., E.B., Ž.P.T.; writing—review and editing, Ž.V.-H., N.K.; supervision, Ž.V.-H., N.K.; funding acquisition, Ž.V.-H., J.L., D.K., N.K. All authors have read and agreed to the published version of the manuscript.

Funding: The research was partially funded by Slovenian ARRS program No P3-0323 and P3-0054.

Acknowledgments: The authors would like to thank all medical nurses from the Department of Nuclear Medicine and Center for Kidney Transplantation of the Department of Nephrology at the University Medical Center Ljubljana for their cooperation and care of our patients.

Conflicts of Interest: The authors declare no conflict of interest.

Abbreviations

CKD	chronic kidney disease
CKD-T	chronic kidney disease of transplanted kidney
^{51}CrEDTA	chromium-51-ethylenediaminetetraacetic acid
GFR	glomerular filtration rate
eGFR	estimated GFR
eGFR CKD EPI creatinine	eGFR with Chronic Kidney Disease Epidemiology Collaboration study formula with s-Creatinine
eGFR CKD EPI CysC	eGFR with Chronic Kidney Disease Epidemiology Collaboration study formula with s-CysC
eGFR CKD EPI creatinine CysC	eGFR with Chronic Kidney Disease Epidemiology Collaboration study formula with s-Creatinine and s-CysC
mGFR ^{51}CrEDTA	measured GFR with ^{51}CrEDTA
IF/TA	interstitial fibrosis/tubular atrophy
KTRs	kidney transplant recipients
miRNA	microRNA
RNA	ribonucleic acid
s-Creatinine	serum creatinine concentration
s-CysC	serum cystatin C concentration
s-Urea	serum urea concentration
s-Uromodulin	serum uromodulin concentration

References

1. Tamm, I.; Horsfall, F.L., Jr. Characterization and separation of an inhibitor of viral hemagglutination present in urine. *Proc. Soc. Exp. Biol. Med.* **1950**, *74*, 106–108. [CrossRef] [PubMed]
2. Vyletal, P.; Bleyer, A.J.; Kmoch, S. Uromodulin biology and pathophysiology—An update. *Kidney Blood Press. Res.* **2010**, *33*, 456–475. [CrossRef] [PubMed]
3. Prajczer, S.; Heidenreich, U.; Pfaller, W.; Kotanko, P.; Lhotta, K.; Jennings, P. Evidence for a role of uromodulin in chronic kidney disease progression. *Nephrol. Dial. Transplant.* **2010**, *25*, 1896–1903. [CrossRef]
4. Scherberich, J.E.; Gruber, R.; Nockher, W.A.; Christensen, E.I.; Schmitt, H.; Herbst, V.; Block, M.; Kaden, J.; Schlumberger, W. Serum uromodulin—A marker of kidney function and renal parenchymal integrity. *Nephrol. Dial. Transplant.* **2018**, *33*, 284–295. [CrossRef] [PubMed]

5. Steubl, D.; Block, M.; Herbst, V.; Nockher, W.A.; Schlumberger, W.; Satanovskij, R.; Angermann, S.; Hasenau, A.L.; Stecher, L.; Heemann, U.; et al. Plasma Uromodulin Correlates With Kidney Function and Identifies Early Stages in Chronic Kidney Disease Patients. *Medicine* **2016**, *95*, e3011. [CrossRef] [PubMed]
6. Bostom, A.; Steubl, D.; Garimella, P.S.; Franceschini, N.; Roberts, M.B.; Pasch, A.; Ix, J.H.; Tuttle, K.R.; Ivanova, A.; Shireman, T.; et al. Serum Uromodulin: A Biomarker of Long-Term Kidney Allograft Failure. *Am. J. Nephrol* **2018**, *47*, 275–282. [CrossRef]
7. Steubl, D.; Block, M.; Herbst, V.; Schlumberger, W.; Nockher, A.; Angermann, S.; Schmaderer, C.; Heemann, U.; Renders, L.; Scherberich, J. Serum uromodulin predicts graft failure in renal transplant recipients. *Biomarkers* **2017**, *22*, 171–177. [CrossRef]
8. Reznichenko, A.; van Dijk, M.C.; van der Heide, J.H.; Bakker, S.J.; Seelen, M.; Navis, G. Uromodulin in renal transplant recipients: Elevated urinary levels and bimodal association with graft failure. *Am. J. Nephrol.* **2011**, *34*, 445–451. [CrossRef]
9. Khan, Z.; Suthanthiran, M.; Muthukumar, T. MicroRNAs and Transplantation. *Clin. Lab. Med.* **2019**, *39*, 125–143. [CrossRef]
10. Wilflingseder, J.; Reindl-Schwaighofer, R.; Sunzenauer, J.; Kainz, A.; Heinzel, A.; Mayer, B.; Oberbauer, R. MicroRNAs in kidney transplantation. *Nephrol. Dial. Transplant.* **2015**, *30*, 910–917. [CrossRef]
11. Janszky, N.; Susal, C. Circulating and urinary microRNAs as possible biomarkers in kidney transplantation. *Transplant. Rev.* **2018**, *32*, 110–118. [CrossRef] [PubMed]
12. Kriegel, A.J.; Liu, Y.; Fang, Y.; Ding, X.; Liang, M. The miR-29 family: Genomics, cell biology, and relevance to renal and cardiovascular injury. *Physiol. Genomics* **2012**, *44*, 237–244. [CrossRef] [PubMed]
13. Taibi, F.; Metzinger-Le Meuth, V.; M'Baya-Moutoula, E.; Djelouat, M.; Louvet, L.; Bugnicourt, J.M.; Poirot, S.; Bengrine, A.; Chillon, J.M.; Massy, Z.A.; et al. Possible involvement of microRNAs in vascular damage in experimental chronic kidney disease. *Biochim. Biophys. Acta* **2014**, *1842*, 88–98. [CrossRef]
14. Metzinger-Le Meuth, V.; Burtey, S.; Maitrias, P.; Massy, Z.A.; Metzinger, L. microRNAs in the pathophysiology of CKD-MBD: Biomarkers and innovative drugs. *Biochim. Biophys. Acta Mol. Basis Dis.* **2017**, *1863*, 337–345. [CrossRef]
15. Fourdinier, O.; Schepers, E.; Metzinger-Le Meuth, V.; Glorieux, G.; Liabeuf, S.; Verbeke, F.; Vanholder, R.; Brigant, B.; Pletinck, A.; Diouf, M.; et al. Serum levels of miR-126 and miR-223 and outcomes in chronic kidney disease patients. *Sci. Rep.* **2019**, *9*, 4477. [CrossRef] [PubMed]
16. Testa, U.; Pelosi, E.; Castelli, G.; Labbaye, C. miR-146 and miR-155: Two Key Modulators of Immune Response and Tumor Development. *Non-Coding RNA* **2017**, *3*, 22. [CrossRef]
17. Milhoransa, P.; Montanari, C.C.; Montenegro, R.; Manfro, R.C. Micro RNA 146a-5p expression in Kidney transplant recipients with delayed graft function. *J. Bras. Nefrol.* **2019**, *41*, 242–251. [CrossRef]
18. Huang, X.L.; Zhang, L.; Li, J.P.; Wang, Y.J.; Duan, Y.; Wang, J. MicroRNA-150: A potential regulator in pathogens infection and autoimmune diseases. *Autoimmunity* **2015**, *48*, 503–510. [CrossRef]
19. De Candia, P.; Torri, A.; Pagani, M.; Abrignani, S. Serum microRNAs as Biomarkers of Human Lymphocyte Activation in Health and Disease. *Front. Immunol.* **2014**, *5*, 43. [CrossRef]
20. Yuan, X.; Berg, N.; Lee, J.W.; Le, T.T.; Neudecker, V.; Jing, N.; Eltzschig, H. MicroRNA miR-223 as regulator of innate immunity. *J. Leukoc. Biol.* **2018**, *104*, 515–524. [CrossRef]
21. Metzinger-Le Meuth, V.; Metzinger, L. miR-223 and other miRNA's evaluation in chronic kidney disease: Innovative biomarkers and therapeutic tools. *Non-Coding RNA Res.* **2019**, *4*, 30–35. [CrossRef]
22. Li, S.; Chen, H.; Ren, J.; Geng, Q.; Song, J.; Lee, C.; Cao, C.; Zhang, J.; Xu, N. MicroRNA-223 inhibits tissue factor expression in vascular endothelial cells. *Atherosclerosis* **2014**, *237*, 514–520. [CrossRef] [PubMed]
23. O'Callaghan, J.M.; Knight, S.R. Noninvasive biomarkers in monitoring kidney allograft health. *Curr. Opin. Organ. Transplant.* **2019**, *24*, 411–415. [CrossRef] [PubMed]
24. Naesens, M.; Anglicheau, D. Precision Transplant Medicine: Biomarkers to the Rescue. *J. Am. Soc. Nephrol.* **2018**, *29*, 24–34. [CrossRef] [PubMed]
25. Buron, F.; Hadj-Aissa, A.; Dubourg, L.; Morelon, E.; Steghens, J.P.; Ducher, M.; Fauvel, J.P. Estimating glomerular filtration rate in kidney transplant recipients: Performance over time of four creatinine-based formulas. *Transplantation* **2011**, *92*, 1005–1011. [CrossRef] [PubMed]
26. Fedak, D.; Kuzniewski, M.; Fugiel, A.; Wieczorek-Surdacka, E.; Przepiorkowska-Hoyer, B.; Jasik, P.; Miarka, P.; Dumnicka, P.; Kapusta, M.; Solnica, B.; et al. Serum uromodulin concentrations correlate with glomerular filtration rate in patients with chronic kidney disease. *Pol. Arch. Med. Wewn.* **2016**, *126*, 995–1004. [CrossRef]

27. Gibson, T. Hyperuricemia, gout and the kidney. *Curr. Opin. Rheumatol.* **2012**, *24*, 127–131. [CrossRef]
28. Millan, O.; Budde, K.; Sommerer, C.; Aliart, I.; Rissling, O.; Bardaji, B.; Matz, M.; Zeier, M.; Silva, I.; Guirado, L.; et al. Urinary miR-155-5p and CXCL10 as prognostic and predictive biomarkers of rejection, graft outcome and treatment response in kidney transplantation. *Br. J. Clin. Pharmacol.* **2017**, *83*, 2636–2650. [CrossRef]
29. Delanaye, P.; Mariat, C. The applicability of eGFR equations to different populations. *Nat. Rev. Nephrol.* **2013**, *9*, 513–522. [CrossRef]
30. Inker, L.A.; Eckfeldt, J.; Levey, A.S.; Leiendecker-Foster, C.; Rynders, G.; Manzi, J.; Waheed, S.; Coresh, J. Expressing the CKD-EPI (Chronic Kidney Disease Epidemiology Collaboration) cystatin C equations for estimating GFR with standardized serum cystatin C values. *Am. J. Kidney Dis.* **2011**, *58*, 682–684. [CrossRef]
31. Levin, A.; Stevens, P.E.; Bilous, R.W.; Coresh, J.; De Francisco, A.L.M.; De Jong, P.E.; Griffith, K.E.; Hemmelgarn, B.R.; Iseki, K.; Lamb, E.J.; et al. Kidney disease: Improving Global Outcomes (KDIGO) CKD Work Group. KDIGO 2012 Clinical Practice Guideline for the Evaluation and Management of Chronic Kidney Disease. *Kidney Int. Suppl.* **2013**, *3*, 1–150.
32. Blaufox, M.D.; Aurell, M.; Bubeck, B.; Fommei, E.; Piepsz, A.; Russell, C.; Taylor, A.; Thomsen, H.S.; Volterrani, D. Report of the Radionuclides in Nephrourology Committee on renal clearance. *J. Nucl. Med.* **1996**, *37*, 1883–1890. [PubMed]
33. Latham, G.J. Normalization of microRNA quantitative RT-PCR data in reduced scale experimental designs. *Methods Mol. Biol.* **2010**, *667*, 19–31. [PubMed]

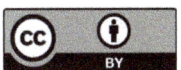

© 2020 by the authors. Licensee MDPI, Basel, Switzerland. This article is an open access article distributed under the terms and conditions of the Creative Commons Attribution (CC BY) license (http://creativecommons.org/licenses/by/4.0/).

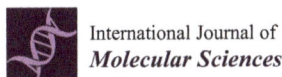

Review

Urinary Biomarkers for Diagnosis and Prediction of Acute Kidney Allograft Rejection: A Systematic Review

Francesco Guzzi [1,2,*], Luigi Cirillo [1,2], Elisa Buti [2], Francesca Becherucci [2], Carmela Errichiello [2], Rosa Maria Roperto [2], James P. Hunter [3] and Paola Romagnani [1,2]

1. Department of Experimental and Clinical Biomedical Sciences "Mario Serio", University of Florence, 50134 Florence, Italy; luigi.cirillo@unifi.it (L.C.); paola.romagnani@unifi.it (P.R.)
2. Nephrology and Dialysis Unit, Meyer Children's University Hospital, 50139 Florence, Italy; elisa.buti@meyer.it (E.B.); francesca.becherucci@meyer.it (F.B.); carmela.errichiello@meyer.it (C.E.); rosa.roperto@meyer.it (R.M.R.)
3. Nuffield Department of Surgical Sciences, Oxford Transplant Centre, Churchill Hospital, University of Oxford, Oxford OX3 7LJ, UK; james.hunter@nds.ox.ac.uk
* Correspondence: francesco.guzzi@gmail.com

Received: 29 August 2020; Accepted: 18 September 2020; Published: 19 September 2020

Abstract: Noninvasive tools for diagnosis or prediction of acute kidney allograft rejection have been extensively investigated in recent years. Biochemical and molecular analyses of blood and urine provide a liquid biopsy that could offer new possibilities for rejection prevention, monitoring, and therefore, treatment. Nevertheless, these tools are not yet available for routine use in clinical practice. In this systematic review, MEDLINE was searched for articles assessing urinary biomarkers for diagnosis or prediction of kidney allograft acute rejection published in the last five years (from 1 January 2015 to 31 May 2020). This review follows the Preferred Reporting Items for Systematic Reviews and Meta-analysis (PRISMA) guidelines. Articles providing targeted or unbiased urine sample analysis for the diagnosis or prediction of both acute cellular and antibody-mediated kidney allograft rejection were included, analyzed, and graded for methodological quality with a particular focus on study design and diagnostic test accuracy measures. Urinary C-X-C motif chemokine ligands were the most promising and frequently studied biomarkers. The combination of precise diagnostic reference in training sets with accurate validation in real-life cohorts provided the most relevant results and exciting groundwork for future studies.

Keywords: kidney transplantation; kidney graft; T-cell-mediated rejection; antibody-mediated rejection; diagnostic test accuracy

1. Introduction

The growing call for precision medicine justifies a trend shift towards the implementation of new prognostic and diagnostic biomarkers in many fields of medicine. Progress in molecular and biomarker technology now permits the possibility to tailor and customize clinical and therapeutic approaches to the specific needs of a single patient, for a variety of medical conditions. Kidney diseases are no exception, with biomarkers constantly gaining more ground in the management of acute kidney injury (AKI), glomerulopathies, and chronic kidney disease (CKD) [1–3]. Also, in the setting of kidney transplantation, precision medicine is rapidly moving forward, with biomarkers a significant part of this trend. In kidney transplantation, biomarkers have been studied for early recognition and diagnosis of disease recurrence, delayed graft function (DGF), infections, and acute and chronic allograft rejection [4]. Since the 1970s, biomarkers have been studied for organ quality assessment prior to transplantation [5,6] and post-transplant evaluation [7]. However, in clinical practice, few genuine biomarkers have emerged, and clinicians still largely rely on serum creatinine and proteinuria monitoring. Novel biomarkers could be of great help not only for early recognition of allograft disease, but also for monitoring disease activity, optimizing the need for invasive biopsies, predicting the effectiveness and safety of a certain treatment, and tailoring the management of each single patient to their specific needs [4,8].

Despite near-optimal immunosuppressive regimens and accurate therapy compliance, kidney transplants still suffer from potentially preventable acute rejection (AR) episodes. AR early identification is important for preserving nephron mass and aiding long-term allograft survival [9]. The gold standard for AR diagnosis is histological examination of a kidney biopsy. The biopsy can then be interpreted with the help of the Banff classification (created in the 1990s and periodically revised), which describes acute lesions according to two mechanistic pathways: T-cell-mediated rejection (TCMR) and antibody-mediated rejection (ABMR) [10]. However, a biopsy is an invasive procedure, may not be straightforward to perform and can be complicated by major bleeding. In addition, potential sampling errors, inter-observer variability, and elevated costs make allograft biopsy impractical for continuous monitoring of the graft over time. Urine samples, as a readily available and direct product of the allograft, with minimal influence from systemic inflammation, are a more desirable source for AR biomarkers. Very recently, narrative reviews explored the use of biomarkers in the diagnosis of AR [11,12]. However, to our knowledge, the most recent systematic review assessing urinary biomarkers' ability for allograft AR diagnosis in kidney transplant patients included papers published until 2015 [7]. The most relevant articles and findings in the field before 2015 have been also thoroughly summarized elsewhere [13–15]. Up to 2015, no urinary biomarker was validated in sufficiently robust trials to be translated into clinical practice independent of traditional surveillance and diagnostic methods.

The aim of this systematic review is to perform a methodical analysis and to summarize important results coming from the most recent literature (2015–present) evaluating urinary biomarkers and their performance as diagnostic and/or predictive tools for kidney allograft acute rejection.

2. Results

2.1. Included Studies

The original literature search yielded a total of 314 citations. Of these, 251 studies were discarded after evaluation of title and abstract in the eligibility process. The remaining 63 studies were reviewed full-text for inclusion in the study. Twenty-five studies were excluded, as detailed in Figure 1.

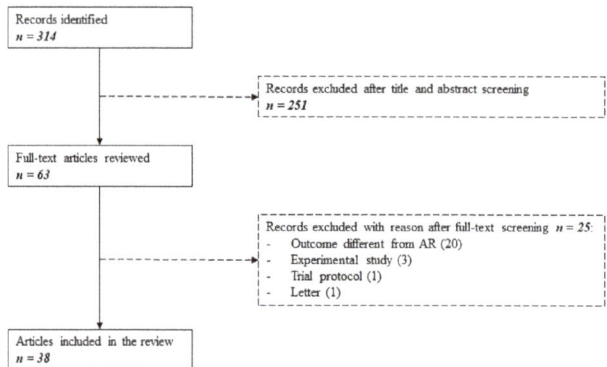

Figure 1. Search flowchart as per PRISMA guidelines. Three hundred fourteen studies were identified searching MEDLINE between January 2015 and May 2020. After evaluating for eligibility and inclusion, 38 articles were selected.

The main reason for exclusion was the evaluation of a different outcome instead of AR (e.g., chronic or late rejection, graft dysfunction, graft failure). Experimental studies, one trial protocol, and one letter were also excluded. A total of 38 remaining articles, published between 1 January 2015 and 31 May 2020, were finally included. No additional articles were included from the reference lists.

2.2. Study Characteristics

Table 1 summarizes the most relevant characteristics of each of the 38 included studies. Twenty-nine were single center studies, while nine were multicenter collaborations. Among the 32 studies assessing urinary biomarkers in the diagnosis of acute rejection, the majority of them, 18/32, were designed as case-control, while 14/32 as cross-sectional studies. Among the six studies assessing the ability of urinary biomarkers to predict acute rejection at variable time-points before the episode, five studies analyzed prospectively collected data and one study analyzed retrospectively collected data. Population characteristics, patient selection protocols, inclusion and exclusion criteria, as well as sample size, were heterogeneous between studies. Sample size varied from 15 to 396 kidney transplant patients, and occasionally more than one urine sample was obtained from the same patient. Although all of the included studies were published after January 2015, some of them enrolled patients transplanted from the early 2000's. Table 1 also highlights the year of study population enrolment to help the identification of possibly overlapping populations and to assess the appropriateness of the Banff classification used in each study. The majority of the included studies applied up to date Banff classification, with ten studies apparently using the 1997 version or not reporting the year. Using an outdated classification could be a source of bias mostly for studies assessing ABMR, as discussed later. For one study, the application of the Banff classification was not clearly stated. Studies were also heterogeneous in terms of the considered outcome. Among the 38 included studies, 15 specifically addressed TCMR only, whereas just two exclusively focused on ABMR. Sixteen studies assessed the combination of TCMR and ABMR, while five studies did not specify the characteristics of the observed acute rejection (Table 1).

Table 1. Description of the study characteristics. The table summarizes the main characteristics of the 38 included studies.

Ref	Study Design	Single/Multicenter	Patients (n)	Enrolment (years)	Urinary Biomarker(s)	Ref. Standard	Outcome
Tinel [16]	Cross-sectional	Single center	329	2011–2016	CXCL9, CXCL10	Banff '15	TCMR, ABMR
Yang [17]	Cross-sectional	Multicenter	364	2010–2018	Q score	Banff '17	TCMR, ABMR
Kalantari [18]	Case-control	Single center	22	2016–2018	Unbiased metabolomics [1]	Banff '17	TCMR
Verma [19]	Case-control	Single center	53	N/R	RNA-Seq signature	Banff '17	TCMR
Goerlich [20]	Case-control	Single center	39	2016–2017	T cells, TEC, PDX	Banff '13	TCMR, ABMR
Banas [21]	Cross-sectional	Single center	109	2011–2012	Unbiased metabolomics [2]	Banff '09	TCMR, ABMR
Tajima [22]	Cross-sectional	Single center	80	2014–2016	LC3, CCL2, LFABP, NGAL, HE4	Banff '09	TCMR, ABMR
Kolling [23]	Case-control	Single center	93	N/R	Circular RNAs	Banff '09	TCMR
Sigdel [24]	Cross-sectional	Multicenter	150	2000–2016	uCRM score	Banff '09	TCMR, ABMR
Kim [25]	Case-control	Multicenter	23	N/R	Unbiased metabolomics [3]	Banff '07	TCMR
Ciftci [26] *	Prospective	Single center	85	2014–2017	CXCL9, CXCL10	Banff '13	TCMR, ABMR
Banas [27]	Case-control	Single center	358	2008–2010; 2015–2016	Unbiased metabolomics [2]	Banff '97	TCMR
Lim [28]	Case-control	Multicenter	47	2013–2015	Exosome proteins	Banff '07	TCMR
Chen [29]	Case-control	Single center	49	2006–2009	CXCL13	Banff '97	TCMR, ABMR
Barabadi [30] §	Cross-sectional	Single center	91	2013–2015	FOXP3	Banff '13	AR
Mockler [31] *§	Prospective	Single center	38	N/R	CCL2	Banff '13	TCMR
Ciftci [32] *	Prospective	Single center	65	2013–2015	TNFα	Banff '97	AR
Park [33]	Case-control	Single center	44	N/R	Exosome proteins	Banff (N/R)	TCMR
Millan [34] *	Prospective	Multicenter	80	N/R	miR-155-5p, CXCL10	Banff '97	TCMR

Table 1. Cont.

Ref	Study Design	Single/Multicenter	Patients (n)	Enrolment (years)	Urinary Biomarker(s)	Ref. Standard	Outcome
Seo [35]	Case-control	Multicenter	88	2013–2015	CTOT4 formula	Banff (N/R)	TCMR, ABMR
Gandolfini [36] §	Case-control	Multicenter	56	N/R	CXCL9	Banff '13	TCMR
Chen [37]	Case-control	Single center	156	2006–2009	sTim3	Banff '97	TCMR, ABMR
Domenico [38] §	Case-control	Single center	49	N/R	miRNA-142-3p	Banff '07	AR
Lee [39] §	Case-control	Single center	34	N/R	Donor-derived cfDNA	unclear	AR
Seeman [40] §	Case-control	Single center	15	2013–2014	NGAL	Banff '07	TCMR, ABMR
Blydt-H. [41]	Cross-sectional	Multicenter	59	2002–N/R	ABMR score	Banff '13	ABMR
Belmar V. [42] *	Retrospective	Single center	86	2012–2015	Albumin	Banff (N/R)	ABMR
Raza [43]	Cross-sectional	Single center	300	2009–2014	CCL2	Banff '97	TCMR
Galichon [44]	Cross-sectional	Multicenter	108	N/R	CTOT4 formula	Banff '09	TCMR, ABMR
Sigdel [45]	Cross-sectional	Single center	396	2000–2011	Unbiased proteomics	Banff '07	TCMR, ABMR
Garcia-C. [46] §	Cross-sectional	Single center	50	N/R	IL10, IFNγ	Banff '09	TCMR, ABMR
Ho [47] §	Cross-sectional	Single center	133	N/R	MMP7, CXCL10	Banff '07	TCMR
A. Elaziz [48]	Cross-sectional	Single center	54	2011–2014	PD1, FOXP3	Banff '07	TCMR
Lorenzen [49]	Cross-sectional	Single center	93	N/R	LncRNAs	Banff '09	TCMR
Rabant [50] *	Prospective	Single center	300	2010–2012	CXCL9, CXCL10	Banff '07	TCMR, ABMR
Rabant [51]	Cross-sectional	Single center	244	2011–2013	CXCL9, CXCL10	Banff '07	TCMR, ABMR
Blydt-H. [52]	Cross-sectional	Single center	51	2002–N/R	CXCL10	Banff '07	TCMR
Sigdel [53] §	Case-control	Single center	30	2000–2009	Exosome proteins	Banff '07	AR

Unbiased metabolomics: [1] (NAD, NADP, nicotinic acid, MNA, GABA, cholesterol sulfate, homocysteine); [2] (alanine, citrate, lactate, urea); [3] (guanidoacetic acid, methylimidazoleacetic acid, dopamine, 4-guanidinobutyric acid, and L-tryptophan). * Prediction study; § Diagnostic Test Accuracy analysis not present. N/R, not reported.

2.3. Biomarkers

The included studies were split into diagnostic and prediction studies. To be considered a diagnostic study, the collection of a urine sample should be performed on the day that AR was suspected or when per-protocol biopsies were planned. There were a few exceptions to this rule where sample collection occasionally occurred up to seven days before biopsy. For prediction studies, urine samples were collected at any time point post-transplant and, in this analysis, these ranged from day one up to six months post-transplantation. Among the various techniques for targeted analysis of known urinary biomarkers, ELISA and RT-PCR were the most frequently utilized. Mass spectrometry, nuclear magnetic resonance spectroscopy, liquid chromatography, RNA expression, and transcriptome analysis by RNA-Seq were employed for unbiased metabolomics, proteomics, and genomic profiling and for detection and identification of urinary exosome proteins. All biomarkers are detailed per category in Table 2.

In accordance with previous studies, the most extensively assessed urinary biomarkers were C-X-C motif chemokine ligand 9 (CXCL9) and 10 (CXCL10), usually adjusted for urinary creatinine concentration. In detail, 12/38 (32%) studies either addressed CXCL9 and CXCL10 alone, in combination, or in the context of particular scores or formulas [16,17,24,26,34–36,44,47,50–52]. Other directly targeted cytokines and interleukins were chemokine ligand 2 (CCL2), also known as monocyte chemoattractant protein 1 [22,31,43], CXCL13 [29], interleukin 10 (IL10) with interferon gamma (IFNγ) [46] and tumor necrosis factor alpha (TNFα) [32].

Table 2. Urinary biomarkers. Table illustrating all urinary biomarkers divided per category and in alphabetic order. Specific formulas and scores are also detailed.

Category	Biomarkers
Cytokines	
Chemokines	CCL2, CXCL9, CXCL10, CXCL13
Other	IFNγ, IL10, TNFα
Metabolites	
Nucleotides	NAD, NADP
Amino acids and Organic acids	Alanine, Citrate, GABA, 4-Guanidinobutyric Acid, Guanidoacetic Acid, Homocysteine, Lactate, Methylimidazoleacetic Acid, Nicotinic Acid, L-Tryptophan
Other small molecules	Cholesterol Sulfate, Dopamine, MNA, Urea
Proteins	Albumin, LFAPB, HE4, LC3, MMP7, NGAL, sTIM3, Urinary extracellular vesicle (exosome) proteins (HPX, TSPAN1)
RNAs	Circular RNAs, FOXP3 mRNA, LncRNAs, PD1 mRNA, RNA-seq
micro RNAs	miR-142-3p, miR-155-5p
Urinary Cells	CD4+/CD8+ T cells, CD10+/EPCAM+ cells, PDX+ cells, TEC
Scores and Formulas	
ABMR score [41]	Signature of 133 unique metabolites
CTOT-4 formula [54]	CD3ε mRNA + CXCL10 mRNA + 18S rRNA
Q score [17]	Cell-free DNA + Clusterin + Creatinine + CXCL10 + Methylated Cell-free DNA + Total Urinary Protein
uCRM score [24]	11 genes expression score on urinary cell pellet (including CXCL9 and CXCL10)

Unbiased metabolomic analysis and untargeted profiling revealed multiple urinary metabolites as potential biomarkers of AR: nicotinamide adenine dinucleotide (NAD), nicotinamide adenine dinucleotide phosphate (NADP), nicotinic acid, 1-methylnicotinamide (MNA), gamma-aminobutyric acid (GABA), cholesterol sulfate, homocysteine [18], the combination of alanine, citrate, lactate, and urea [21,27], and the combination of guanidoacetic acid, methylimidazoleacetic acid, dopamine, 4-guanidinobutyric acid, and L-tryptophan [25].

Urinary proteins of interest were neutrophil gelatinase-associated lipocalin (NGAL) [22,40], liver-type fatty acid-binding protein (LFABP) [22], human epididymis protein 4 (HE4) [22], matrix metalloproteinase 7 (MMP7) [47], soluble T cell immunoglobulin mucin domain 3 (sTIM3) [37]. The presence and diagnostic performance of urinary extracellular vesicle (exosome) proteins, derived from inflammatory cells and collected with the help of nano-membrane or immune-magnetic capture, was investigated by three studies [28,32,52].

Direct RT-PCR was used to identify targeted RNAs like programmed cell death protein1 (PD1) mRNA, forkhead box P3 (FOXP3) mRNA, and micro (mi) RNAs (miR-142-3p, miR-155-5p) [30,34,38,48], while genome-wide or transcriptome analysis were applied for the unbiased identification of circular and long noncoding RNAs [23,49].

The amount of urinary CD4+ and CD8+ T cells, tubular epithelial cells (TEC), podocalyxin (PDX)-positive, CD10+ or epithelial cell adhesion molecule (EPCAM)-positive cells was determined by flow cytometry and compared with biopsy results [20].

Two studies [35,44] investigated the diagnostic accuracy of the *CTOT4 formula* (CXCL10 mRNA, CD3ε mRNA, 18S rRNA), previously validated by the CTOT-4 (clinical trials in organ transplantation-4) multicenter study group [54]. CXCL10 was also included in newly derived scores such as the *Q score*, composed of six DNA, protein, and metabolite urinary biomarkers (cell-free DNA, methylated cell-free DNA, clusterin, total protein, creatinine, and CXCL10) [17], while CXCL9 and CXCL10 genes were included in the *uCRM score* [24]. Finally, the *ABMR score* comprised more than 130 unique metabolites [41].

2.4. Quality Assessment

Studies reporting diagnostic test accuracy (DTA) analysis (29/38) were graded for risk of bias and applicability concerns according to the QUADAS-2 tool (Table 3). Risk of bias was frequently high for patient selection (14/29, 48%) and index test (23/29, 79%).

Table 3. QUADAS-2 tool assessment for DTA studies. Table illustrating risk of bias and applicability concerns evaluation as per QUADAS-2 tool for 29 studies providing diagnostic test accuracy data.

Ref	Risk of Bias				Applicability Concerns		
	Patient Selection	Index Test	Reference Standard	Flow and Timing	Patient Selection	Index Test	Reference Standard
Tinel [16]	☺	☺	☺	☺	☺	☺	☺
Yang [17]	☺	☹	☺	☺	☺	☺	☺
Kalantari [18]	☹	☹	☺	?	☹	☹	☺
Verma [19]	☹	☹	☺	☺	☹	☺	☺
Goerlich [20]	☹	☹	☺	☺	☹	☺	☺
Banas [21]	☺	☹	☺	?	☺	☺	☺
Tajima [22]	☺	☹	☺	☺	☹	☺	☺
Kolling [23]	☹	☹	☺	☺	☺	☺	☺
Sigdel [24]	☺	☹	☺	☺	☺	☺	☺
Kim [25]	☹	☹	☺	☺	☺	☺	☺
Ciftci [26] *	☹	☹	☺	?	☹	☺	☺
Banas [27]	☹	☹	☺	☺	☺	☺	☺
Lim [28]	☹	☹	☺	☺	☹	☺	☺
Chen [29]	☹	☹	?	☺	☹	☺	☺
Ciftci [31] *	☹	☹	?	?	☹	☺	☺
Park [33]	☹	☺	☺	☺	☹	☺	☺
Millan [34] *	?	☹	☺	?	☹	☺	☺
Seo [35]	☹	☹	☺	☹	☹	☺	☺
Chen [37]	☹	☹	?	☺	☹	☺	☺
Blydt-H. [41]	☺	☹	☺	☺	☺	☺	☺
Belm.V. [42] *	☹	☹	?	☺	☺	☺	☺
Raza [43]	☹	☹	☺	☹	☺	☺	☺
Galichon [44]	☺	☹	?	☺	☺	☺	☺
Sigdel [45]	☺	☹	☺	☺	☺	☺	☺
A. Elaziz [48]	?	☹	☺	☺	☺	☺	☺
Lorenzen [49]	☺	☹	☺	☺	☺	☺	☺
Rabant [50] *	☺	☹	☺	☺	☺	☺	☺
Rabant [51]	☺	☹	☺	☺	☺	☺	☺
Blydt-H. [52]	☺	☹	☺	☹	☺	☺	☺

*, Prediction study; ☺, Low Risk; ☹, High Risk; ?, Unclear Risk.

The most frequent reasons for high risk of bias were the selection of the study population by case-control design, which was the case for the majority of the studies, the exclusion of the typical confounding of a real-life setting, the absence of threshold definition and independent validation. For example, when control patients were selected among stable patients without performing allograft biopsy, or only among normal histology patients, and the obtained thresholds were not tested in a randomly selected validation group, the study was highlighted for high risk of bias in patient selection and index test (Table 3). This then raised the possibility of an increased risk of over-fitting association and unrealistic DTA performance and, therefore, concerns for applicability. The ideal control patients were randomly (or in a cross-sectional fashion) selected, all having had an allograft biopsy (per indication or per protocol) with various histological diagnosis (e.g., normal histology; acute tubular necrosis, ATN; interstitial fibrosis and tubular atrophy, IFTA; chronic allograft nephropathy, CAN; BK virus nephropathy, BKVN; recurrence of the primary disease on the allograft). Only 5/29 studies were found to have a low risk of bias in both patient selection and index test. Allograft histology, according to Banff classification, was the reference standard for AR diagnosis, with histology grading usually assigned in a blinded fashion with respect to the index test results. Since urinary samples were frequently obtained for all included patients, prior to a diagnostic allograft biopsy, and all included patients were evaluated in the DTA analysis, a low risk of bias was frequently identified in the flow and timing domain. The QUADAS-2 tool does not include publication bias (PB) as one of the variables and, in the context of this review, it is difficult to formally assess PB. Given the broad variety of different biomarkers that were assessed and the absence of a meta-analysis, performing formal PB assessment such as Egger's test, Deek's test or the construction of a funnel plot was not possible. It is also recognized that the assessment of PB in data synthesis of DTA data is challenging with limited reliability [55].

2.5. Summary of the Results

Tables 4–6 provide a detailed summary of each study results. When DTA analysis was available (29 studies), the results are summarized in Table 4 for diagnostic studies (24/38) and Table 5 for prediction studies (5/38). Descriptive results from the remaining nine studies are briefly reported in Table 6. For each DTA study, the particular outcome of interest and characteristics of the control population are reported with sample size for each group included in the final DTA analysis. The urinary biomarker of interest, thresholds (when available) and test design (training, validation, or particular comparisons between groups) are also detailed. For prediction studies, time from transplantation to urinary biomarker analysis is also reported (between 1 day to 6 months post-transplantation). Sensitivity, specificity, positive and negative predictive values (PPV, NPV), and area under the receiver operating characteristic curve (AUC) are reported as measures of diagnostic test accuracy when available (Tables 4 and 5) and results are in bold text when arising from validation cohorts. Results confirmation in at least one validation cohort was available in less than one third of studies (7/29, 24%). Of these, two were case-control studies [25,33], while the others were the previously mentioned five cross-sectional studies with the lowest risk of bias score [16,17,21,41,45]. Sensitivity and specificity values were highly variable between studies, ranging from 9% to 100% and from 34% and 100%, respectively. PPV and NPV were also variable, ranging from 15% to 98% and from 32% to 100%, respectively.

Table 4. Summary of the study results—Diagnostic studies with DTA. This table shows the outcome of diagnostic studies. Outcome and control group for the DTA analysis are reported (sample size when available), followed by test design, studied urinary biomarker(s), and thresholds when provided.

Ref.	Outcome (n)	Control Group (n)	Test Design, Biomarkers, Thresholds	Diagnostic Test Accuracy (95%CI)				
				Sens.	Spec.	PPV	NPV	AUC–Accuracy(%)
Tinel [16]	TCMR (17), ABMR (64), mixed (14)	ALL-B (normal, 21; IFTA, 154; BKVN, 23; ATN, 11; recurrent disease, 9; other, 78)	CXCL9 + CXCL10 for AR	62%	72%	41%	86%	**0.70 (0.64–0.76)**
			CXCL9 + CXCL10 for TCMR	79%	74%	21%	98%	**0.81 (0.73–0.89)**
		ALL-B (normal, 170; bAR, 50;	CXCL9 + CXCL10 for ABMR	72%	54%	28%	88%	**0.67 (0.61–0.74)**
			Training: AR vs normal (Q score ≥ 32)	95%	100%	-	-	0.99 (0.99–1.00)
Yang [17]	TCMR + ABMR (103)	BKVN, 9)	Validation 1: AR vs normal	91%	92%	-	-	**0.98 (0.96–1.00)**
			Validation 2: AR vs normal	100%	96%	-	-	**1.00 (1.00–1.00)**
			All AR vs All normal	95%	96%	87%	98%	**0.99(0.98–0.99)**
			All AR vs ALL-B	-	-	-	-	**0.96 (0.94–0.98)**
Kalantari [18]	TCMR (7)	DYS-B (normal, 15)	Unbiased metab.¹	67–71%	40–100%			0.51–0.71
Verna [19]	TCMR (22)	ALL-B (normal, 28)	13-gene urinary cell signature	-	-			0.92 (0.85–0.99)
Goerlich [20]	TCMR (14) + ABMR (7)	DYS-B (normal, 18)	T cells + total TEC					0.90
			T cells + CD10+ TEC					0.89
			T cells + ECPAM+ TEC					0.91
			T cells + PDX+ cells					0.89
Banas [21]	TCMR + ABMR + mixed	ALL-B (normal) + STA	Unbiased metab.²	-	-	-	-	0.75 (0.68–0.83)
			Score = 3.0	91% (79–98)	34% (30–38)	-	-	-
	+ bAR	+ (IFTA + other)	Score = 13.0	48% (33–63)	89% (86–91)	-	-	-
Tajima [22]	TCMR + ABMR (subclinical, 11)	STA-B (normal or borderline AR, 69)	LC3 (517.9 pg/mg)	64% (31–89)	78% (67–87)	32%	93%	**0.71 (0.64–0.79)**
			CCL2 (226.0 pg/mg)	82% (48–98)	57% (44–68)	23%	95%	0.73 (0.55–0.90)
			L-FABP (7.6 ng/mg)	9% (0–41)	88% (78–94)	15%	100%	0.69 (0.54–0.84)
			NGAL (12.8 ng/mg)	100% (72–100)	48% (36–60)	23%	100%	0.61 (0.45–0.77)
Kolling [23]	TCMR (11; subclinical, 51)	STA-B (normal, 31)	HE4 (789.1 ng/mg)	100% (72–100)	54% (41–66)	26%	100%	0.72 (0.59–0.84)
			hsa_circ_0001334 (2.41)	70% (59–80)	92% (64–100)	98%	32%	0.81 (0.70–0.92)
Sigdel [24]	TCMR + ABMR (45)	ALL-B (normal, 43; bAR, 19; BKVN, 43)	AR vs normal (uCRM score = 3.63)	95%	98%	-	-	0.85 ($p < 0.0001$)
								0.99, $p < 0.0001$

Table 4. Cont.

Ref.	Outcome (n)	Control Group (n)	Test Design, Biomarkers, Thresholds	Diagnostic Test Accuracy (95%CI)				
				Sens.	Spec.	PPV	NPV	AUC–Accuracy(%)
Kim [25]	TCMR (14)	STA-B (normal, 17)	AR vs normal + bAR	87%	98%	-	-	-
			AR vs normal + bAR + BKVN	77%	98%	-	-	96.6%
			Unbiased metab.³	-	-	-	-	-
			Training: TCMR (10) vs STA-B (13)	90%	85%	-	-	0.93 (0.72–1.00) – 87%
			Validation: TCMR (4) vs STA-B (4)	-	-	-	-	62.5%
Banas [27]	TCMR	ALL-B (normal) + STA (extended)	Unbiased metab.², train (180)	-	-	-	-	0.76 (0.69–0.82)
			Test (178) strict/extended cohort	-	-	-	-	0.72 (0.58–0.86)/ 0.74 (0.62–0.86)
Lim [28]	TCMR (25)	STA-B (normal, 22)	TSPAN1 + HPX	64%	73%	-	-	0.74
Chen [29]	TCMR (37) + ABMR (12)	ALL-B (normal, 58; CAN, 29; ATN, 10)	CXCL13 for AR vs. normal	84%	79%	-	-	0.82 (0.73–0.90)
			CXCL13 for AR vs. CAN + ATN	-	-	-	-	0.63 (0.52–0.75)
			iKEA	-	-	-	-	-
Park [33]	TCMR (22)	DYS-B (normal, 22)	Training: TCMR (15) vs normal (15)	93%	88%	-	-	0.91 ± 0.02 - 90%
			Validation: TCMR (7) vs normal (7)	64%	100%	-	-	**0.84 ± 0.11 - 71%**
Seo [35]	TCMR (27) + ABMR (13)	STA-B (normal, 17); STA (22)	CTOT4 formula	-	-	-	-	0.72 (0.60–0.83)
			CXCL10 mRNA	-	-	-	-	0.72 (0.60–0.83)
			CD3ε mRNA	-	-	-	-	0.71 (0.60–0.83)
			18S rRNA	-	-	-	-	0.47 (0.33–0.60)
Chen [37]	TCMR (37) + ABMR (12)	STA-B (normal, 58)	sTim-3 (1.836 ng/mmol)	90%	83%	-	-	0.88 (0.81–0.95)
Blydt-H. [41]	ABMR (10)	ALL-B (normal, TCMR, transplant glomerulopathy, IFTA, other, 49)	ABMR score = 0.23	78%	83%	40%	96%	0.84 (0.77–0.91)
			ABMR score with top 10 metabolites	-	-	-	-	0.80 (0.73–0.88)
Raza [43]	TCMR (acute, 101; borderline, 47; vascular, 17)	DYS-B (normal, 47; IFTA, 46) + STA (42)	Validation	-	-	-	-	**0.76 (0.67–0.84)**
			CCL2 (198 pg/mL)	87%	62%	-	-	0.81 (0.76–0.86)
Galichon [44]	TCMR (11) + bAR (3) + ABMR (28) + mixed (9)	ALL-B (56)	CTOT4 formula	-	-	-	-	0.72 (0.61–0.82)
			CXCL10 mRNA	-	-	-	-	0.76 (0.66–0.86)
			CD3ε mRNA	-	-	-	-	0.67 (0.56–0.78)
			18S rRNA	-	-	-	-	0.63 (0.53–0.74)

Table 4. *Cont.*

Ref.	Outcome (n)	Control Group (n)	Test Design, Biomarkers, Thresholds	Diagnostic Test Accuracy (95%CI)				
				Sens.	Spec.	PPV	NPV	AUC–Accuracy(%)
Sigdel [45]	TCMR + ABMR (42)	ALL-B (normal, 47; CAN, 46; BKVN, 16)	Unbiased proteomics (11 peptides) Validation: AR (20) vs normal (27), CAN (15), BKVN (16)	-	-	-	-	**0.94 (0.93–0.95)**
A. Elaziz [48]	TCMR (31)	STA-B (normal, 23)	PD1 mRNA (2.6) FOXP3 mRNA (1.5) PD1 + FOXP3 mRNA	80% 83% 94%	84% 90% 97%	- - -	- - -	0.81 0.91 0.98
Lorenzen [49]	TCMR (11; subclinical 51)	STA-B (normal, 31)	RNA L328 (9.556)	49%	96%	49%	93%	0.76 ($p < 0.001$)
Rabant [51]	TCMR (10) + ABMR (37) + mixed (31)	DYS-B (203)	CXCL9 CXCL10	58% 59%	85% 83%	59% 58%	84% 84%	0.71 (0.64–0.78) 0.74 (0.68–0.80)
Blydt-H. [52]	TCMR (subclinical, 17; clinical, 9)	ALL-B (normal, 21; IFTA, 31)	CXCL10, subclinical (4.82 ng/mL) Clinical (4.72 ng/mL)	59% 77%	67% 60%	- -	- -	0.81 (0.70–0.92) 0.88 (0.73–1.0)

Results from a validation group are shown in **bold**. Unbiased metabolomics: [1] (NAD, NADP, nicotinic acid, MNA, GABA, cholesterol sulfate, homocysteine); [2] (alanine, citrate, lactate, urea); [3] (guanidoacetic acid, methylimidazoleacetic acid, dopamine, 4-guanidinobutyric acid, and L-tryptophan). ALL, all patients irrespectively of allograft function (-B, biopsied); DYS, dysfunctional graft patients (-B, biopsied); STA, stable graft patients (-B, biopsied).

Table 5. Summary of the study results—Predictive studies with DTA. This table shows the outcome of prediction studies. Outcome and control group for the DTA analysis are reported (sample size when available), followed by the studied urinary biomarker(s), thresholds and time from transplant to test.

Ref.	Outcome (n)	Control Group (n)	Biomarkers, Thresholds and Time Post-Transplant	Diagnostic Test Accuracy (95%CI)				
				Sens.	Spec.	PPV	NPV	AUC
Ciftci [26]	TCMR (9) + ABMR (6)	STA (70)	CXCL9, 1 day - 3 months	70–85%	37–88%	60–71%	71–90%	0.71–0.95
			CXCL10, 1 day - 3 months	78–82%	58–85%	59–73%	74–87%	0.75–0.97
			TNF-α (12.08 pg/mL), 1 day	71%	57%	-	-	0.74 (0.51–0.97)
Ciftci [32]	AR (9)	STA (56)	TNF-α (11.03), 7 days	100%	84%	-	-	0.95 (0.88–1.00)
			TNF-α (9.85), 1 month	100%	83%	-	-	0.91 (0.81–1.00)
			TNF-α (9.13), 3 months	100%	71%	-	-	0.83 (0.75–0.98)
			TNF-α (7.42), 6 months	100%	62%	-	-	0.82 (0.69–0.95)
Millan [34]	TCMR (8)	STA (72)	miR-155-5p (0.51), 1wk-6m	85%	86%	88%	100%	0.88 (0.78–0.97)
			CXCL10 (84.73 pg/mL),1wk-6m	84%	80%	90%	85%	0.87 (0.81–0.92)
			CXCL10:Cr (0.43), 1wk-6m	72%	73%	90%	96%	0.75 (0.67–0.83)
Belm.V. [42]	ABMR (subclinical)	ALL-B	Albuminuria (> 30 mg/g), 6m	-	-	-	-	0.75 (0.55–0.95)
Rabant [50]	AR (TCMR + ABMR + mixed, 76)	ALL-B	CXCL9:Cr (1.78 ng/mmoL),10d	61%	50%	24%	84%	0.58 (0.47–0.68)
			CXCL9:Cr (0.96), 1 month	81%	35%	23%	89%	0.50 (0.37–0.62)
			CXCL9:Cr (1.67), 3 months	57%	62%	18%	91%	0.57 (0.39–0.75)
			CXCL10:Cr (4.80), 10 days	57%	52%	23%	83%	0.54 (0.43–0.65)
			CXCL10:Cr (2.79), 1 month	83%	51%	29%	93%	0.72 (0.61–0.80)
			CXCL10:Cr (5.32), 3 months	54%	77%	25%	92%	0.68 (0.55–0.80)

ALL, all patients irrespectively of allograft function (-B, biopsied); STA, stable graft patients (-B, biopsied).

2.5.1. Acute Rejection Diagnosis

Among studies with the lowest risk of bias, only three studies [16,17,45] yielded a very good (0.8–0.9) or excellent (> 0.9) performance as diagnostic AUC (Table 4). All of these studies provided diagnostic accuracy measure for the diagnosis of AR, considering both TCMR and ABMR as outcome of interest. Tinel et al. found that the combination of urinary CXCL9 and CXCL10 could distinguish AR patients among almost three-hundred heterogeneous patients with an AUC of 0.70 [16]. These results strengthened the good performance previously described, among dysfunctional allografts, separately for CXCL9 (AUC 0.71) and CXCL10 (AUC 0.74) by Rabant and colleagues [51]. Yang et al. separately validated the so-called Q score in two validation cohorts for the diagnosis of AR. A Q score ≥ 32 maintained an excellent diagnostic performance (AUC 0.96) also when validated in the entire study population (n = 364), with high PPV and NPV (87–98%) [17]. Banas et al., after identifying a urinary metabolite signature with good diagnostic performance for TCMR [27], validated it in a cohort of 109 patients for the diagnosis of AR with and AUC of 0.71 [21]. Through unbiased metabolomics, Sigdel et al. identified a signature of eleven urinary peptides able to segregate AR patients from normal histology, chronic allograft nephropathy and BK virus nephropathy patients with an excellent AUC of 0.94 in validation cohort [45]. The same authors proved a urine cell sediment gene expression-based score (*uCRM score*) able to diagnose AR with 96.6% accuracy and potentially quantify the degree of injury [24].

Table 6. Summary of the study results—Studies with no DTA. This table describes the main results from studies with no DTA. Sample size is reported for the outcome and control group when available.

Ref.	Outcome (n)	Control Group (n)	Biomarkers, Thresholds and Main Results
Barabadi [30]	AR (27)	ALL-B (normal, 45; CAN, 19)	FOXP3 mRNA expression was significantly higher in AR (**$p < 0.001$**)
Mockler [31] *	TCMR (5; borderline, 3)	STA-B	There was no significant association between 6 months post-transplant CCL2 and TCMR changes ($p = 0.46$)
Gandolfini [36]	TCMR (22)	ALL-B (normal, 19)	CXCL9 > 200 pg/mL in TCMR, 100-200 in dysfunction graft, and < 100 pg/mL in stable graft (**$p < 0.01$**)
Domenico [38]	AR (23)	ALL-B (ATN, 18; normal, 8)	mirRNA 142-3p was significantly higher in AR compared to stable graft (**$p < 0.001$**); not compared to ATN ($p = 0.079$)
Lee [39]	AR (8)	STA (8); DYS-B (ATN, 8; other, 4)	Donor-derived cfDNA was not significantly different between groups ($p = 0.95$)
Seeman [40]	TCMR (2) + ABMR (2)	DYS-B (11)	NGAL was not significantly different between groups ($p = 0.48$)
Garcia-C. [46]	AR (9)	ALL-B (fibrosis, 31; other, 10)	IL10 and IFNγ were not significantly different between groups ($p = 0.95$, $p = 0.1$)
Ho [47]	TCMR (17; subclinical, 17)	ALL-B (normal, 22)	MMP7 and CXCL10 were significantly elevated in subclinical (**$p = 0.01$, $p < 0.0001$**) and clinical (**$p < 0.001$**) TCMR
Sigdel [53]	AR (10)	DYS-B (IFTA, BKVN, 20)	Ten urinary exosomal proteins were significantly increased in AR (**$p < 0.05$**)

Statistically significant ($p < 0.05$) results are shown in **bold**. * Prediction study. ALL, all patients irrespectively of allograft function (-B, biopsied); DYS, dysfunctional graft patients (-B, biopsied); STA, stable graft patients (-B, biopsied).

2.5.2. T-Cell-Mediated Rejection Diagnosis

The previously mentioned study by Tinel et al. also provided separate outcome analysis for CXCL9 and CXCL10, with the best performance for TCMR diagnosis with a NPV of 98% and a very good AUC of 0.81 [16]. Also of note, CCL2, at a threshold level of 198 pg/mL, yielded very good performance (AUC 0.81) for TCMR identification among a population of 300 normal and dysfunctional grafts in the study by Raza et al. [43]. Urinary exosome proteins were investigated in two case-control studies for the diagnosis of TCMR. Lim et al. found significantly higher urinary tetraspanin-1 (TSPAN1) and hemopexin (HPX) expression levels in TCMR patients with good diagnostic performance (AUC 0.74) [28], while Park et al. reported the initial results of an optimized integrated kidney exosome analysis (iKEA) able to distinguish TCMR from normal histology patients, with a very good performance (AUC 0.84) in a small validation cohort [33].

2.5.3. Antibody-Mediated Rejection Diagnosis

The study from Blydt-Hansen et al. was the only one to specifically evaluate the diagnostic performance for ABMR diagnosis [41]. The authors tested and validated the use of the *ABMR score*, with a good sensitivity (78%) and specificity (83%), NPV of 96%, a good performance (AUC 0.76 in validation), and the ability to provide a stratification from negative—indeterminate—to positive ABMR patients [41].

2.5.4. Acute Rejection, TCMR, and ABMR Prediction

Among prediction studies (Table 5), high risk of bias was often identified for patient selection and index test. However, good performances for AR prediction were obtained by three months post-transplant for CXCL9 and CXCL10 levels [26], and seven days and one month post-transplant for TNF-alpha levels [32]. The well-conducted study by Rabant et al. found both urinary CXCL9 and CXCL10, adjusted for urinary creatinine concentration, to have high NPV (89 to 93%) for AR at one and three months post-transplantation. CXCL10 yielded the best predictive performance (AUC 0.72) at one month post-transplantation, at the threshold of 2.79 ng/mmoL [50]. For TCMR prediction, post-transplant CXCL10 and miR-155-5p levels yielded positive results [34], while for ABMR prediction six months albuminuria was investigated [42].

3. Discussion

With this systematic review, we critically summarize the results of the last five years research, the latest advances, and highlight the most frequent limitations of studies assessing urinary biomarkers for the diagnosis or prediction of acute allograft rejection. We focused on study design, distinction between TCMR and ABMR setting, evaluation of confounding (e.g., DGF, infections, calcineurin inhibitors nephrotoxicity), comparison with the gold standard of diagnosis (both for cases and controls), and presence of estimates of the biomarker(s) performance in validation.

The main finding was the strengthening in evidence for the clinical utility of urinary C-X-C motif chemokine ligands (in particular for the diagnosis of TCMR) alone or in combination with other biomarkers as in the *Q score* (cell-free DNA, methylated cell-free DNA, clusterin, total protein, creatinine, and CXCL10) or in the CTOT-4 formula. CXCL9 and CXCL10 had AUC ranging from 0.67–0.88 with a NPV ranging from 84–98% for AR diagnosis and AUC ranging from 0.50–0.97 with a NPV ranging from 71–96% for AR prediction. Signatures of urinary peptides and metabolites identified through unbiased proteomic and metabolomics, and a cluster of urinary cell pellet genes (*uCRM score*) were also established for the diagnosis of AR, net of some limitations for their introduction in clinical practice. Confounding outcomes need always to be considered due to potential overlap in diagnosis. For example, urinary chemokines are also elevated in allograft BK virus nephropathy (as discussed below), urinary NGAL was proposed as early predictor of DGF [56], and as a biomarker of CNI toxicity [57], while urinary miRNAs dysregulation has been linked to interstitial inflammation and tubular atrophy [58]. For the first time Tinel and colleagues demonstrated that considering (instead of excluding) potential confounding factors (i.e., urinary tract infection and BK virus reactivation) in a diagnostic multi-parametric model could optimize its performance [16]. A model combining eight parameters (recipient age, sex, eGFR, DSA presence, signs of urinary tract infection, BKV blood viral load, CXCL9, and CXCL10) could reach AR diagnosis with high accuracy (AUC: 0.85, 0.80–0.89), paving the way for new studies combining urinary biomarkers with clinical characteristics to reach the highest clinical relevance and provide targeted therapy for our patients.

Up to 2015, almost ninety non-redundant molecules were identified as urinary biomarkers of AR, participating in different pathways such as complement activation, antigen presentation, and inflammation signaling [15]. Urine was the most frequent matrix of choice for these analyses, and studies were often limited by small sample size and case-control design, no histology in the control cohorts, lack of confounding adjustment, lack of a validation set, and technical difficulties with procedure standardization and costs [15]. Although serum creatinine levels and proteinuria monitoring are well established biomarkers used by transplant physicians to suspect AR, they lack both sensitivity and specificity, and they are of little help in the prediction phase, in detecting subclinical rejection, and in differential diagnosis between AR, infections, drug toxicity, and acute tubular necrosis [14,59]. In a study of 281 consecutive biopsies, indicated by an increase in serum creatinine levels, only 27.8% revealed any sign of AR [51]. Conversely, subclinical rejection (i.e., rejection without clinical dysfunction) was found in over 40% of patients with normal renal function in the presence of anti-HLA de novo donor-specific antibodies (DSA) [60]. Proteinuria is common after kidney transplant and, although widely used as a biomarker of renal disease and despite its value as an independent predictor of long-term graft survival, it could also be sign of post-transplant primary disease recurrence (e.g., focal-segmental glomerulosclerosis), infections (e.g., CMV), immunosuppressive medication toxicity, or systemic (e.g., new-onset diabetes) and urologic complications (e.g., ureteral stenosis) [59,61]. DSA monitoring is currently considered the primary biomarker for ABMR but, despite the increasing ability to detect low level of DSAs, their positive predictive value is low, so that up to 60% of patients showing de novo DSA do not show any sign of AR at biopsy [60].

Continuous advances in molecular techniques and the "-omics" sciences have helped to identify many potential new blood and urine biomarkers for the diagnosis and prediction of kidney allograft AR in the last two decades. Of note, elevated pretransplant serum CXCL9 and CXCL10 levels were found to be associated to increased risk of early and severe AR and graft failure [62–64]. Subsequently, among urine-derived proteins, a 2012 study found CXCL9 and CXCL10 to be considerably elevated in patients experiencing either AR (clinical or subclinical) or BK virus infection (86% sensitivity and 80% specificity for CXCL9; 80% sensitivity and 76% specificity for CXCL10), but they were not able to distinguish between the two conditions [65]. These results were reinforced by the 2013 CTOT-1 study, which found that low urine CXCL9 measured at 6 months post-transplant identified a subset of patients at low-risk for AR development (92% NPV for Banff ≥1A TCMR) and predicted allograft stability up to 24 months post-transplant (93-99% NPV) [66]. With the help of mass spectroscopy, elevated beta2-microglobulin levels were identified as strongly correlated with AR (83% sensitivity, 80% specificity, 89% PPV, 71% NPV) and then validated by ELISA in the urine of AR patients [67]. Cytotoxic proteins perforine and granzyme B urine mRNAs were proposed to noninvasively diagnose AR (respectively with 83% sensitivity, 83% specificity, and 79% sensitivity, 77% specificity) [68] and Treg marker FOXP3 was shown to predict reversal of AR (90% sensitivity, 73% specificity) [69]. T-cell immunoglobulin-3 domain, mucin domain mRNA expression (Tim-3, also known as hepatitis A virus cellular receptor 2) in urinary cells was found to be able to discriminate AR from other causes of acute graft dysfunction (calcineurin inhibitor nephrotoxicity or interstitial fibrosis and tubular atrophy) with an AUC of 0.96, 89% PPV and 94% NPV [70]. A 2013 multicenter study from the CTOT-4 study group later identified a 3-gene urinary mRNA signature (CD3ε mRNA, CXCL10 mRNA, 18S rRNA) able to discriminate acute TCMR from no rejection in indication biopsies, with an AUC of 0.74, 79% sensitivity and 78% specificity in a validation set [54]. Also, noncoding miRNAs (e.g., miRNA-10a, miRNA-10b, miRNA-210), although limited by the easy degradation, proved to be detectable in the urine, and in particular low miRNA-210 levels discriminated patients affected by AR from stable control transplant patients (74% sensitivity, 52% specificity) [71].

Our systematic analysis of the more recent literature details the accuracy of a variety of urinary biomarkers for allograft AR with the objective of allowing transplant physicians early diagnosis and prediction of rejection episodes, and differential diagnosis with other causes of allograft dysfunction. A correct histologic diagnosis of AR is essential during the process of new biomarkers validation and the Banff criteria are considered the gold standard for biopsy evaluation. The diagnostic criteria for TCMR have essentially undergone no major change in the last decade with lymphocytic infiltrate of tubules (tubulitis) and larger vessels (vasculitis) being the main descriptive features. The severity of these lesions is graded according to the degree of lymphocytic infiltrate per high-powered field. On the other hand, ABMR criteria has continuously evolved in recent years–thus highlighting the great importance of applying an up to date classification in this setting–with the recognition of its variable histologic presentation [72,73]. Original criteria established in 2000s included active tissue injury, immunohistologic evidence of peritubular capillary complement split-product C4d deposition and circulating DSA. Subsequent studies demonstrating the presence of ABMR also in lacking detectable C4d staining biopsies [74], pushed the Banff Working Group in 2013 to the major change in the ABMR criteria, removing the requirement for C4d detection [75]. The most recent changes in 2017 included removing the requirement for documented circulating DSA in the setting of positive C4d staining and microvascular inflammation and included the use of AMR-associated gene transcripts panels [10].

The ideal biomarker should be readily available, accurate, inexpensive, standardized, repeatable, and noninvasive and would be useful to reduce the need for protocol biopsy and enable early targeted intervention. The chance of finding an ideal biomarker with high sensitivity, specificity, PPV and NPV is small. However, not all biomarkers need to be highly sensitive and highly specific at the same time, depending on the clinical question they are going to answer. Therefore, targeting specific populations and accepting lower predictive values in certain variables may be a better strategy. For example, to confirm the need for allograft biopsy in a population at high risk for AR (thus providing biopsy to the correct patients), a test with high sensitivity, and low false negative rate, would be the most useful. On the contrary, to propose diagnostic biopsies in a population at low risk for AR (thus avoiding unnecessary per-protocol biopsies), a test with high specificity, and low false positive rate, would be the test of choice. Also, TCMR and ABMR are different clinical entities and it is unrealistic, on current evidence, to hope for a biomarker that will accurately predict AR in both forms in a typical population of transplant patients with possible confounding.

Our systematic review has some limitations. The heterogeneity of the included studies did not permit to detail the many facets of individual study results, especially the more complex ones, to stick with the systematic review question. For space restraints, tables only report the major findings of each study, limited to urinary biomarkers. A narrative synthesis of the most promising results was applied to improve readability and a meta-analysis could not be performed. From our work, overall good quality studies emerged, many with DTA analysis and some comprising a thorough validation process yielding a very good to excellent diagnostic performance. Although specific forms of bias were assessed using QUADAS-2 publication bias could not be formally assessed and the authors acknowledge this can overestimate the weight of positive results. Weaknesses of the included studies were often the use of small cohorts obtained by case-control selection yielding inflated predictive values, the exclusion of confounding, unclear or out of date Banff classification application, the absence of validation cohorts, and lack of hypothesis-driven approach. In fact, the biomarker discovery process should not only consist of a training phase (i.e., a case-control study), but also comprise independent validation in a prospective study and confrontation with real-life clinical setting.

4. Materials and Methods

4.1. Literature Search

This review follows the Preferred Reporting Items for Systematic Reviews and Meta-Analysis (PRISMA) guidelines [76]. The objective of the study, search strategy, inclusion and exclusion criteria, and study evaluation method were planned in advance, refined, and approved by all authors. MEDLINE was searched from 1 January 2015 to 31 May 2020. Key terms like "kidney", "renal", "transplant/transplantation", "urine/urinary", "marker/biomarker", and "rejection" were combined in the search strategy. Additional relevant articles were searched from scanning reference lists of included studies and added if not detected by the original literature search.

4.2. Selection Process

The first screening by title and abstract was separately performed by two authors (F.G., L.C.) in the eligibility process. Original articles were selected if they assessed one, more, or a combination of urinary biomarker(s) and their performance in diagnosis or prediction of kidney allograft AR. Abstracts, reviews, studies assessing biomarkers from other matrix (e.g., blood samples or histology staining), and studies specifically evaluating different outcomes (e.g., chronic rejection, infection, or allograft survival) were excluded. In the inclusion process, selected articles were then independently full-text reviewed by two authors (F.G., L.C.). Any disagreement between the two investigators was discussed and solved with the help of all authors.

4.3. Data Collection and Analysis

Data from each of the included studies were collected with the help of a pre-specified spreadsheet and extraction table refined by all authors. Study design, single or multicenter patient collection, sample size, years of enrollment, urinary biomarker(s) of interest (i.e., index test), the Banff classification used for histological AR diagnosis (i.e., reference standard) and the addressed outcome(s) were collected in a descriptive table. Studies were distinguished between diagnostic and predictive. Diagnostic studies were usually collecting urine samples on the day of the diagnostic biopsy while predictive studies were analyzing urine samples collected before AR development. Studies that reported DTA data, such as sensitivity, specificity, PPV, NPV, and AUC were evaluated for risk of bias and applicability concern using the Quality Assessment Tool for Diagnostic Accuracy Studies-2 (QUADAS-2), a tool for quality evaluation of diagnostic accuracy studies [77]. The most important items for a positive evaluation included; a cross-sectional study design; avoiding patient selection bias and inappropriate exclusion; the definition of the index test (biomarker) threshold in a training set and its validation in a separate set of patients; and compliance with the correct histological definition of AR as a standard reference for all patients included in the analysis. Due to the great heterogeneity of the included studies, a meta-analysis was not performed, and a narrative synthesis of the results was preferred.

5. Conclusions

In recent years, numerous studies joined the challenging quest for urinary biomarkers in diagnosis and prediction of acute kidney allograft rejection. Authors must face the difficult task to allow for mediating between the need for a precise setting and reference standard diagnosis (to develop the most precise biomarkers), and the need for their validation in the most heterogeneous population of kidney allograft patients (to increase clinical utility). Urinary chemokines CXCL9 and CXCL10, alone or in combination with others, are the most frequently used and the most promising biomarkers, but multi-parametric clinical and laboratory models could represent the best strategy for future studies. Remarkable advances have been made on the path of allowing a more precise allocation of resources, helping clinicians to move from the standard protocol/indication biopsy dichotomy, to reduce unnecessary immunosuppression, and to improve kidney allograft outcomes in the long-term.

Author Contributions: Conceptualization, investigation, resources, F.G. and L.C.; methodology, data curation, formal analysis, visualization F.G.; writing—original draft preparation, F.G. and L.C.; writing—review and editing, E.B., F.B., C.E., R.M.R., J.P.H.; supervision J.P.H., P.R.; funding acquisition, P.R. All authors made a significant contribution to the content of this manuscript as per ICJME recommendations. All authors have read and agreed to the published version of the manuscript.

Funding: This research received no external funding.

Acknowledgments: We thank the Meyer Children's Hospital and the Meyer Children's Hospital Foundation.

Conflicts of Interest: The authors declare no conflict of interest.

Abbreviations

ABMR	Antibody-mediated rejection
AKI	Acute kidney injury
AR	Acute rejection
ATN	Acute tubular necrosis
AUC	Area under the ROC curve
BKVN	BK virus nephropathy
CAN	Chronic allograft nephropathy
CCL2	Chemokine ligand 2
cfDNA	Cell free DNA
CKD	Chronic kidney disease
CTOT	Clinical trials in organ transplantation
CXCL	C-X-C motif chemokine ligands
DGF	Delayed graft function
DSA	Donor-specific antibodies
DTA	Diagnostic test accuracy
EPCAM	Epithelial cell adhesion molecule
FOXP3	Forkhead box P3
GABA	Gamma-aminobutyric acid

HE4	Human epididymis protein 4
HPX	Hemopexin
IFNγ	Interferon gamma
IFTA	Interstitial fibrosis and tubular atrophy
iKEA	Integrated kidney exosome analysis
IL	Interleukin
LC3	Microtubule-associated protein 1A/1B-light chain 3
LFABP	Liver-type fatty acid-binding protein
MMP7	Matrix metalloproteinase 7
MNA	1-methylnicotinamide
NAD	Nicotinamide adenine dinucleotide
NADP	Nicotinamide adenine dinucleotide phosphate
NGAL	Neutrophil gelatinase-associated lipocalin
NPV	Negative predictive value
PB	Publication bias
PD1	Programmed cell death protein 1
PDX	Podocalyxin
PPV	Positive predictive value
PRISMA	Preferred reporting items for systematic reviews and meta-analysis
QUADAS	Quality assessment tool for diagnostic accuracy studies
Sens	Sensitivity
Spec	Specificity
sTIM3	Soluble T cell immunoglobulin mucin domain 3
TCMR	T-cell mediated rejection
TEC	Tubular epithelial cells
TNFα	Tumor necrosis factor alpha
TSPAN1	Tetraspanin 1
uCRM	Urinary common rejection module

References

1. Ronco, C.; Bellomo, R.; Kellum, J.A. Acute kidney injury. *Lancet* **2019**, *394*, 1949–1964. [CrossRef]
2. Yang, J.Y.C.; Sarwal, R.D.; Fervenza, F.C.; Sarwal, M.M.; Lafayette, R.A. Noninvasive Urinary Monitoring of Progression in IgA Nephropathy. *Int. J. Mol. Sci.* **2019**, *20*, 4463. [CrossRef] [PubMed]
3. Kwan, B.; Fuhrer, T.; Zhang, J.; Darshi, M.; Van Espen, B.; Montemayor, D.; de Boer, I.H.; Dobre, M.; Hsu, C.-Y.; Kelly, T.N.; et al. Metabolomic Markers of Kidney Function Decline in Patients With Diabetes: Evidence From the Chronic Renal Insufficiency Cohort (CRIC) Study. *Am. J. Kidney Dis.* **2020**. S0272-6386(20)30572-2. [CrossRef] [PubMed]
4. Naesens, M.; Anglicheau, D. Precision Transplant Medicine: Biomarkers to the Rescue. *J. Am. Soc. Nephrol.* **2018**, *29*, 24–34. [CrossRef]
5. Guzzi, F.; Knight, S.R.; Ploeg, R.J.; Hunter, J.P. A systematic review to identify whether perfusate biomarkers produced during hypothermic machine perfusion can predict graft outcomes in kidney transplantation. *Transpl. Int.* **2020**, *33*, 590–602. [CrossRef]
6. Jochmans, I.; Pirenne, J. Graft quality assessment in kidney transplantation: Not an exact science yet! *Curr. Opin. Organ Transplant.* **2011**, *16*, 174–179. [CrossRef]
7. Jamshaid, F.; Froghi, S.; Cocco, P.D.; Dor, F.J. Novel non-invasive biomarkers diagnostic of acute rejection in renal transplant recipients: A systematic review. *Int. J. Clin. Pract.* **2018**, *72*, e13220. [CrossRef]
8. Wiebe, C.; Ho, J.; Gibson, I.W.; Rush, D.N.; Nickerson, P.W. Carpe diem-Time to transition from empiric to precision medicine in kidney transplantation. *Am. J. Transplant.* **2018**, *18*, 1615–1625. [CrossRef]
9. Thierry, A.; Thervet, E.; Vuiblet, V.; Goujon, J.-M.; Machet, M.-C.; Noel, L.-H.; Rioux-Leclercq, N.; Comoz, F.; Cordonnier, C.; François, A.; et al. Long-term impact of subclinical inflammation diagnosed by protocol biopsy one year after renal transplantation. *Am. J. Transplant.* **2011**, *11*, 2153–2161. [CrossRef]
10. Haas, M.; Loupy, A.; Lefaucheur, C.; Roufosse, C.; Glotz, D.; Seron, D.; Nankivell, B.J.; Halloran, P.F.; Colvin, R.B.; Akalin, E.; et al. The Banff 2017 Kidney Meeting Report: Revised diagnostic criteria for chronic active T cell-mediated rejection, antibody-mediated rejection, and prospects for integrative endpoints for next-generation clinical trials. *Am. J. Transplant.* **2018**, *18*, 293–307. [CrossRef]

11. Singh, N.; Samant, H.; Hawxby, A.; Samaniego, M.D. Biomarkers of rejection in kidney transplantation. *Curr Opin Organ Transplant* **2019**, *24*, 103–110. [CrossRef] [PubMed]
12. Quaglia, M.; Merlotti, G.; Guglielmetti, G.; Castellano, G.; Cantaluppi, V. Recent Advances on Biomarkers of Early and Late Kidney Graft Dysfunction. *Int. J. Mol. Sci.* **2020**, *21*, 5404. [CrossRef] [PubMed]
13. Anglicheau, D.; Naesens, M.; Essig, M.; Gwinner, W.; Marquet, P. Establishing Biomarkers in Transplant Medicine: A Critical Review of Current Approaches. *Transplantation* **2016**, *100*, 2024–2038. [CrossRef]
14. Lo, D.J.; Kaplan, B.; Kirk, A.D. Biomarkers for kidney transplant rejection. *Nat. Rev. Nephrol.* **2014**, *10*, 215–225. [CrossRef] [PubMed]
15. Gwinner, W.; Metzger, J.; Husi, H.; Marx, D. Proteomics for rejection diagnosis in renal transplant patients: Where are we now? *World J. Transplant* **2016**, *6*, 28–41. [CrossRef] [PubMed]
16. Tinel, C.; Devresse, A.; Vermorel, A.; Sauvaget, V.; Marx, D.; Avettand-Fenoel, V.; Amrouche, L.; Timsit, M.-O.; Snanoudj, R.; Caillard, S.; et al. Development and validation of an optimized integrative model using urinary chemokines for noninvasive diagnosis of acute allograft rejection. *Am. J. Transplant.* **2020**. [CrossRef]
17. Yang, J.Y.C.; Sarwal, R.D.; Sigdel, T.K.; Damm, I.; Rosenbaum, B.; Liberto, J.M.; Chan-On, C.; Arreola-Guerra, J.M.; Alberu, J.; Vincenti, F.; et al. A urine score for noninvasive accurate diagnosis and prediction of kidney transplant rejection. *Sci. Transl. Med.* **2020**, *12*, eaba2501. [CrossRef]
18. Kalantari, S.; Chashmniam, S.; Nafar, M.; Samavat, S.; Rezaie, D.; Dalili, N. A Noninvasive Urine Metabolome Panel as Potential Biomarkers for Diagnosis of T Cell-Mediated Renal Transplant Rejection. *OMICS A J. Integr. Biol.* **2020**, *24*, 140–147. [CrossRef]
19. Verma, A.; Muthukumar, T.; Yang, H.; Lubetzky, M.; Cassidy, M.F.; Lee, J.R.; Dadhania, D.M.; Snopkowski, C.; Shankaranarayanan, D.; Salvatore, S.P.; et al. Urinary cell transcriptomics and acute rejection in human kidney allografts. *JCI Insight* **2020**, *5*, e131552. [CrossRef]
20. Goerlich, N.; Brand, H.A.; Langhans, V.; Tesch, S.; Schachtner, T.; Koch, B.; Paliege, A.; Schneider, W.; Grützkau, A.; Reinke, P.; et al. Kidney transplant monitoring by urinary flow cytometry: Biomarker combination of T cells, renal tubular epithelial cells, and podocalyxin-positive cells detects rejection. *Sci. Rep.* **2020**, *10*, 796. [CrossRef]
21. Banas, M.C.; Neumann, S.; Pagel, P.; Putz, F.J.; Krämer, B.K.; Böhmig, G.A.; Eiglsperger, J.; Schiffer, E.; Ruemmele, P.; Banas, B. A urinary metabolite constellation to detect acute rejection in kidney allografts. *EBioMedicine* **2019**, *48*, 505–512. [CrossRef] [PubMed]
22. Tajima, S.; Fu, R.; Shigematsu, T.; Noguchi, H.; Kaku, K.; Tsuchimoto, A.; Okabe, Y.; Masuda, S. Urinary Human Epididymis Secretory Protein 4 as a Useful Biomarker for Subclinical Acute Rejection Three Months after Kidney Transplantation. *Int. J. Mol. Sci.* **2019**, *20*, 4699. [CrossRef]
23. Kölling, M.; Haddad, G.; Wegmann, U.; Kistler, A.; Bosakova, A.; Seeger, H.; Hübel, K.; Haller, H.; Mueller, T.; Wüthrich, R.P.; et al. Circular RNAs in Urine of Kidney Transplant Patients with Acute T Cell-Mediated Allograft Rejection. *Clin. Chem.* **2019**, *65*, 1287–1294. [CrossRef] [PubMed]
24. Sigdel, T.K.; Yang, J.Y.C.; Bestard, O.; Schroeder, A.; Hsieh, S.-C.; Liberto, J.M.; Damm, I.; Geraedts, A.C.M.; Sarwal, M.M. A urinary Common Rejection Module (uCRM) score for non-invasive kidney transplant monitoring. *PLoS ONE* **2019**, *14*, e0220052. [CrossRef] [PubMed]
25. Kim, S.-Y.; Kim, B.K.; Gwon, M.-R.; Seong, S.J.; Ohk, B.; Kang, W.Y.; Lee, H.W.; Jung, H.-Y.; Cho, J.-H.; Chung, B.H.; et al. Urinary metabolomic profiling for noninvasive diagnosis of acute T cell-mediated rejection after kidney transplantation. *J. Chromatogr. B Analyt. Technol. Biomed. Life Sci.* **2019**, *1118–1119*, 157–163. [CrossRef] [PubMed]
26. Ciftci, H.S.; Tefik, T.; Savran, M.K.; Demir, E.; Caliskan, Y.; Ogret, Y.D.; Oktar, T.; Sanlı, O.; Kocak, T.; Ozluk, Y.; et al. Urinary CXCL9 and CXCL10 Levels and Acute Renal Graft Rejection. *Int. J. Organ Transplant. Med.* **2019**, *10*, 53–63.
27. Banas, M.; Neumann, S.; Eiglsperger, J.; Schiffer, E.; Putz, F.J.; Reichelt-Wurm, S.; Krämer, B.K.; Pagel, P.; Banas, B. Identification of a urine metabolite constellation characteristic for kidney allograft rejection. *Metabolomics* **2018**, *14*, 116. [CrossRef] [PubMed]
28. Lim, J.-H.; Lee, C.-H.; Kim, K.Y.; Jung, H.-Y.; Choi, J.-Y.; Cho, J.-H.; Park, S.-H.; Kim, Y.-L.; Baek, M.-C.; Park, J.B.; et al. Novel urinary exosomal biomarkers of acute T cell-mediated rejection in kidney transplant recipients: A cross-sectional study. *PLoS ONE* **2018**, *13*, e0204204. [CrossRef]
29. Chen, D.; Zhang, J.; Peng, W.; Weng, C.; Chen, J. Urinary C-X-C motif chemokine 13 is a noninvasive biomarker of antibody-mediated renal allograft rejection. *Mol. Med. Rep.* **2018**, *18*, 2399–2406. [CrossRef]

30. Barabadi, M.; Shahbaz, S.K.; Foroughi, F.; Hosseinzadeh, M.; Nafar, M.; Yekaninejad, M.S.; Amirzargar, A. High Expression of FOXP3 mRNA in Blood and Urine as a Predictive Marker in Kidney Transplantation. *Prog. Transplant.* **2018**, *28*, 134–141. [CrossRef]
31. Mockler, C.; Sharma, A.; Gibson, I.W.; Gao, A.; Wong, A.; Ho, J.; Blydt-Hansen, T.D. The prognostic value of urinary chemokines at 6 months after pediatric kidney transplantation. *Pediatr. Transplant.* **2018**, *22*, e13205. [CrossRef] [PubMed]
32. Senturk Ciftci, H.; Demir, E.; Savran Karadeniz, M.; Tefik, T.; Yazici, H.; Nane, I.; Savran Oguz, F.; Aydin, F.; Turkmen, A. Serum and Urinary Levels of Tumor Necrosis Factor-Alpha in Renal Transplant Patients. *Exp. Clin. Transplant.* **2018**, *16*, 671–675. [CrossRef] [PubMed]
33. Park, J.; Lin, H.-Y.; Assaker, J.P.; Jeong, S.; Huang, C.-H.; Kurdi, A.; Lee, K.; Fraser, K.; Min, C.; Eskandari, S.; et al. Integrated Kidney Exosome Analysis for the Detection of Kidney Transplant Rejection. *ACS Nano* **2017**, *11*, 11041–11046. [CrossRef] [PubMed]
34. Millán, O.; Budde, K.; Sommerer, C.; Aliart, I.; Rissling, O.; Bardaji, B.; Matz, M.; Zeier, M.; Silva, I.; Guirado, L.; et al. Urinary miR-155-5p and CXCL10 as prognostic and predictive biomarkers of rejection, graft outcome and treatment response in kidney transplantation. *Br. J. Clin. Pharmacol.* **2017**, *83*, 2636–2650. [CrossRef]
35. Seo, J.-W.; Moon, H.; Kim, S.-Y.; Moon, J.-Y.; Jeong, K.H.; Lee, Y.-H.; Kim, Y.-G.; Lee, T.-W.; Ihm, C.-G.; Kim, C.-D.; et al. Both absolute and relative quantification of urinary mRNA are useful for non-invasive diagnosis of acute kidney allograft rejection. *PLoS ONE* **2017**, *12*, e0180045. [CrossRef]
36. Gandolfini, I.; Harris, C.; Abecassis, M.; Anderson, L.; Bestard, O.; Comai, G.; Cravedi, P.; Cremaschi, E.; Duty, J.A.; Florman, S.; et al. Rapid Biolayer Interferometry Measurements of Urinary CXCL9 to Detect Cellular Infiltrates Noninvasively After Kidney Transplantation. *Kidney Int. Rep.* **2017**, *2*, 1186–1193. [CrossRef]
37. Chen, D.; Peng, W.; Jiang, H.; Yang, H.; Wu, J.; Wang, H.; Chen, J. Noninvasive detection of acute renal allograft rejection by measurement of soluble Tim-3 in urine. *Mol. Med. Rep.* **2017**, *16*, 915–921. [CrossRef]
38. Domenico, T.D.; Joelsons, G.; Montenegro, R.M.; Manfro, R.C. Upregulation of microRNA 142-3p in the peripheral blood and urinary cells of kidney transplant recipients with post-transplant graft dysfunction. *Braz. J. Med. Biol. Res.* **2017**, *50*, e5533. [CrossRef]
39. Lee, H.; Park, Y.-M.; We, Y.-M.; Han, D.J.; Seo, J.-W.; Moon, H.; Lee, Y.-H.; Kim, Y.-G.; Moon, J.-Y.; Lee, S.-H.; et al. Evaluation of Digital PCR as a Technique for Monitoring Acute Rejection in Kidney Transplantation. *Genomics Inform.* **2017**, *15*, 2–10. [CrossRef]
40. Seeman, T.; Vondrak, K.; Dusek, J.; Simankova, N.; Zieg, J.; Hacek, J.; Chadimova, M.; Sopko, B.; Fortova, M. Urinary Neutrophil Gelatinase-Associated Lipocalin Does Not Distinguish Acute Rejection from Other Causes of Acute Kidney Injury in Pediatric Renal Transplant Recipients. *Clin. Lab.* **2017**, *63*, 111–114. [CrossRef]
41. Blydt-Hansen, T.D.; Sharma, A.; Gibson, I.W.; Wishart, D.S.; Mandal, R.; Ho, J.; Nickerson, P.; Rush, D. Urinary Metabolomics for Noninvasive Detection of Antibody-Mediated Rejection in Children After Kidney Transplantation. *Transplantation* **2017**, *101*, 2553–2561. [CrossRef] [PubMed]
42. Belmar Vega, L.; Rodrigo Calabia, E.; Gómez Román, J.J.; Ruiz San Millán, J.C.; Martín Penagos, L.; Arias Rodríguez, M. Relationship Between Albuminuria During the First Year and Antibody-Mediated Rejection in Protocol Biopsies in Kidney Transplant Recipients. *Transplant. Proc.* **2016**, *48*, 2950–2952. [CrossRef] [PubMed]
43. Raza, A.; Firasat, S.; Khaliq, S.; Khan, A.R.; Mahmood, S.; Aziz, T.; Mubarak, M.; Naqvi, S.A.A.; Rizvi, S.A.H.; Abid, A. Monocyte Chemoattractant Protein-1 (MCP-1/CCL2) Levels and Its Association with Renal Allograft Rejection. *Immunol. Investig.* **2017**, *46*, 251–262. [CrossRef]
44. Galichon, P.; Amrouche, L.; Hertig, A.; Brocheriou, I.; Rabant, M.; Xu-Dubois, Y.-C.; Ouali, N.; Dahan, K.; Morin, L.; Terzi, F.; et al. Urinary mRNA for the Diagnosis of Renal Allograft Rejection: The Issue of Normalization. *Am. J. Transplant.* **2016**, *16*, 3033–3040. [CrossRef]
45. Sigdel, T.K.; Gao, Y.; He, J.; Wang, A.; Nicora, C.D.; Fillmore, T.L.; Shi, T.; Webb-Robertson, B.-J.; Smith, R.D.; Qian, W.-J.; et al. Mining the human urine proteome for monitoring renal transplant injury. *Kidney Int.* **2016**, *89*, 1244–1252. [CrossRef] [PubMed]

46. García-Covarrubias, L.; Ventura, E.; Soto, V.; González, E.; García, A.; Aguilar, J.C.; Torres, J.M.; Hinojosa, H.; Fragoso, P.; De Los Santos, J.; et al. Lack of Association Between Elevated Urinary Levels of Interleukin-10 and Interferon Gamma With the Presence of Inflammation in Kidney Transplant Recipients. *Transplant. Proc.* **2016**, *48*, 583–587. [CrossRef]
47. Ho, J.; Rush, D.N.; Krokhin, O.; Antonovici, M.; Gao, A.; Bestland, J.; Wiebe, C.; Hiebert, B.; Rigatto, C.; Gibson, I.W.; et al. Elevated Urinary Matrix Metalloproteinase-7 Detects Underlying Renal Allograft Inflammation and Injury. *Transplantation* **2016**, *100*, 648–654. [CrossRef]
48. Abd Elaziz, M.M.; Bakry, S.; M Abd ElAal, A.E.; Rashed, L.; Hesham, D. Validation of Urinary PD-1 and FOXP3 mRNA in a Cohort of Egyptian Renal Allograft Recipients. *Ann. Transplant.* **2016**, *21*, 17–24. [CrossRef]
49. Lorenzen, J.M.; Schauerte, C.; Kölling, M.; Hübner, A.; Knapp, M.; Haller, H.; Thum, T. Long Noncoding RNAs in Urine Are Detectable and May Enable Early Detection of Acute T Cell-Mediated Rejection of Renal Allografts. *Clin. Chem.* **2015**, *61*, 1505–1514. [CrossRef]
50. Rabant, M.; Amrouche, L.; Morin, L.; Bonifay, R.; Lebreton, X.; Aouni, L.; Benon, A.; Sauvaget, V.; Le Vaillant, L.; Aulagnon, F.; et al. Early Low Urinary CXCL9 and CXCL10 Might Predict Immunological Quiescence in Clinically and Histologically Stable Kidney Recipients. *Am. J. Transplant.* **2016**, *16*, 1868–1881. [CrossRef]
51. Rabant, M.; Amrouche, L.; Lebreton, X.; Aulagnon, F.; Benon, A.; Sauvaget, V.; Bonifay, R.; Morin, L.; Scemla, A.; Delville, M.; et al. Urinary C-X-C Motif Chemokine 10 Independently Improves the Noninvasive Diagnosis of Antibody-Mediated Kidney Allograft Rejection. *J. Am. Soc. Nephrol.* **2015**, *26*, 2840–2851. [CrossRef] [PubMed]
52. Blydt-Hansen, T.D.; Gibson, I.W.; Gao, A.; Dufault, B.; Ho, J. Elevated urinary CXCL10-to-creatinine ratio is associated with subclinical and clinical rejection in pediatric renal transplantation. *Transplantation* **2015**, *99*, 797–804. [CrossRef] [PubMed]
53. Sigdel, T.K.; Ng, Y.W.; Lee, S.; Nicora, C.D.; Qian, W.-J.; Smith, R.D.; Camp, D.G., II; Sarwal, M.M. Perturbations in the urinary exosome in transplant rejection. *Front. Med. (Lausanne)* **2014**, *1*, 57. [CrossRef] [PubMed]
54. Suthanthiran, M.; Schwartz, J.E.; Ding, R.; Abecassis, M.; Dadhania, D.; Samstein, B.; Knechtle, S.J.; Friedewald, J.; Becker, Y.T.; Sharma, V.K.; et al. Urinary-cell mRNA profile and acute cellular rejection in kidney allografts. *N. Engl. J. Med.* **2013**, *369*, 20–31. [CrossRef] [PubMed]
55. van Enst, W.A.; Ochodo, E.; Scholten, R.J.P.M.; Hooft, L.; Leeflang, M.M. Investigation of publication bias in meta-analyses of diagnostic test accuracy: A meta-epidemiological study. *BMC Med. Res. Methodol.* **2014**, *14*, 70. [CrossRef]
56. Li, Y.M.; Li, Y.; Yan, L.; Wang, H.; Wu, X.J.; Tang, J.T.; Wang, L.L.; Shi, Y.Y. Comparison of urine and blood NGAL for early prediction of delayed graft function in adult kidney transplant recipients: A meta-analysis of observational studies. *BMC Nephrol.* **2019**, *20*, 291. [CrossRef]
57. Tsuchimoto, A.; Shinke, H.; Uesugi, M.; Kikuchi, M.; Hashimoto, E.; Sato, T.; Ogura, Y.; Hata, K.; Fujimoto, Y.; Kaido, T.; et al. Urinary Neutrophil Gelatinase-Associated Lipocalin: A Useful Biomarker for Tacrolimus-Induced Acute Kidney Injury in Liver Transplant Patients. *PLoS ONE* **2014**, *9*, e110527. [CrossRef]
58. Zununi Vahed, S.; Omidi, Y.; Ardalan, M.; Samadi, N. Dysregulation of urinary miR-21 and miR-200b associated with interstitial fibrosis and tubular atrophy (IFTA) in renal transplant recipients. *Clin. Biochem.* **2017**, *50*, 32–39. [CrossRef]
59. Naesens, M.; Lerut, E.; Emonds, M.-P.; Herelixka, A.; Evenepoel, P.; Claes, K.; Bammens, B.; Sprangers, B.; Meijers, B.; Jochmans, I.; et al. Proteinuria as a Noninvasive Marker for Renal Allograft Histology and Failure: An Observational Cohort Study. *J. Am. Soc. Nephrol.* **2016**, *27*, 281–292. [CrossRef]
60. Bertrand, D.; Gatault, P.; Jauréguy, M.; Garrouste, C.; Sayegh, J.; Bouvier, N.; Caillard, S.; Lanfranco, L.; Galinier, A.; Laurent, C.; et al. Protocol Biopsies in Patients with Subclinical De Novo DSA After Kidney Transplantation: A multicentric study. *Transplantation* **2020**, *104*, 1726–1737. [CrossRef]
61. Diena, D.; Messina, M.; De Biase, C.; Fop, F.; Scardino, E.; Rossetti, M.M.; Barreca, A.; Verri, A.; Biancone, L. Relationship between early proteinuria and long term outcome of kidney transplanted patients from different decades of donor age. *BMC Nephrol.* **2019**, *20*, 443. [CrossRef] [PubMed]
62. Rotondi, M.; Rosati, A.; Buonamano, A.; Lasagni, L.; Lazzeri, E.; Pradella, F.; Fossombroni, V.; Cirami, C.; Liotta, F.; La Villa, G.; et al. High pretransplant serum levels of CXCL10/IP-10 are related to increased risk of renal allograft failure. *Am. J. Transplant.* **2004**, *4*, 1466–1474. [CrossRef] [PubMed]

63. Lazzeri, E.; Rotondi, M.; Mazzinghi, B.; Lasagni, L.; Buonamano, A.; Rosati, A.; Pradella, F.; Fossombroni, V.; La Villa, G.; Gacci, M.; et al. High CXCL10 expression in rejected kidneys and predictive role of pretransplant serum CXCL10 for acute rejection and chronic allograft nephropathy. *Transplantation* **2005**, *79*, 1215–1220. [CrossRef] [PubMed]
64. Rotondi, M.; Netti, G.S.; Lazzeri, E.; Stallone, G.; Bertoni, E.; Chiovato, L.; Grandaliano, G.; Gesualdo, L.; Salvadori, M.; Schena, F.P.; et al. High pretransplant serum levels of CXCL9 are associated with increased risk of acute rejection and graft failure in kidney graft recipients. *Transpl. Int.* **2010**, *23*, 465–475. [CrossRef] [PubMed]
65. Jackson, J.A.; Kim, E.J.; Begley, B.; Cheeseman, J.; Harden, T.; Perez, S.D.; Thomas, S.; Warshaw, B.; Kirk, A.D. Urinary chemokines CXCL9 and CXCL10 are noninvasive markers of renal allograft rejection and BK viral infection. *Am. J. Transplant.* **2011**, *11*, 2228–2234. [CrossRef] [PubMed]
66. Hricik, D.E.; Nickerson, P.; Formica, R.N.; Poggio, E.D.; Rush, D.; Newell, K.A.; Goebel, J.; Gibson, I.W.; Fairchild, R.L.; Riggs, M.; et al. Multicenter validation of urinary CXCL9 as a risk-stratifying biomarker for kidney transplant injury. *Am. J. Transplant.* **2013**, *13*, 2634–2644. [CrossRef] [PubMed]
67. Oetting, W.S.; Rogers, T.B.; Krick, T.P.; Matas, A.J.; Ibrahim, H.N. Urinary beta2-microglobulin is associated with acute renal allograft rejection. *Am. J. Kidney Dis.* **2006**, *47*, 898–904. [CrossRef]
68. Li, B.; Hartono, C.; Ding, R.; Sharma, V.K.; Ramaswamy, R.; Qian, B.; Serur, D.; Mouradian, J.; Schwartz, J.E.; Suthanthiran, M. Noninvasive diagnosis of renal-allograft rejection by measurement of messenger RNA for perforin and granzyme B in urine. *N. Engl. J. Med.* **2001**, *344*, 947–954. [CrossRef]
69. Muthukumar, T.; Dadhania, D.; Ding, R.; Snopkowski, C.; Naqvi, R.; Lee, J.B.; Hartono, C.; Li, B.; Sharma, V.K.; Seshan, S.V.; et al. Messenger RNA for FOXP3 in the urine of renal-allograft recipients. *N. Engl. J. Med.* **2005**, *353*, 2342–2351. [CrossRef]
70. Manfro, R.C.; Aquino-Dias, E.C.; Joelsons, G.; Nogare, A.L.; Carpio, V.N.; Gonçalves, L.F.S. Noninvasive Tim-3 messenger RNA evaluation in renal transplant recipients with graft dysfunction. *Transplantation* **2008**, *86*, 1869–1874. [CrossRef]
71. Lorenzen, J.M.; Volkmann, I.; Fiedler, J.; Schmidt, M.; Scheffner, I.; Haller, H.; Gwinner, W.; Thum, T. Urinary miR-210 as a mediator of acute T-cell mediated rejection in renal allograft recipients. *Am. J. Transplant.* **2011**, *11*, 2221–2227. [CrossRef] [PubMed]
72. Cooper, J.E. Evaluation and Treatment of Acute Rejection in Kidney Allografts. *CJASN* **2020**, *15*, 430–438. [CrossRef] [PubMed]
73. Haas, M. Evolving criteria for the diagnosis of antibody-mediated rejection in renal allografts. *Curr. Opin. Nephrol. Hypertens.* **2018**, *27*, 137–143. [CrossRef]
74. Sis, B.; Jhangri, G.S.; Bunnag, S.; Allanach, K.; Kaplan, B.; Halloran, P.F. Endothelial gene expression in kidney transplants with alloantibody indicates antibody-mediated damage despite lack of C4d staining. *Am. J. Transplant.* **2009**, *9*, 2312–2323. [CrossRef]
75. Haas, M.; Sis, B.; Racusen, L.C.; Solez, K.; Glotz, D.; Colvin, R.B.; Castro, M.C.R.; David, D.S.R.; David-Neto, E.; Bagnasco, S.M.; et al. Banff 2013 meeting report: Inclusion of c4d-negative antibody-mediated rejection and antibody-associated arterial lesions. *Am. J. Transplant.* **2014**, *14*, 272–283. [CrossRef] [PubMed]
76. Moher, D.; Liberati, A.; Tetzlaff, J.; Altman, D.G. PRISMA Group Preferred reporting items for systematic reviews and meta-analyses: The PRISMA statement. *BMJ* **2009**, *339*, b2535. [CrossRef]
77. Whiting, P.F.; Rutjes, A.W.S.; Westwood, M.E.; Mallett, S.; Deeks, J.J.; Reitsma, J.B.; Leeflang, M.M.G.; Sterne, J.A.C.; Bossuyt, P.M.M. QUADAS-2 Group QUADAS-2: A revised tool for the quality assessment of diagnostic accuracy studies. *Ann. Intern. Med.* **2011**, *155*, 529–536. [CrossRef]

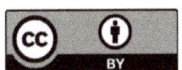

© 2020 by the authors. Licensee MDPI, Basel, Switzerland. This article is an open access article distributed under the terms and conditions of the Creative Commons Attribution (CC BY) license (http://creativecommons.org/licenses/by/4.0/).

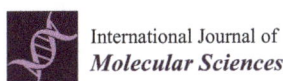

Review

Recent Advances on Biomarkers of Early and Late Kidney Graft Dysfunction

Marco Quaglia [1], Guido Merlotti [1], Gabriele Guglielmetti [1], Giuseppe Castellano [2] and Vincenzo Cantaluppi [1,*]

[1] Nephrology and Kidney Transplantation Unit, Center for Translational Research on Autoimmune and Allergic Disease (CAAD), Department of Translational Medicine, University of Piemonte Orientale (UPO), AOU Maggiore della Carità, via Gen. P. Solaroli, 17-28100 Novara, Italy; marco.quaglia@med.uniupo.it (M.Q.); guido.merlotti@maggioreosp.novara.it (G.M.); g.guglielmetti@maggioreosp.novara.it (G.G.)

[2] Nephrology, Dialysis and Transplant Unit, Department of Medical and Surgical Sciences, University of Foggia, 71121 Foggia, Italy; giuseppe.castellano@unifg.it

* Correspondence: vincenzo.cantaluppi@med.uniupo.it

Received: 2 July 2020; Accepted: 27 July 2020; Published: 29 July 2020

Abstract: New biomarkers of early and late graft dysfunction are needed in renal transplant to improve management of complications and prolong graft survival. A wide range of potential diagnostic and prognostic biomarkers, measured in different biological fluids (serum, plasma, urine) and in renal tissues, have been proposed for post-transplant delayed graft function (DGF), acute rejection (AR), and chronic allograft dysfunction (CAD). This review investigates old and new potential biomarkers for each of these clinical domains, seeking to underline their limits and strengths. OMICs technology has allowed identifying many candidate biomarkers, providing diagnostic and prognostic information at very early stages of pathological processes, such as AR. Donor-derived cell-free DNA (ddcfDNA) and extracellular vesicles (EVs) are further promising tools. Although most of these biomarkers still need to be validated in multiple independent cohorts and standardized, they are paving the way for substantial advances, such as the possibility of accurately predicting risk of DGF before graft is implanted, of making a "molecular" diagnosis of subclinical rejection even before histological lesions develop, or of dissecting etiology of CAD. Identification of "immunoquiescent" or even tolerant patients to guide minimization of immunosuppressive therapy is another area of active research. The parallel progress in imaging techniques, bioinformatics, and artificial intelligence (AI) is helping to fully exploit the wealth of information provided by biomarkers, leading to improved disease nosology of old entities such as transplant glomerulopathy. Prospective studies are needed to assess whether introduction of these new sets of biomarkers into clinical practice could actually reduce the need for renal biopsy, integrate traditional tools, and ultimately improve graft survival compared to current management.

Keywords: renal transplant; biomarkers; extracellular vesicles; acute rejection; chronic rejection; chronic allograft dysfunction; calcineurin-inhibitor nephrotoxicity; Polyomavirus associated nephropathy; immunosuppression

1. Introduction

General Features and Meaning of a Biomarker

A biomarker has been defined as "a characteristic that is objectively measured and evaluated as an indicator of a normal biological process, pathogenic process or pharmacological response to a therapeutic intervention" [1,2].

Transplanted kidney is currently monitored through a complex of clinical (e.g., GFR, proteinuria), immunological (e.g., DSA), instrumental (e.g., resistive index at Doppler ultrasound), and histological parameters. Overall these "traditional biomarkers" have many limits related not only to disease, but also to both nephrologists' and pathologists' skills. Even histological examination through renal biopsy, which remains the diagnostic golden standard criterion despite its invasiveness, is hampered by many drawbacks: low sensitivity (e.g., failure to detect subclinical acute rejection), low specificity due to heterogeneity of processes underlying the same lesion (e.g., uncertain interpretation of interstitial fibrosis-tubular atrophy, IFTA), lack of standardization (poor reproducibility, elevated inter-observer variability due to expertise-dependence) and of quantitative thresholds, sampling errors (e.g., failure to detect focal disorders such as Polyomavirus associated nephropathy, PVAN) [3].

New biomarkers have been the focus of intense research over the last decade to overcome these limits and improve allograft monitoring. Most of them are derived from "OMICs" revolution [4] and can be considered the cornerstone of precision medicine, which is based on a proactive approach and aims at predicting and preventing pathological processes by providing earlier and more extensive information than traditional ones [5].

In general, biomarkers can be classified into seven categories with different meaning and aims [5], outlined in Table 1.

Table 1. Biomarkers categories and their meaning in renal transplant.

Type of Biomarker	Meaning in Renal Transplant
Susceptibility or risk biomarker	It estimates the risk of developing a condition (e.g., AR) in a stable graft without any clinical sign of dysfunction
Diagnostic biomarker	It identifies patients with a disease or a subset of it (e.g., AR type)
Prognostic biomarker	It estimates the likelihood of a clinical event or of disease progression, staging severity of disease (e.g., severe rejection with risk of graft loss)
Predictive biomarker	It estimates the likelihood of achieving a favorable response from a therapy (e.g., Eculizumab for complement-fixing DSA)
Monitoring biomarker	It is serially measured in order to detect a change in evolution of disease or signs of drug toxicity, or to detect exposure to immunosuppressive drugs (e.g., TAC levels)
Pharmacodynamic/response biomarker	It verifies that a biological response has occurred after a drug exposure (e.g., DSA MFI after treatment of ABMR)
Safety biomarker	It estimates presence and severity of drug-related toxicity (e.g., CNI nephrotoxicity)

A plethora of new, non-invasive biomarkers measured in either urine or peripheral blood have been studied over the last years, mainly with a diagnostic and prognostic meaning, with different degrees of preclinical and clinical success. Some of them have been validated in independent cohorts and may be already employed in clinical decision-making when kidney biopsy is contraindicated or inconclusive. Other biomarkers, mainly represented by gene expression signatures, have been assessed in kidney tissue and appear to significantly expand information provided by traditional histology [6].

Different pathological processes can cause early and late KTx dysfunction and are outlined in Figure 1.

We herein reviewed the current literature on potential biomarkers in three main settings of KTx: ischemia reperfusion injury (IRI) and DGF, AR, and CAD. The latter includes biomarkers for chronic rejection, chronic Calcineurin-Inhibitor (CNI) nephrotoxicity, and PVAN.

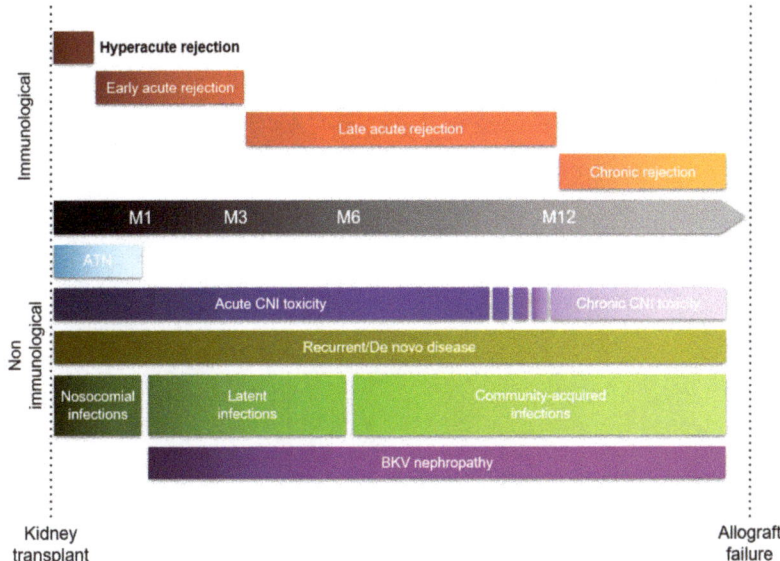

Figure 1. Timeline of early and late causes of graft dysfunction.

2. IRI and DGF

DGF is a common complication of KTx, which affects short and long-term outcomes, including risk of acute rejection and graft survival. It is often caused by IRI due to long cold ischemia time, especially in kidney from "extended-criteria" donors (ECD) and donation after cardiac death (DCD). The most commonly employed definition for DGF relies on the need for dialysis in the first week after KTx.

Biomarkers measured in the immediate post-Tx would be extremely useful to identify patients at risk of DGF and prevent this common complication, for example delaying start of CNI [7].

Ideally, biomarkers predicting DGF should be available either before KTx, in the donor, or immediately after it, in the recipient. The first option is especially interesting in the current era of increasingly higher risk ECDs [8], as accurate tools to assess kidney quality are needed to help allocate them to the most adequate recipient, or even discard them when considered unsuitable [9].

A lot of potential biomarkers of DGF have been studied and some of them have already been validated in independent cohorts (Tables 2 and 3). Some biomarkers have been analyzed in donor's biological fluids or in the graft (e.g., preservation fluid) before KTx, whereas most of them were studied in the recipient after KTx.

2.1. Donor-Related Biomarkers

Donor-related biomarkers can be measured in donor biological fluids, in graft preservation fluid, or in the perfusate of machine-perfused kidneys.

Table 2. Potential biomarkers for DGF.

Biomarker	Source	Main Features	Author
Mitochondrial DNA	Donor plasma	It predicts DGF in DCD donors	Han F. et al. [10]
Complement C5a	Donor urine	It predicts DGF	Schroppel B. et al. [11]
miRNA	Graft preservation fluid	Several miRNAs proposed as biomarkers of DGF; miR-505-3p validated in DCD grafts	Gomez-Dos-Santos V. et al. [12] Roest H. et al. [13]
LDH, NGAL and MMP-2	Perfusate of machine-perfused kidneys	Different levels according to type of donor (DCD vs. DBD vs. LD), reflecting degree of IRI	Moser M. et al. [14]
Exosomal mRNA for NGAL and NGAL	Perfusate of machine-perfused kidneys	They predict DGF	Cappuccilli M. et al. [15]
πGST	Perfusate of machine-perfused kidneys	It predicts DGF	Hall I. et al. [16]
Furosemide stress test	—	Clinical test: non-responsive patients are at increased risk of DGF in the following days	Udomkarnjananun S. et al. [17]
miR182-5p, miR-21-3p	Recipient's serum and urine	They predict DGF	Wilflingseder J. et al. [18]
miR146a-5p	Recipient's peripheral blood and renal tissue	Increased in both DGF and AR	Milhoransa P. et al. [19]
miR-9, miR-10a, miR-21, miR-29a, miR-221, miR-429	Recipient's urine (first 5 days after KTx)	This panel predicts DGF (validated in an independent cohort)	Khalid U. et al. [20]
NGAL	Recipient's serum/plasma and urine (first days after KTx)	Both bNGAL and uNGAL predict DGF and 1-year graft function, but bNGAL is more accurate. Urine NGAL predicts DGF also in KTx from LD.	Cappuccilli M. et al. [15] Maier H. et al. [21] Ramirez-Sandoval J. et al. [22] Li Y. et al. [23] Sahraei Z. et al. [24]
Corin	Recipient's plasma	It is reduced in DGF	Hu X. et al. [25]
TLR-4 surface expression	Recipient's circulating monocytes	It is reduced in DGF and associated with poor graft function at follow-up	Zmonarski S. et al. [26]
Amylase	Recipient's serum	It increases in DGF	Comai G. et al. [27]
Fascin and Vimentin	Graft biopsy in recipient	Expression of these EndMT biomarkers on microvasculature correlated with long-term graft function after DGF	Xu-Dubois Y-C. et al. [28]

2.1.1. Donor Biological Fluids

Elevated donor plasma mitochondrial DNA levels independently predicted DGF and correlated with 1-year graft survival in a cohort of DCD [10].

Following organ procurement, the role of innate immune system, such as Complement in IRI, has been extensively investigated. By generating effector molecules (C4b, C4d, C3b, iC3b, C3dg, and C3d) and anaphylatoxins (C3a, C5a), Complement can recruit granulocytes, monocytes, and other inflammatory cells to the site of ischemic injury and regulate activation of tubular epithelial cells and pericytes within the kidney. In addition, Complement factors can directly damage renal parenchymal cells by inducing tubular apoptosis, endothelial-to-mesenchymal transition (EndMT), pericytes-to-mesenchymal transition, and accelerated senescence [28–31]. EndMT deeply modifies endothelial cells, which acquires a mesenchymal phenotype and new properties, such as capacity to produce extracellular matrix (EM) and induce fibrosis. Biomarkers of EndMT have been the focus of recent research in different KTx areas and will be discussed in detail in following sections on recipient-related DGF biomarkers (Section 2.2.4) and on chronic rejection-IFTA within the setting of CAD (Section 4.1.3).

Consistently, donor urinary C5a levels were independently associated with recipient post-transplant DGF, providing a potential rationale for complement-blocking therapies to prevent DGF in high risk patients [11].

2.1.2. Graft Preservation Fluid

Other studies have recently focused on analysis of potential biomarkers within graft preservation fluids, especially during hypothermic machine perfusion, with the rationale that their concentration may reflect organ viability and correlate with post-transplant renal function [12].

Cell-free microRNAs (miRNAs) show promise as biomarkers in several KTx settings. These are short non-coding RNAs that play a pivotal role in regulation of gene expression through epigenetic, transcriptional, and post-transcriptional mechanisms. They can be isolated, quantified and profiled by multiple platforms which can also characterize their target genes [32]. They have been studied in graft preservation fluid and proposed as viability biomarkers (miR-486-5p, miR-144-3p, miR-142-5p, and miR-144-5p) [12]; however, only miR-505-3p has been demonstrated to be an independent predictor of DGF in DCD grafts with high accuracy (AUC = 0.83) and was confirmed in a validation cohort [13].

Of note, a significant percentage of miRNAs do not circulate free but are carried by EVs that have been detected in preservation fluid. These structures contain both donor-derived RNAs and selected miRNA which could be associated with graft function during the first seven post-operative days [33].

General features of EVs and their role as biomarkers of DGF will be discussed in more detail in the following paragraphs.

2.1.3. Perfusate of Machine-Perfused Kidneys

Proteomic analysis of perfusate from machine cold perfusion of graft was compared between different types of donor kidneys. LDH, neutrophil gelatinase-associated lipocalin (NGAL), and matrix metalloproteinase-2 levels were highest in DCD kidneys, followed by DBD and living-donor (LD) kidneys. Other molecules, such as periredoxin-2 and α-1 antitripsin, were also significantly different across the three groups, probably reflecting different degrees of IRI [14,15]. Exosomal mRNA for NGAL and NGAL concentration in the perfusate of machine-perfused kidneys were associated with DGF also in another study [15]. The α and π iso-enzymes of glutathione S-transferase (GST) levels, measured from perfusate solution at the start and the end of machine perfusion, were analyzed in 428 KTx recipients. While levels of both iso-enzymes significantly increased during this procedure, only πGST levels at the end of machine perfusion were independently associated with DGF [16].

All the above-mentioned molecules represent potential biomarkers and therapeutic targets that may be useful in the setting of DGF, but still need to be validated.

2.2. Recipient-Related Biomarkers

2.2.1. Furosemide Stress Test

Furosemide stress test (FST) is a simple test to predict DGF in the post-transplant period. FST non-responsive patients (urine volume < 350 cc after 4 h of Furosemide infusion) are at risk of developing DGF in the following days [17].

2.2.2. miRNAs

miRNAs, which we already analyzed as donor-derived biomarkers, have been the focus of several studies also in KTx recipients, representing both a biomarker and a potential therapeutic target [34–36]. MiR 182-5p and miR-21-3p in recipient's serum and urine correlated with DGF in one study [18]. MiR 146a-5p has been studied in renal tissue and peripheral blood during DGF. It was significantly increased in renal biopsy of patients with DGF as compared to stable recipients and those with AR and a similar trend was found in peripheral blood samples [19].

A urinary panel of six miRNAs (miR-9; miR-10a; miR-21; miR-29a; miR-221; miR-429) was consistently elevated in the first urine passed after Tx and in urine samples collected daily across the following five post-operative days in patients who developed DGF (ROC AUC = 0.94). This panel was validated in an independent cohort [20].

In experimental IRI studies in mice, the expression of miR-139-5p in renal tissues of the IRI group was 40% lower than that of the sham-operated one. A set of candidate genes involved in regeneration and repair of kidney tissue, EM degradation and inflammation was also shown to be markedly overexpressed in this setting and may provide new biomarkers in the future [37].

2.2.3. Neutrophil Gelatinase-Associated Lipocalin (NGAL) and Other Biomarkers

NGAL has been the focus of many studies as a tubular injury biomarker for early prediction of DGF in KTx recipients. It has been studied both in graft perfusion fluid and in recipient's blood and urine.

Increased release from ischemia-injured tubular cells has been proved to discriminate patients at risk for AKI. Blood NGAL (bNGAL)—performed on serum/plasma—and urine NGAL (uNGAL) were shown to predict DGF in the early post-operative period, whereas its meaning as a perfusion fluid biomarker has already been discussed [15,21].

In one study on 50 KTx recipients from ECD, bNGAL levels at day 1 were significantly higher in the DGF group; of interest, NGAL accurately discriminated between slow and immediate graft function even within the non-DGF group. Furthermore, bNGAL levels preceded decrease in serum creatinine and allowed earlier TAC introduction in a "sequential" immunosuppressive protocol, shortening CNI-free window as compared to standard, creatinine-based management. Thus, bNGAL may help avoid unnecessary CNI underexposure in patients in which renal function is about to recover. The same study also shed light on NGAL function as a growth factor for tubular epithelial cells. In vitro, either hypoxia or TAC exposure induced its release from tubular epithelial cells and NGAL stimulated their regeneration after IRI and acute nephrotoxicity through an autocrine loop. However, chronic tubular stimulation by NGAL also appeared to promote epithelial-to-mesenchymal transition (EMT) and progression toward CKD. This pathological process will be discussed in detail in the following Section 4.1.3 concerning mechanisms of chronic rejection and IFTA. Overall these data suggest that NGAL levels might even predict a maladaptive repair with increased risk of progression from DGF to chronic loss of graft function [38].

Consistently, a more recent study prospectively assessed dynamic profile of bNGAL and uNGAL in 170 consecutive recipients within 7 days of Tx and found that their level on post-operative day 2 could accurately predict DGF. Multivariate analyses revealed donor age, serum and urinary NGAL were each independently associated with DGF ($p < 0.001$) [21].

A metanalysis first demonstrated that elevated serum and urine NGAL levels can predict DGF and 1-year graft function [22]; a second, more recent one, including 1036 patients from 14 studies, confirmed that both bNGAL—performed on serum/plasma—and uNGAL were robust biomarkers for DGF (AUC 0.91 and 0.95, respectively), with superior predictive value of bNGAL over uNGAL [23].

Of interest, urine NGAL post-operative modification in the first 24 hours were associated not only with DGF but also with worse renal outcomes at 2 years in terms of graft function and survival in LD KTx [24].

Several other biomarkers have been proposed in the setting of DGF.

A urinary tissue inhibitor of metalloproteinases-2 (TIMP-2), a validated biomarker for AKI, was reported to predict the occurrence and duration of DGF in DCD KTx recipients [39].

In a transcriptomic study on IRI mice, Corin was one of the most downregulated among more than 2200 differentially expressed genes and protein level of renal Corin was markedly reduced in IRI. Consistently, also plasma Corin concentrations were reduced in a small sample of recipients with DGF as compared to uncomplicated KTx recipients [25].

Expression of Toll-like (TLR-4) expression on circulating monocytes was reported to be lower in DGF patients and associated with poor graft function at follow-up [26].

An increase in serum Amylase (>20%), especially if associated with increased Resistive Index (>0.7) predicted a higher incidence of DGF, longer hospital stay, and worse renal function at discharge in another study [27].

2.2.4. BioMarkers of EndMT

In a recent study biomarkers of partial microvasculature EndMT (Fascin and Vimentin) and of tubular EMT (Vimentin) were analyzed with immunoistochemistry in renal biopsies performed in early post-transplant due to DGF, showing ATN lesions. Extent of ATN was correlated with short and long-term (2 year) graft dysfunction only in the presence of partial EndMT (pEndMT) biomarkers expression, suggesting that early endothelial cell activation can identify patients at risk of incomplete recovery after DGF [28]. EndMt will be discussed in detail in the following Section 4.1.3 concerning mechanisms of chronic rejection and IFTA.

2.2.5. EVs

EVs is a general term which includes membrane structures of different size, released by cells after fusion of endosomes with the plasma membrane (exosomes), shed from plasma membrane (microvesicles), or released during apoptosis (apoptotic bodies). EVs are then taken up by neighboring or distant target cells (paracrine or endocrine effect) [40] and mediate a wide range of physiological and pathological processes, including renal disease [41]. EVs also exert pleiotropic, immunomodulatory roles in KTx [42]. Their bioactive cargo includes graft antigens, costimulatory/inhibitory molecules, cytokines, growth factors and, as discussed before, functional miRNAs that modulate expression of recipient cell target genes. Recent studies dissected this complex content, suggesting that some of these molecules may be potential biomarkers of DGF, paralleling recovery of renal and endothelial function. Even though initial evidence on dynamics of circulating EVs after KTx needs to be confirmed [43], this area of research appears to be promising.

Plasma and urinary EVs investigated as possible biomarkers of DGF in KTx are outlined in Table 3 [44–50].

Table 3. Extracellular vescicles (EVs) as potential biomarkers of DGF.

Type of EV	Main Features	Author
Plasma Endothelial EVs	EVs level and their procoagulant activity progressively decrease after KTx, paralleling renal function recovery	Al-Massarani G et al. [44,45]
Plasma Endothelial and platelet EVs	Endothelial and platelet EVs size and level progressively decrease after KTx, paralleling renal function recovery	Martins S et al. [46]
Urinary EVs	NGAL expression in urinary EVs correlated with DGF	Alvarez S et al. [47]
Urinary CD 133+ EVs	Decreased level in recipients with DGF and vascular damage	Dimuccio V et al. [48]
Acquaporin-1 containing EVs	Decreased urinary Acquaporin-1-containing EVs in DGF	Sonoda H et al. [49] Asvapromtada S et al. [50]

3. AR

Potential biomarkers of acute antibody-mediated rejection (ABMR) and T-cell mediated rejection (TCMR) are reported in detail in Tables 4–6.

Table 4. Potential biomarkers for acute rejection (AR).

Biomarker	Type of Rejection	Main Features	Author
Three-gene signature (CTOT 04 study)	TCMR	It increases up to 20 days before histological diagnosis	Suthanthiran M et al. [51]
Seven-gene signature (KALIBRE study)	TCMR	It increases 7 weeks before histological diagnosis and decreased after treatment	Christakoudi S et al. [52]
Seventeen-gene signature (GoCAR study)	TCMR	It identifies subclinical TCMR and correlates with long-term graft survival	Zhang W et al. [53]
Eight-gene signature	ABMR	It correlates with histological features of acute and chronic ABMR	Van Loon E et al. [54]
Panel of gene signature (CTOT 08 study)	TCMR and ABMR	It correlates with clinical and histological outcomes and with de novo DSA; useful to identify immunologically quiescent patients	Friedewald J et al. [55]
Nineteen-gene signature	TCMR and ABMR	It includes TCMR genes. Analysis performed on RNA extracted from archival fresh frozen paraffin-embedded renal biopsy tissue.	Sigdel T et al. [56]
kSORT (AART study)	TCMR and ABMR	Rejection predicted 3 months before histological diagnosis in 64% of patients with stable graft function.	Roedder S et al. [57] Zhang W et al. [53]
ENDATs	ABMR	Analysis of endothelial transcripts predicts ABMR with excellent accuracy (AUC = 0.92).	Sis B et al. [58] Adam B et al. [59]
Complement fragments	ABMR	Levels correlate with ABMR	Stites E et al. [60]
Innate immunity genes	TCMR	Unbiased transcriptome analysis identifies increased expression of innate immune system genes	Mueller F et al. [61]
CXCL9	TCMR and ABMR	High NPP (99.3%): low levels at 6 months predict low risk of rejection until 24 months. Highly accurate for ABMR diagnosis when associated with DSA.	Hricik D et al. [62] Rabant M et al. [63] Faddoul G et al. [64] Mühlbacher J et al. [65]
CXCL10	ABMR and mixed	High NPP (99%). It predicts rejection at 1 month post-KTx in stable graft.	Rabant M et al. [66]
dd-cfDNA	ABMR and TCMR	Due to elevated negative NPP, it could help rule out especially ABMR and play a role for surveillance after a rejection episode or in sensitized patients	Bloom R et al. [67–72]
Allogenic circulating B- and T-cell assays	ABMR and TCMR	Useful to predict subclinical forms of rejection and DSA	Hricik D et al. [73] Crespo E et al. [74] Gorbacheva V et al. [75]
Peripheral blood miRNAs	TCMR	miR-15b, miR-16, miR-103a, miR-106A, miR107 predict vascular TCMR	Matz M et al. [76]
Peritransplant soluble CD30 (sCD30)	TCMR	Strong association between sCD30 and TCMR	Trailin A et al. [77] Mirzakhani M et al. [78]
CD154-positive T cytotoxic memory cells	TCMR	Association with TCMR and its histological severity in steroid-free regimen	Ashokkumar C et al. [79]
CD 200 and CD200R1	TCMR and ABMR	Increased pre-transplant CD200R1/CD200 ratio identifies recipients at increased risk of AR and worse renal function	Oweira H et al. [80]
CD45RC	TCMR	Pre-transplant expression of CD45RC on circulating CD8+ T predicts AR	Lemerle M et al. [81]
N-glycan	ABMR and TCMR	N-glycan levels (integrated within a clinical score) predict rejection-free survival in KTx from LD	Soma O et al. [82]
HSP-90	ABMR and TCMR	It discriminates AR from other causes of graft dysfunction	Maehana T et al. [83]
Heparan Sulfate	TCMR	It predicts DGF	Barbas A et al. [84]

3.1. Transcriptomic Studies

3.1.1. Urine and Peripheral Blood Transcriptomics

The CTOT 04 trial has analyzed mRNA transcripts in urinary sediment cells and identified a three-gene signature (CD3ε mRNA, CXCL10 mRNA, and 18S rRNA) predicting TCMR up to 20 days before biopsy-proven diagnosis [51]. A more recent study by the same group analyzed gene expression in urinary cells and renal biopsies during AR and identified unique and shared gene signatures associated with biological pathways involved in TCMR and ABMR. Furthermore, they demonstrated the enrichment of biopsy gene signature in urinary cells and of immune cell types in urine compared with renal tissue. These findings support the hypothesis that urine gene expression patterns can reflect and even amplify ongoing renal tissue immune pathways and may help diagnose rejection and monitor its dynamics [85]. This is consistent with evidence from previous studies suggesting that graft can sort renal tissue infiltrating cells in urine as an in vivo flow cytometer [86].

Several studies have tried to identify a peripheral blood gene expression signature to diagnose subclinical AR at an early stage.

Christakoudi S et al. analyzed expression of 22 literature-based genes in peripheral blood samples of patients from Kidney Allograft Immune Biomarkers of Rejection Episodes (KALIBRE) study and identified a seven-gene TCMR-signature (IFN-γ, IP-10, ITGA4, MARCH8, RORc, SEMA7A, WDR40A) which allowed diagnosis of AR 7 weeks before renal biopsy and correlated with response to therapy [52].

Zhang W et al. focused on patients with subclinical TCMR (protocol biopsy at third month) in KTx recipients from Genomics of Chronic Allograft Rejection (GoCAR) study [87] and identified a 17-gene peripheral blood signature which characterized ongoing subclinical TCMR and predicted an increased risk of clinical TCMR at 24 months and decreased graft survival [53].

A peripheral blood mRNA assay based on eight genes (CXCL-10, FCGR1A, FCGR1B, GBP1, GBP4, IL15, KLRC1, TIMP1) was developed in a multicenter, prospective study and correlated with histological features of acute and chronic ABMR (microvascular inflammation, transplant glomerulopathy) but not of TCMR. Diagnostic accuracy was high (ROC AUC 79.9% $p < 0.0001$), even in the setting of stable graft function [54].

A blood molecular biomarker based on multiple gene expression signatures was designed to distinguish "immunological quiescence" from subclinical AR in a multicenter study (CTOT-08). This correlated with clinical (AR, renal function) and histological outcomes (IFTA) and with de novo DSA. This biomarker was validated with surveillance biopsies data and proved to be especially useful in ruling out subclinical rejection (NPP: 78–88%) [55].

In a multi-center "Assessment of Acute Rejection in renal Transplant (AART)" study, peripheral blood transcriptome analysis identified a 17-gene signature called "Kidney Solid Organ Response test" (kSORT), which predicted both TCMR and ABMR up to 3 months before histological diagnosis in an independent prospective cohort. This tool is characterized by a high accuracy in predicting AR, especially when compared with performance of other biomarkers in the same setting (AUC = 0.94; sensitivity: 83%, specificity: 90.6%; PPV: 93,2%) [57,88].

kSORT has also been used in association with an IFNγ Elispot in the ESCAPE study, resulting in a higher PPP (AUC > 0.85) for subclinical TCMR and ABMR [74].

Peripheral blood transcriptomic analysis allowed to build a classification model capable of discriminating ABMR from accommodation in ABO-incompatible kidney transplants [89].

A blood test (TruGraf v1) has been developed to study a set of microarray-based gene expression in order to discriminate patients with a stable graft and immunological quiescence ("Transplant Excellence") from those with renal dysfunction or AR. This tool was proposed as a tool to avoid unnecessary surveillance biopsies on the basis of high accuracy in detecting AR (74%) and high NPP (90%) [90]. The value of serial TruGraf testing to confirm immunoquiescence and avoid surveillance biopsies has been confirmed in a recent study [91].

3.1.2. Renal Tissue Transcriptomics

Sigdel T et al. analyzed tissue expression of selected 19 target genes, including those previously identified in tissue common rejection module (tCRM). Interestingly, they employed RNA extracted from archival fresh frozen paraffin-embedded renal biopsy tissue. Eight genes were related to specific cellular infiltrates, whereas the others reflected a "graft inflammation score" based on tCRM. This set of genes allowed to distinguish biopsies of stable grafts from those of recipients with AR and even borderline inflammation [56].

Molecular patterns such as upregulation of intrarenal complement regulatory genes discriminate accommodation from subclinical antibody-mediated rejection in AB0-incompatible KTx [92].

An intra-graft mRNA transcriptomic landscape of TCMR has been outlined through computational analysis and has shown an increased expression of innate immunity genes, such as genes for pattern recognition receptors, and a decreased expression of calcineurin, suggesting inadequate immunosuppression, as compared to stable graft [61].

Real time central molecular assessment of changes in mRNA expression in graft tissue through microarrays is the basis of "molecular microscope diagnostic system", which predicted risk of AR and graft failure with greater precision than conventional biopsy. Pathogenesis-based transcripts sets (PBTs) which segregate together and characterize different processes (e.g., IGF-gamma expression, T cell infiltrates), were employed to define "classifiers" which predict molecular phenotype, quantifying its likelihood with a score. Of importance, this approach has been validated in several independent cohorts [93,94].

Other studies have shown that endothelial associated transcripts (ENDATs) in biopsies of DSA-positive patients can reveal ABMR even in the absence of C4d positivity [58] and that ABMR-related endothelial genes RNA transcripts are expressed before histological onset of lesions, allowing excellent identification (AUC = 0.92) and potentially early, preemptive treatment of rejection [59].

Finally, single-cell transcriptomics can comprehensively describe cell types and states in a human kidney biopsy and was employed to analyze immune response in mixed rejection: 16 distinct cell types were identified, including different sub-clusters of activated endothelial cells [95]. This cell-based approach may provide a wealth of new biomarkers for ABMR in the future [96].

3.2. Complement-Related Biomarkers

Complement system is deeply involved in ABMR and can therefore provide potential biomarkers related to this process.

The C4d deposition has been considered the gold standard for ABMR diagnosis for several years, indicating activation of Classical pathway of Complement; however, all Complement pathways have been proved to be involved in ABMR, leading to recruitment and activation of leukocytes such as Natural Killer cells, monocytes/macrophages, and lymphocytes [97].

Bobka S. et al. also demonstrated an increased Complement activation in pre-transplant biopsies from diabetic, hypertensive, or smoking donors, suggesting a predictive value of Complement activation in donor biopsies for later outcome [98]. Expression of these Complement components at time of diagnosis of ABMR was associated with higher serum creatinine and more severe morphological changes. As further evidence, C5 blockade prevented ABMR and stabilized long-term renal function.

In addition, EVs shed by endothelial cell expressing C4d (CD144$^+$ C4d$^+$) are increased in ABMR and correlate with its severity and response to treatment [99] and plasma levels of complement activation fragments C4a and Ba are increased in ABMR [60]. Single nucleotide polymorphisms (SNP) of complement C3 gene have also been found to correlate with ABMR [100]. Upregulation of intrarenal complement regulatory genes and complement transcripts in peripheral blood of ABO-incompatible KTx has already been discussed in "Transcriptomic Studies" [92]. Altogether, these data support the use of Complement Factors as potential biomarkers in ABMR.

3.3. Urinary and Serum Chemokines

IFN-γ induced urinary C-X-C motif chemokine ligand 9 (CXCL9) and 10 (CXCL10) chemokines are associated with Th-1 immune response and involved in T cell recruitment in inflammatory processes. They are promising as biomarkers for TCMR and ABMR [62,66].

Low levels are associated with immunological quiescence, as shown by their very high NPP, which makes them an ideal tool to rule out rejection, including subclinical ones, and to identify transplant recipients at low immunological risk [63]. This was especially evident for CXCL 9 (CTOT-01 study), which was associated with acute TCMR within the first year.

However, a subsequent study with a longer follow-up (CTOT-17) showed that changes in eGFR between 3 or 6 months and 24 months better predicted 5-year graft loss than CXCL-9 measurement [64].

Association of urinary CXCL10-to-creatinine ratio with DSA improved identification of ABMR and prediction of graft loss. In a recent study, higher blood and urine levels of both CXCL9 and CXCL10 were found in ABMR, but urinary CXCL9 was the most accurate biomarker of rejection (AUC of ROC: 0.77) and—if measured in combination with immunodominant DSA mean fluorescence intensity (MFI)—it allowed a net reclassification increase of 73% compared to DSA MFI alone [65].

Interestingly, even CXCL9 and CXCL10 baseline recipient's serum levels assessed before KTx may predict AR [101,102].

Additionally, urinary CXCR3—the receptor for CXCL9 and CXCL10, expressed on activated T-lymphocytes—was shown to detect subclinical inflammation and correlate with evolution towards chronic damage; of interest, its level decreased after immunosuppression intensification [103].

In another study, serum concentration of chemokine CXCL13, a B lymphocyte chemoattractant, was significantly higher in TCMR than in stable graft and in borderline rejection; furthermore, a marked increase (>5-fold) was found in patients developing AR within first post-transplant week and correlated with entity of B cell infiltration in renal biopsy. A similar correlation was found in a mouse model of TCMR, indicating that CXCL13 serum levels may be a marker of B cell-involvement in TCMR, identifying a severe subset of this type of rejection [104].

On the whole, growing evidence points to a role of urinary and serum chemokines as biomarkers of both types of AR.

3.4. Other Potential Urinary Biomarkers

Other urinary molecules have been proposed as markers of AR.

High urinary π-GST values at postoperative day 1 discriminated AR (sensitivity, 100%; specificity, 66.6%) as well as between DGF from normal-functioning grafts (sensitivity, 100%; specificity, 62.6%). Similarly, α-GST values > 33.97 ng/mg uCrea identified AR, with a lower sensitivity (77.7%) but optimal specificity (100%) [105].

Urinary untargeted metabolomic profiling led to identification of a panel of five potential biomarkers (guanidoacetil acid, methylimidazolacetic acid, dopamine, 4-guanidobutyric acid, and L-tryptophan), which discriminated between TCMR and stable graft (ROC curve AUC: sensitivity 90%; specificity 84.6%) [106].

3.5. dd-cfDNA

Small fragments of cell-free DNA, released from graft cells into the recipient circulation due to cell death or injury, have been proposed as biomarkers of AR.

While dd-cf DNA represents on average 0.34% of total cf-DNA in plasma of stable KTx recipients, levels are increased during AR and, to a lesser extent, acute pyelonephritis and ATN.

A kinetic pilot study of dd-cfDNA after Tx showed high median level in the immediate post-Tx hours (around 20%), rapidly decreasing on the first day (around 5%) and then stabilizing below 1% [107].

In the DART (Diagnosing Active Rejection in Kidney Transplant Recipients) trial, Bloom RD et al. first reported higher dd-cfDNA levels in patients with acute (TCMR Banff > IB and ABMR) and chronic active rejection and identified a 1% threshold to discriminate these patients from stable ones. This test was characterized by elevated NPP (84%) and a lower PPP (61%), suggesting that <1% percentage of dd-cfDNA could be used to rule out rejection, especially ABMR. Coexistence of DSA increased PPP to 85%. Furthermore, dd-cfDNA levels not only increased before changes in serum creatinine but also decreased after rejection treatment, suggesting that longitudinal monitoring of this biomarker could be useful after a rejection episode, possibly limiting need for surveillance biopsies [67].

In a subsequent work, Huang E et al. [68] demonstrated that a lower dd-cfDNA threshold of 0.74% could reliably identify ABMR—but not TCMR—in a group of immunologically high-risk patients undergoing indication biopsies, increasing NPP to 100%.

However, other authors suggested comparable performance of dd-cfDNA in diagnosing ABMR and TCMR, using a different quantification methodology [69].

Absolute quantification of dd-cfDNA (copies/mL) showed superior performance in discriminating BPAR as compared to dd-cfDNA percentage and also seemed to identify a subset of patients with inadequate Tacrolimus levels and subclinical immunological damage in a prospective observational study [70].

Of interest, dd-cfDNA diagnostic capacity for ABMR appears to improve when applied to DSA-positive recipients, suggesting a preferential employment in monitoring highly sensitized patients [71].

Determination of dd-cfDNA can be unreliable in case of recent (within 1 month) whole blood transfusion and falsely positive within 24 h of a renal biopsy; it should also not be employed to monitor a second KTx as release from previous graft could alter its levels. Falsely positive results can also occur in the case of ATN and acute pyelonephritis and type of donor also affects levels (higher levels in cadaveric vs. LD), probably reflecting difference in degree of initial ischemic damage and inflammation [72].

Despite these issues, dd-cfDNA remains a promising biomarker and it has been proposed as a surrogate diagnostic ABMR criterion in DSA-negative forms [108].

Furthermore, recent studies suggest that dd-cfDNA determination could also have a broader meaning beyond AR diagnosis, reflecting graft injury and consequently exerting a negative impact on several long-term outcomes [109]. Of interest, a multicentric study on patients with initial TCMR (TCMR 1A and borderline lesions) showed that dd-cfDNA levels above 0.5% were effective in stratifying risk of eGFR decline, de novo DSA development and further AR episodes [110]. Consistently, emerging evidence indicates that levels of dd-cfDNA increase before onset of de novo DSA (both HLA-DSA and non-HLA DSA) and eGFR decline [73], suggesting that dd-cf DNA itself is immunogenic and can trigger subclinical inflammation, initiating an immune response [75].

Urinary levels of cell-free mitochondrial DNA during early post-transplant phase have also been reported to correlate with AR, DGF and short-term renal function [76].

3.6. Allogenic Circulating B-Cell and T-Cell Assays

Peripheral circulating donor HLA-specific memory B cells quantified by enzyme-linked immunospot (ELISPOT) [77] and serum B-cell activating factor level on post-operative day 7 [78] both predicted ABMR, especially in DSA-positive recipients.

Pre-transplant T cell alloreactivity can be assessed with a donor-specific IFN-γ ELISPOT which measures IFN-γ release by recipient T cells in response to donor antigens. IFN-γ ELISPOT intensity appears to correlate with development of subclinical TCMR, ABMR, and DSA [79,80].

3.7. Peripheral Blood miRNAs

General features and meaning of miRNAs have already been dealt with in the paragraph on DGF biomarkers. A panel of five peripheral blood miRNAs—miR-15b, miR-16, miR-103a, miR-106A, miR107—was shown to improve sensitivity of diagnosis of vascular TCMR [81].

3.8. Immune Cells Biomarkers

Peri-transplant soluble CD30 (sCD30), a marker of activated T-cell mediated immunity, has been reported to predict early AR [82].

A recent metanalysis on 18 studies (1453 total patients) has confirmed a strong association between sCD30 and AR, especially for KTx from deceased donors [83].

CD154-positive T cytotoxic memory cells were associated with acute TCMR and its histological severity in a small cohort of KTx recipients receiving steroid-free TAC after alemtuzumab induction [84].

Pre-transplant, baseline levels of CD200 (a protein belonging to immunoglobulin superfamily) and CD200R1 (its myeloid-cell specific receptor, which mediates inhibitory signals) have been analyzed in a monocentric cohort of 125 KTx recipients; an increased pre-transplant CD200R1/CD200 ratio identified recipients at increased risk of AR and worse renal function at the 3rd and 6th month after KTx [111].

Additionally, pre-transplant expression of CD45RC on circulating CD8+ T lymphocytes predicted AR (mainly TCMR); a percentage of CD8+CD45RC T cells above 58.4% was independently associated with a 4-fold increase in the risk of AR [112].

3.9. Non-HLA DSA

Donor human leukocyte antigen (HLA)-specific antibodies were initially identified as a major cause of ABMR. This type of DSA has been extensively studied and represents an established, "traditional" biomarker of ABMR, which is beyond the scope of this review [113,114].

In more recent years, preformed and de novo non-HLA specific DSA targeting G-protein coupled receptors expressed on graft glomerular endothelium have been the focus of intense research, as they may account for a significant proportion of HLA-DSA negative acute and chronic ABMR [115–117]. They include a wide range of autoantibodies against different antigens, all of which represent potential biomarkers for ABMR [118] (Table 5).

Antibodies against type 1 receptor for Angiotensin 2 (AT1R) and Endothelin type A receptor (ETAR) are the most studied non-HLA, activating antibodies and appear to exert their effect either alone or in synergy with DSA. After binding to their receptors, these autoantibodies phenotypically modify and activate endothelial cell by triggering different intracellular pathways. They probably represent a bridge between allo- and autoimmunity within rejection, as these two components can interact and amplify one another [119]. Pre-transplant antibodies against AT1R and ETAR may identify a subset of patients at higher risk for acute and chronic rejection and graft loss, independent of HLA-directed alloimmune response [120,121], possibly even in a setting of low-immunological risk such as KTx from LD [122–124]. Pre-transplant antibodies against AT1R have also been associated with more severe microvascular inflammation histological lesions as compared to negative patients [125].

Anti-vimentin antibodies detected before KTx, probably reflecting previous endothelial damage occurred during hemodialysis, have also been associated with graft dysfunction [126].

Anti-Perlecan/LG3 antibodies are produced as a consequence of Perlecan release from injured endothelial cells [127]. They are highly prevalent in hypersensitized patients [128] and have been associated with acute ABMR, DGF, and reduced long term survival [129,130].

Anti-endothelial cell antibodies (AECA), which include a wide range of autoantibodies against several surface antigens, may also prove to be a source of rejection biomarkers [131,132].

In general, AECA have been associated with acute and chronic rejection and with early graft dysfunction in different types of solid organ transplant, including heart and kidney. De novo AECA seem to be more strongly associated with ABMR than preformed ones [133].

Identification of their target antigens is complex, and their precise meaning must still be elucidated for most of them, as they could represent biomarkers of past vascular injury or, on the contrary, be active contributors to microvascular inflammation [134].

However, some specific types of AECA have already been clinically characterized and show promise as biomarkers of endothelial injury. Their antigenic targets are Endoglin, Fms-like tyrosine kinase-3 ligand (FLT3-L), EGF-like repeats and discoidin I-like domains 3 (EDIL-3), and intercellular adhesion molecule 4 (ICAM-4), all involved in endothelial cell activation and leukocyte adhesion and margination. AECA have been associated with de novo DSA, ABMR, and early transplant glomerulopathy [131]. More recently, also anti-keratin-1 (KRT-1) antibodies were found to be associated with an increased risk of AR [132].

Finally, development of antibodies directed against tissue-specific self-antigens, such as Fibronectin (FN) and Collagen type IV (Col IV), increases the risk of AR in pancreas-kidney transplantation (PKT) [135] and transplant glomerulopathy in KTx [136]. These autoantibodies probably reflect breakdown of tolerance towards self-antigens, as suggested by detection of self-Ag-specific IFN-γ and IL-17 secreting T-cells in the same patients. Therefore, they could provide a biomarker of a tissue-specific autoimmune component of rejection.

In the near future, improved identification and characterization of non-HLA DSAs may help better classification of ABMR subphenotypes and provide diagnostic and prognostic biomarkers and potentially even indication for preemptive specific therapies in this subset of patients [124].

Table 5. Non-HLA DSA as a potential biomarker for antibody-mediated rejection (ABMR).

Biomarker	Main Features	Author
Anti-AT1R	Pre-transplant levels associated with, acute and chronic ABMR, severity of microvascular inflammation, graft dysfunction, and graft loss	Dragun D et al. [119] Philogene MC Hum Imm 2019 [120] Sas-Strozik et al. [121] Shinae Y et al. [122] DF Pinelli et al. [123] MA Lim et al. [125]
Anti-ETAR	Pre-transplant levels associated with acute and chronic ABMR graft dysfunction and graft loss	Philogene MC et al. Hum Imm 2019 [120] Shinae Y et al. [122] DF Pinelli et al. [123] Jackson AM et al. [131]
Anti-Vimentin	Pre-transplant levels associated with graft dysfunction	Dyvanian T et al. [126]
Anti-Perlecan	Highly prevalent in hypersensitized patients. Pre-transplant levels associated with increased risk of DGF, acute ABMR, and reduced long-term function	Dieudè M et al. [127] Riesco L et al. [128] Padet L et al. [129] Yang B et al. [130]
AECA	They include a variety of antibodies against endothelial antigens (Endoglin, FLT-3, EDIL-3, ICAM-4, KTR-1) and correlate with increased risk of ABMR	Jackson AM et al. [131] Guo X et al. [132] Sanchez Zapardiel E et al. [133]
Anti-FN and Col-IV	De novo development increases risk of AR (PKT) and transplant glomerulopathy (KTx)	Angaswamy N et al. [135] Gunasekeran M et al. [136]

3.10. Other Biomarkers

Another potential biomarker is serum N-glycan determination, performed at days 1 and 7 post-Tx and integrated in a clinical score (including age, gender, and immunological risk factors). A higher sum of scores at days 1 and 7 (>0.5) predicted graft rejection (AUC = 0.87) and correlated with long-term rejection-free survival in a cohort of LD Tx recipients [137].

Heat shock protein 90 (HSP-90), a molecular chaperon protein released into serum by damaged cells, was found to be significantly elevated in plasma of KTx with AR as compared to stable graft and other pathological conditions (chronic rejection, CNI nephrotoxicity, Polyomavirus nephropathy) and returned to baseline after immunosuppressive treatment [2,138].

Heparan Sulfate plasma levels are increased in TCMR compared to stable graft, due to release from EM during graft T-cell infiltration [2,139].

Many other urinary and plasmatic proteins could be potential biomarkers of rejection but deserve to be further studied: among these, C-C motif chemokine ligand 2 (CCL2), NGAL, IL-18, cystatin C, KIM-1, T-cell immunoglobulin and mucine domains-containing protein 3 (TIM3), alpha-1 antitrypsin (A1AT), alpha-2 antiplasmin (A2AP), serum amyloid A (SAA), and apolipoprotein CIII (APOC3) [2,140,141].

3.11. EVs

General features and meaning of EVs have already been dealt with in the paragraph on DGF biomarkers.

EVs represent a versatile tool given the huge variety of mediators included in their cargo. Therefore, potential applications of plasma and urinary EVS as biomarkers have also been studied in AR, as outlined in Table 6. In some studies, EVs levels have been considered as biomarkers themselves [99], whereas a set of specific molecules included in their cargo proved to be a potential biomarker of AR in others [142–146].

Table 6. EVs as potential biomarkers of AR.

Type of EV	Type of Rejection	Main Features	Author
Plasma C4d+CD144+ endothelial EVs	ABMR	Levels correlate with ABMR presence and severity and decrease after successful treatment	Tower C et al. [99]
Plasma endothelial EVs	ABMR	A combination score based on 4 mRNA transcripts overexpressed in EVs of patients with ABMR predicts imminent rejection in HLA-sensitized patients	Zhang H et al. [142]
Plasma endothelial EVs	ABMR	Levels increase in ABMR and decrease after treatment in the early post-transplant; however, they are also influenced by renal function recovery	Qamri Z et al. [143]
Urinary EVs	TCMR	A total of 11 protein enriched in urinary EV in patients with TCMR	Sigdel T et al. [144]
Urinary EVs	TCMR	A total of 17 protein enriched in urinary EV in patients with TCMR; Tetraspanin-1 and Hemopexin proposed as biomarkers	Lim J et al. [145]
Urinary EVs	TCMR	High levels of CD3 + EVs released by T-cell in urine are strongly associated with TCMR	Park J et al. [146]

4. Chronic Allograft Dysfunction (CAD)

Chronic allograft dysfunction is the main cause of long-term graft loss [147].

Different entities can be accounted for this picture, with chronic ABMR (cABMR) playing a predominant role in most cases [148].

However, other components can be represented by CNI nephrotoxicity, PVAN, de novo or relapsing glomerulonephritis. Many studies have focused on biomarkers for late graft dysfunction as a global entity, while others have tried to identify specific biomarkers to dissect each of these components.

In general, defining specific biomarkers for CAD is difficult, because molecular fingerprints of acute and chronic rejection are overlapping, partly reflecting similar mechanisms. Some authors propose a "threshold effect", with AR developing when intensity of alterations is high and chronic rejection expressing a less important degree of alterations [2]. For example, Complement is not only involved in ABMR, as described in a previous paragraph, but also plays a pivotal role as mediator of tubular senescence [28,30,149] and interstitial fibrosis, premature aging phenomena that characterize progression to chronic damage [150]. C3a, C5a, and the terminal C5b-9 complex can each amplify damage during CKD progression. Anaphylatoxins bind to their specific receptors inducing pro-inflammatory and fibrogenic activity on tubular and endothelial cells [151,152], pericytes [153], and resident fibroblasts, whereas C5b-9 complex can regulate production of pro-fibrotic and pro-inflammatory cytokines [97]. Collectively, these data indicate that uncontrolled Complement activation may result in maladaptive tissue repair with irreversible development of renal fibrosis and aging. Identification of biomarkers of CAD is therefore challenging due to coexistence of acute and chronic processes, but it would be extremely useful for a differential diagnosis [154].

4.1. Chronic Rejection and IFTA

Potential biomarkers for chronic rejection and IFTA are outlined in Table 7. IFTA is found in around 25% of 1-year biopsies and correlates with decreased graft survival when histological evidence of inflammation is present.

Table 7. Potential biomarkers for chronic rejection and interstitial fibrosis-tubular atrophy (IFTA).

Biomarker	Main Features	Author
Set of genes related to fibrosis (i.e., TGFβ), extracellular matrix deposition and immune response	Upregulated in IFTA	Mas V et al. [155]
4-gene urinary signature (mRNA for vimentin, NKCC2, E-cadherin, and 18S rRNA)	It predicts evolution of chronic rejection towards IFTA	Lee J. et al. [86]
13-gene renal tissue signature (GoCAR study)	It predicts CAD at the 12th month even with normal histology at the 3rd month	O'Connell P. et al. [87]
85-gene renal tissue signature	Associated with IFTA	Li L. et al. [156]
Urinary mi-R21 and mi-R200b	Increased expression predicts IFTA and CAD	Zununi V. et al. [157]
Plasmatic miR-150, miR-192, miR-200b, and miR-423-3p	Highly accurate in identifying IFTA (AUC = 0.87; sensitivity = 78%; specificity = 91%)	Zununi V. et al. [158]
Plasmatic miR-21, miR-142-3p, miR-155, and mi-R 21	Upregulated in IFTA; mi-R 21 correlates with GFR	Zununi V. et al. [159]
miR-145-5p expression in blood cells	Downregulated in IFTA; It can discriminate it from acute and borderline rejection	Matz M. et al. [160]

4.1.1. Transcriptomic Studies

Growing evidence of highly shared deregulated gene pathways between IFTA and AR suggests a common immunological etiology in most cases of late CAD [154].

Recent studies have focused on upregulation of genes involved in IFTA. Inflammation in IFTA areas ("inflammatory IFTA", i-IFTA) has been identified as pivotal element in prompting development of chronic renal damage, further underlying the relationship between chronic, subclinical immunological activity and irreversible fibrosis [161,162].

Several transcriptomic studies have shed light on specific genes and miRNAs involved in fibrotic evolution of chronic rejection.

In a study by Mas V. et al. an upregulation of genes related to fibrosis (TGFβ), extracellular matrix deposition, and immune response was found [155].

In the already quoted CTOT-04 trial, Lee J. R. et al. identified a four-gene urinary signature (mRNA for vimentin, NKCC2, E-cadherin, and 18S rRNA) which predicted IFTA [86].

In the study of Genomics of Chronic Allograft Rejection (GoCAR), renal biopsy transcriptome expression analysis identified a set of 13 genes which independently predicted development of CAD at the 12th month, despite normal histology at the 3rd month after KTx, in more than 200 prospectively followed patients with stable graft function. This multicenter study was validated in two independent cohorts and first raised hope that allograft injury may be detected before it becomes clinically evident [87].

Halloran et al. employed the "molecular microscope" approach (already discussed in the paragraph on AR) and demonstrated a progressively higher prevalence of IFTA lesions over time and its association with transcripts related to rejection and glomerulonephritis in late biopsies. This suggests a continuing, active tissue response rather than autonomous fibrogenesis and that early abrogation of the immunological process may be critical to block this evolution and preserve long-term graft function [93,161].

Another transcriptomic study employed an 85-gene signature related to IFTA and employed it to test targeted new anti-fibrotic drugs [156].

4.1.2. miRNAs

miRNAs, which we already analyzed as candidate biomarkers in the setting of DGF and AR, are also opening new perspectives in this setting. Recent studies have proposed sets of urinary and renal biopsy miRNAs as prognostic biomarkers of IFTA and CAD [163].

Aberrant urinary mi-R21 and miR200b expression was associated with IFTA and CAD [157].

Plasma circulating levels of miR-150, miR-192, miR-200b, and miR-423-3p were significantly different between patients with IFTA and those with stable renal Tx and accurately identified IFTA (AUC = 0.87; sensitivity = 78%; specificity = 91%) [158].

In another study, plasma expression of miR-21, miR-142-3p, and miR-155 were upregulated in IFTA and mi-R 21 levels were positively correlated with eGFR [159].

On the contrary, miR-145-5p expression in blood cells was significantly downregulated in IFTA and could discriminate it from many other active lesions, such as TCMR, ABMR, borderline-rejection, and from a condition of stable graft function [160].

Another area of active research is that of epigenetic modifications of immunity genes on progression to IFTA: epigenetic mechanisms such as hypomethylation could directly enhance their expression and also indirectly modulate it by regulating miRNAs [164].

4.1.3. Biomarkers of EMT and EndMT

IF is determined by massive deposition of EM, which is mainly produced by activated myofibroblasts probably derived from several cell types, especially renal tubular cells, through EMT.

This process, promoted by several factors such as oxidative stress and mitochondrial dysfunction due to IRI, deeply alters epithelial cell properties, determining loss of polarity and cell–cell adhesion and assumption of a mesenchymal phenotype, characterized by markedly increased production of EM [165].

More recently, activated myofibroblasts have been shown to arise also from renal endothelial cells through a similar process, EndMT, already mentioned in the section on DGF [166].

Both EMT and EndMT lead to abnormal production of EM and consequently play a key role in the pathogenesis of allograft IFTA [161]. Several histological and urinary EMT biomarkers have been proposed (Table 8), whereas more recent, initial evidence on potential EndMT biomarkers in KTx is available. Biomarkers of both processes will be analyzed.

Table 8. Potential biomarkers for epithelial-to-mesenchymal transition (EMT).

Biomarker	Main Features	Author
CD45, VIM, and POSTN	They correlate to each other and with iIFTA and graft loss	Alfieri C et al. [167]
Smurf 1	It is included in a pathway involved in EMT. Its inhibition by Bortezomib may mediate its anti-fibrotic effect.	Zhou J et al. [168]
VIM and β-catenin	Tubular expression correlates with IFTA and long-term eGFR decline	Hazzan M et al. [169]
Senescence biomarkers (e.g., p16INK4a)	They mark SASP, an inflammatory phenotype connected to EMT	Sosa Pena DPM et al. [170].
VIM and CD45 relative to UPK mRNA	This ratio based on urinary mRNAs correlates with VIM expression in renal tissue and may detect EMT and early graft fibrogenesis	Mezni I et al. [171]
Urinary transcriptomic patterns	They are associated with pEMT and subclinical graft injury	Galichon P et al. [172]

(a) Biomarkers of EMT

Histological biomarkers

In a recent study, renal expression of CD45, vimentin (VIM), and periostin (POSTN) correlated with iIFTA and POSTN was the strongest predictor of graft loss. Of interest, its expression was inversely correlated with 25(OH)VitD levels, suggesting that these might influence graft fibrosis [167].

Smad ubiquitination regulatory factor 1 (Smurf1) is part of Smurf1/Akt/mTOR/P70S6K signaling pathway, activated by TNF-α and involved in EMT. Of interest, Bortezomib blunted progression of EMT and IF by inhibiting TNF-α production and consequently expression of Smurf1, suggesting that this could be an EMT biomarker with diagnostic and therapeutic value [168].

Tubular expression of VIM and β-catenin, biomarkers of EMT, in protocol biopsy performed 3 months after KTx, was an independent risk factor for IFTA and eGFR decline up to 4 years post-transplant in CsA-treated recipients [169].

Finally, an interesting area of research is that of cellular senescence. This is associated with an inflammatory, "senescence-associated secretory phenotype" (SASP) which is tightly connected to EMT and CAD. Senescence markers (e.g., $p16^{INK4a}$) could therefore be considered as potential surrogate biomarkers of EMT [170].

Urinary biomarkers

An interesting non-invasive biomarker of EMT is the ratio between VIM and CD45 relative to uroplakin 1a (UPK) urinary mRNA, which has been shown to correlate with intensity of VIM renal expression measured with immunostaining in per-protocol renal biopsies [171].

Other studies adopting a whole transcriptomic analysis approach identified specific urinary transcriptomic patterns associated with pEMT. Unbiased pathway analysis revealed that these patterns expressed increased inflammation and reduced metabolic functions, suggesting that they may be effective to detect subclinical immune response leading to EMT and graft fibrosis [172].

(b) Biomarkers of EndMT

Three biomarkers of EndMT, fascin1, vimentin, and heat shock protein 47, were strongly expressed in endothelial cells of peritubular capillaries in ABMR as compared to stable patients and predicted late graft dysfunction (up to 4 years since ABMR diagnosis) better than histological lesions. These results suggest that they may be reliable in identifying persistent endothelial activation and evolution towards cABMR [173].

In vitro and in vivo experimental studies demonstrated that EndMT may promote IF by targeting the TGF-β/Smad and Akt/mTOR/p70S6K signaling pathways, indicating that components of these pathways may be a potential source of EndMT biomarkers [174].

Finally, E Glover et al. analyzed evidence of miRNAs regulation of EndMT from experimental studies and their potential impact on kidney and other solid organ allograft dysfunction in a recent review. However, clinical studies in humans are needed to confirm their role as EndMT biomarkers [175].

4.2. Chronic CNI Nephrotoxicity

Some other studies identified potential specific biomarkers for chronic CNI nephrotoxicity, which are outlined in Table 9.

Chronic ischemia due to the vasoconstrictive effect of CNI triggers an alteration in expression of proteins involved in pro-inflammatory response and oxidative stress; however, the renal histology of chronic CNI nephrotoxicity is not peculiar (it may in fact merely determine IFTA) and this hampers efforts to identify specific biomarkers [176].

A metabolomic study compared urine from healthy subjects and KTx recipients with biopsy-proven chronic TAC nephrotoxicity and proposed symmetric dimethylarginine and serine as marker of this type of kidney injury (ROC analysis AUC of 0.95 and 0.81, respectively) [177].

uNGAL was proved to correlate with duration of CsA therapy in children with CNI nephrotoxicity [178].

A SNP in the FK-506-binding protein (FKBP), rs6041749 C variant, appeared to enhance FKBP1A gene transcription compared to the T variant and was associated with an increased risk of CAD in a Chinese cohort of TAC-treated KTx recipients, although with an unclear mechanism [179].

Other studies in rat models have reported increased urinary levels of TNAα, LIM-1, and FN in the early phase of CsA nephrotoxicity and late increases of urinary Osteopontin and TGF-β in chronic nephrotoxicity [180].

Decreased expression of Slc12a3 and KS-WNK1, leading to impaired sodium transport in distal tubules and chronic activation of renin-angiotensin system, was associated with CsA and TAC nephrotoxicity in another rat model [181]. Potential biomarkers identified in the last two experimental studies need to be validated in humans.

Table 9. Potential biomarkers for chronic calcineurin-inhibitor (CNI) nephrotoxicity.

Biomarker	Main Features	Author
Urinary symmetric dimethylarginine and serine	Highly accurate for CNI nephrotoxicity (AUC of 0.95 and 0.81, respectively)	Xia T et al. [177]
uNGAL	It correlates with duration of CsA therapy in children with CNI nephrotoxicity	Gacka E et al. [178]
Genetic polymorphism of FK-506-binding protein, rs6041749 C variant	It enhances FKBP1A gene transcription and is associated with an increased risk of CAD in TAC-treated KTx recipients	Wu Z et al. [179]
Increased urinary TNAα, LIM-1, FN Osteopontin, and TGF-β	These markers correlate with different stages of CsA nephrotoxicity in rat models	Carlos C et al. [180]
Decreased renal expression of Slc12a3 and KS-WNK1	These markers correlate with different stages of CNI nephrotoxicity in rat models	Cui Y et al. [181]

4.3. PVAN

Potential biomarkers for PVAN, an important cause of CAD [182], are outlined in Table 10.

Table 10. Potential biomarkers for Polyomavirus-associated nephropathy (PVAN).

Biomarker	Main Features	Author
Urinary exosomal bkv-miR-B1-5p and bkv-miR-B1-5p/miR-16	Excellent diagnostic accuracy for PVAN	Kim M et al. [183]
Urinary CXCL10	Associated with subclinical tubule-interstitial inflammation and viremia	Ho J et al. [184]
IL28B SNP C/T (rs12979860)	Associated with presence of PVAN in viremic patients	Dvir R et al. [185]

Urinary exosomal bkv-miR-B1-5p and bkv-miR-B1-5p/miR-16, two miRNAs encoded by PVAN, have both demonstrated very high discriminative capacity for this complication (ROC AUC 0.98 for each) as compared with that of commonly used surrogate biomarkers, such as plasma viral load [183].

Urinary CXCL10 has been associated with subclinical inflammation within the tubule-interstitial and peritubular capillary spaces and correlated with Polyomavirus viremia [184].

A single nucleotide polymorphism (SNP) of IL28B (C/T polymorphism rs12979860) was associated with presence of PVAN, discriminating these patients from those with viremia without any renal involvement [185].

The search for renal tissue transcriptomic biomarkers of PVAN has not provided any solid result so far. Overlap in pathogenetic mechanisms and gene expression between PVAN and non-viral forms of allograft injury, such as TCMR and iIFTA, makes it difficult to identify peculiar molecular signatures [186].

5. Current Limits and Perspectives of Biomarkers in Renal Transplant

Advances in high-throughput technologies have been providing an avalanche of new potential biomarkers over the last decade. However, in general, their application in clinical practice is currently being restrained by several drawbacks. Most available biomarkers do not meet ideal requirements outlined in Table 11 and certainly require further validation through multicenter studies, as single-center discovery step often inflates their value [187].

Most important, their role and cost-effectiveness should be assessed in prospective randomized trials designed to compare them with standard KTx management with traditional diagnostic tools.

Despite these limits, biomarkers represent the cornerstone of precision medicine, which aims at integrating traditional clinical information and tailoring medical care to select the best treatment for an individual patient [5]. This new frontier will probably deeply change the way we monitor KTx and manage its complications.

Renal biopsy, the traditional gold standard for assessing graft dysfunction, is usually triggered by a change in serum creatinine and/or proteinuria and has a limited diagnostic power for initial injury, when histological changes are minimal or equivocal [3]. By contrast, an ideal biomarker (or a set of biomarkers) should lead to an earlier and more objective diagnosis (Table 11) making it possible to pre-emptively treat histological initial lesions long before they become irreversible, or even before they become visible with traditional tools, marking patterns of molecular alterations which predate histological injury ("molecular rejection"). Biomarkers could decrease the need for renal biopsy to detect subclinical disease (e.g., protocol biopsies) and even substitute for it when contraindicated. Furthermore, while current new potential biomarkers in KTx mainly have a diagnostic/prognostic meaning, the area of monitoring, pharmacodynamic/response, and safety biomarkers (Table 1) is substantially unexplored in this setting and could help us improve long-term management of allograft dysfunction (e.g., follow-up of patients after BPAR, with repeated, non-invasive monitoring biomarkers to rule out persistence of ongoing subclinical rejection; assessment of etiology and degree of activity/chronicity in CAD).

Table 11. Features of an ideal biomarker for kidney transplant (KTx) [1,2,187].

Biomarker Features	Comment
Non-invasive and easy to measure	Urine and blood biomarkers are easily available and can be serially measured, whereas renal tissue biomarkers require renal biopsy with inherent invasiveness and limits. Urine and blood biomarkers may be used when renal biopsy is contraindicated or reduce the need for repeated surveillance biopsies.
Short turn-around time	Results should be available within a time frame which allows rapid, potentially pre-emptive intervention (e.g., diagnosis of subclinical AR)
Easy to interpret	Results should be easy to interpret, and threshold values should be established to help transplant physician in clinical practice
Reproducible and standardized	Results should be validated in multiple independent cohorts with different features (e.g., elderly, or highly sensitized KTx recipients, or different ethnicity) and assay standardization of analytical process performed in order to minimize inter-laboratory and inter-platform variability
Accuracy (sensitivity and specificity)	Biomarker levels should strictly reflect a single specific pathological process, without being influenced by other causes of kidney damage (e.g., AR vs. CNI nephrotoxicity or vs. infections)
Good prognostic performance (PPV and NPV)	Acceptable PPP and NPP. In general, new biomarkers should be preferably tested in subsets of patients at different immunological risk, rather than on the transplant population as a whole, in order to improve their statistical performance (e.g., higher a priori chance of AR in highly sensitized KTx recipients improves PPV compared to standard recipients).
Proof of cause	Reduction of a biomarker level correlates with an improvement in the underlying pathological process assessed with current gold-standard (histological examination with renal biopsy)
Cost-effective	Results should improve clinical management and consequently impact long-term outcomes and related economic aspects, justifying biomarker costs (e.g., a biomarker which detects subclinical AR could improve treatment, prolong graft survival and reduce costs)

Particularly interesting perspectives are immunological risk stratification and identification of low-risk, or even tolerant patients.

Peripheral blood gene expression tests such TruGraf [91] or kSORT [57] have already become commercial and appear accurate in identifying a state of "immunological quiescence" in stable recipients; due to their high NPP they could allow to rule out ongoing subclinical rejection through serial monitoring, as an alternative to surveillance biopsies, and guide immunosuppression minimization in fragile patients at low immunological risk [188].

A further step forward would be to identify biomarkers of operational tolerance, a rare condition characterized by maintenance of stable renal function without any immunosuppressive therapy.

Tolerant patients seem to be depicted by increased expression of B cell associated genes in the blood and urine and by a peculiar B cell repertoire, enriched in naive and transitional B cells. Of interest, this pattern appears to be associated with better long-term graft function [189] and potential biomarkers of this process are beginning to emerge. For example, TCL1A, an oncogene expressed in immature naive and transitional B cells, and promoting their survival, has been associated with immunosuppressive properties of this lymphocyte sub-population and seems to be upregulated in stable, rejection-free KTx recipients [190].

Of interest, Newell et al. identified a B-cell signature formed by a set of three genes which correlated with increased expression of CD20 mRNAs (FoxP3, CD20, CD3, perforin) in urinary sediment of tolerant patients compared to healthy controls (all of them) and to stable KTx (only CD20) [191], whereas Danger et al. showed that a composite score based on a 20-gene signature peripheral blood cells could accurately discriminate operationally tolerant recipients from stable ones, independent of immunosuppressive therapy [192]. All these approaches need to be validated, but they may pave the way for the identification of tolerance biomarkers, with important implications on management of immunosuppressive therapy [193]. The state-of-the-art of this family of biomarkers was recently analyzed in several reviews [2,194,195] and is beyond the scope of this work.

At the other end of the spectrum, biomarkers could be preferably employed to monitor high-immunological risk patients (e.g., sensitized, DSA-positive recipients). Testing biomarkers in this subset helps increase PPP due to a higher a priori risk of AR. A combination of different biomarkers can also increase diagnostic accuracy; for example, association of kSORT with IFNγ ELISPOT improves predictive power for subclinical TCMR and ABMR [74].

Another intriguing perspective is the application of artificial intelligence (AI) models which allows computational analysis and interpretation of large-scale molecular data generation by exploiting machine learning algorithms and neural networks [196,197]. For example, classifiers like artificial neural networks, support vector machines and Bayesian inference have already been employed in pilot studies to screen KTx recipients requiring renal biopsy [198] and AI has proved useful to improve estimation of TAC Area Under the Concentration Over Time Curve [199].

"Molecular microscope" is another important example application of AI to renal tissue transcriptomic analysis [93,94].

In another recent work an unsupervised learning method integrating a wide range of parameters (clinical functional, immunologic, and histologic) was applied to a large cohort of KTx recipients and allowed to classify five transplant glomerulopathy archetypes, each associated with a different allograft 5-year graft survival (ranging from 88% to 22%) [200].

These studies suggest that progress in AI can significantly contribute to a completely new, more accurate disease nosology, integrating complex sets of biomarkers of different nature (from clinical data to molecular aspects) for a subtle characterization of traditional entities.

6. Conclusions

Development of Omics technology and expanding knowledge of new tools, such as EVs and dd-cfDNA, has led to an increased availability of a wide range of new potential biomarkers, which may be applied to all key settings of early and late graft dysfunction. Non-invasive biomarkers measured in urine or blood appear promising in providing very early diagnosis of pathological processes, such as subclinical AR, or in stratifying risk of DGF or of rejection, potentially reducing need for surveillance biopsies to monitor low-risk recipients. Tissue biomarkers have also proved effective in integrating traditional histology, leading to improved disease nosology and more accurate prognosis. Tolerance biomarkers and progress in AI are opening new frontiers, which may revolutionize transplant medicine.

Although larger, multi-center validation studies are needed before combination of biomarkers can be widely implemented in the clinic, the transplant physician should rise to the challenge of becoming familiar with this new landscape, in order to start taking advantage of the various facets of its huge potential.

Author Contributions: M.Q. and V.C. designed and wrote the initial manuscript; G.M. designed Figure and Tables; G.G. organized References; G.C. contributed to specific parts concerning Complement-related biomarkers. All authors critically revised, discussed and edited the article until it reached its current form and agreed to the published version of the manuscript. All authors have read and agreed to the published version of the manuscript.

Funding: This study was (partially) funded by the Italian Ministry of Education, University and Research (MIUR) program "Departments of Excellence 2018–2022", AGING Project—Department of Translational Medicine, University of Piemonte Orientale (UPO) and by local grants of the University of Piemonte Orientale (UPO, FAR) to M.Q. and V.C.

Conflicts of Interest: The authors declare no conflict of interest.

Abbreviations

ABMR	antibody-mediated rejection
cABMR	chronic antibody-mediated rejection
AI	artificial intelligence
AR	acute rejection
ATN	acute tubular necrosis
AT1R	Angiotensin 2 receptor 1
AUC	area under the curve
CAD	chronic allograft dysfunction
CNI	calcineurin inhibitor
Col-IV	Collagen type IV
CsA	Cyclosporin A
DCD	donation after circulatory death
DBD	donation after brain death
DGF	delayed graft function
DSA	donor-specific antibodies
ECD	extended criteria donor
EDIL-3	EGF-like repeats and discoidin I-like domains 3
EM	extracellular matrix
EMT	epithelial-to-mesenchymal transition
ENDATs	endothelial associated transcripts
EndMT	endothelial-to-mesenchymal transition
ETAR	endothelin type A receptor
EVs	extracellular vesicles
FLT3-L	Fms-like tyrosine kinase-3 ligand
FN	Fibronectin
GFR	glomerular filtration rate
GST	glutathione S-transferase
HLA	human leukocyte antigen
HSP	heat shock protein
ICAM-4	intercellular adhesion molecule 4
IFTA	interstitial fibrosis tubular atrophy
iIFTA	inflammatory interstitial fibrosis tubular atrophy
IRI	ischemia-reperfusion injury
kSORT	kidney solid organ response test
KTx	kidney transplant
KTR-3	Keratin-3
FST	furosemide stress test
LD	living-donor
MFI	mean fluorescence intensity
MMP-2	matrix metalloprotein-2
miRNA	microRNA
NGAL	neutrophil gelatinase-associated lipocalin
NPP	negative predictive power
PBTs	pathogenesis-based transcript sets
pEMT	partial epithelial-to-mesenchymal transition
POSTN	Periostin
PVAN	Polyomavirus-associated nephropathy
PPP	Positive predictive power
ROC	receiver operating characteristic
SNP	single nucleotide polymorphism
TAC	Tacrolimus
TCMR	T-cell mediated rejection
tCRM	tissue common rejection module
TIMP-2	tissue inhibitor of metalloproteinases-2
TLR-4	Toll-like receptor 4
VIM	Vimentin

References

1. Califf, R.M. Biomarker definitions and their applications. *Exp. Biol. Med. Maywood NJ* **2018**, *243*, 213–221. [CrossRef] [PubMed]
2. Salvadori, M.; Tsalouchos, A. Biomarkers in renal transplantation: An updated review. *World J. Transplant.* **2017**, *7*, 161–178. [CrossRef] [PubMed]
3. Sarwal, M.; Chua, M.-S.; Kambham, N.; Hsieh, S.-C.; Satterwhite, T.; Masek, M.; Salvatierra, O.J. Molecular heterogeneity in acute renal allograft rejection identified by DNA microarray profiling. *N. Engl. J. Med.* **2003**, *349*, 125–138. [CrossRef]
4. Stapleton, C.P.; Conlon, P.J.; Phelan, P.J. Using omics to explore complications of kidney transplantation. *Transpl. Int.* **2018**, *31*, 251–262. [CrossRef] [PubMed]
5. Naesens, M.; Anglicheau, D. Precision Transplant Medicine: Biomarkers to the Rescue. *J. Am. Soc. Nephrol.* **2018**, *29*, 24–34. [CrossRef] [PubMed]
6. Herath, S.; Erlich, J.; Au, A.Y.M.; Endre, Z.H. Advances in Detection of Kidney Transplant Injury. *Mol. Diagn. Ther.* **2019**, *23*, 333–351. [CrossRef] [PubMed]
7. Nashan, B.; Abbud-Filho, M.; Citterio, F. Prediction, prevention, and management of delayed graft function: Where are we now? *Clin. Transplant.* **2016**, *30*, 1198–1208. [CrossRef]
8. Noble, J.; Jouve, T.; Malvezzi, P.; Süsal, C.; Rostaing, L. Transplantation of Marginal Organs: Immunological Aspects and Therapeutic Perspectives in Kidney Transplantation. *Front. Immunol.* **2019**, *10*, 3142. [CrossRef]
9. Caulfield, T.; Murdoch, B.; Sapir-Pichhadze, R.; Keown, P. Policy Challenges for Organ Allocation in an Era of "Precision Medicine". *Can. J. Kidney Health Dis.* **2020**, *7*, 2054358120912655. [CrossRef]
10. Han, F.; Wan, S.; Sun, Q.; Chen, N.; Li, H.; Zheng, L.; Zhang, N.; Huang, Z.; Hong, L.; Sun, Q. Donor Plasma Mitochondrial DNA Is Correlated with Posttransplant Renal Allograft Function. *Transplantation* **2019**, *103*, 2347–2358. [CrossRef]
11. Schröppel, B.; Heeger, P.S.; Thiessen-Philbrook, H.; Hall, I.E.; Doshi, M.D.; Weng, F.L.; Reese, P.P.; Parikh, C.R. Donor Urinary C5a Levels Independently Correlate with Posttransplant Delayed Graft Function. *Transplantation* **2019**, *103*, e29–e35. [CrossRef] [PubMed]
12. Gómez-Dos-Santos, V.; Ramos-Muñoz, E.; García-Bermejo, M.L.; Ruiz-Hernández, M.; Rodríguez-Serrano, E.M.; Saiz-González, A.; Martínez-Perez, A.; Burgos-Revilla, F.J. MicroRNAs in Kidney Machine Perfusion Fluid as Novel Biomarkers for Graft Function. Normalization Methods for miRNAs Profile Analysis. *Transplant. Proc.* **2019**, *51*, 307–310. [CrossRef] [PubMed]
13. Roest, H.P.; Ooms, L.S.S.; Gillis, A.J.M.; IJzermans, J.N.M.; Looijenga, L.H.J.; Dorssers, L.C.J.; Dor, F.J.M.F.; van der Laan, L.J.W. Cell-free MicroRNA miR-505-3p in Graft Preservation Fluid Is an Independent Predictor of Delayed Graft Function After Kidney Transplantation. *Transplantation* **2019**, *103*, 329–335. [CrossRef] [PubMed]
14. Moser, M.A.J.; Sawicka, K.; Arcand, S.; O'Brien, P.; Luke, P.; Beck, G.; Sawicka, J.; Cohen, A.; Sawicki, G. Proteomic Analysis of Perfusate from Machine Cold Perfusion of Transplant Kidneys: Insights into Protection from Injury. *Ann. Transplant.* **2017**, *22*, 730–739. [CrossRef] [PubMed]
15. Cappuccilli, M.; Capelli, I.; Comai, G.; Cianciolo, G.; La Manna, G. Neutrophil Gelatinase-Associated Lipocalin as a Biomarker of Allograft Function after Renal Transplantation: Evaluation of the Current Status and Future Insights. *Artif. Organs* **2018**, *42*, 8–14. [CrossRef]
16. Hall, I.E.; Bhangoo, R.S.; Reese, P.P.; Doshi, M.D.; Weng, F.L.; Hong, K.; Lin, H.; Han, G.; Hasz, R.D.; Goldstein, M.J.; et al. Glutathione S-transferase iso-enzymes in perfusate from pumped kidneys are associated with delayed graft function. *Am. J. Transplant.* **2014**, *14*, 886–896. [CrossRef]
17. Udomkarnjananun, S.; Townamchai, N.; Iampenkhae, K.; Petchlorlian, A.; Srisawat, N.; Katavetin, P.; Sutherasan, M.; Santingamkun, A.; Praditpornsilpa, K.; Eiam-Ong, S.; et al. Furosemide Stress Test as a Predicting Biomarker for Delayed Graft Function in Kidney Transplantation. *Nephron* **2019**, *141*, 236–248. [CrossRef]
18. Wilflingseder, J.; Sunzenauer, J.; Toronyi, E.; Heinzel, A.; Kainz, A.; Mayer, B.; Perco, P.; Telkes, G.; Langer, R.M.; Oberbauer, R. Molecular pathogenesis of post-transplant acute kidney injury: Assessment of whole-genome mRNA and miRNA profiles. *PLoS ONE* **2014**, *9*, e104164. [CrossRef]
19. Milhoransa, P.; Montanari, C.C.; Montenegro, R.; Manfro, R.C. Micro RNA 146a-5p expression in Kidney transplant recipients with delayed graft function. *Braz. J. Nephrol.* **2019**, *41*, 242–251. [CrossRef]

20. Khalid, U.; Newbury, L.J.; Simpson, K.; Jenkins, R.H.; Bowen, T.; Bates, L.; Sheerin, N.S.; Chavez, R.; Fraser, D.J. A urinary microRNA panel that is an early predictive biomarker of delayed graft function following kidney transplantation. *Sci. Rep.* **2019**, *9*, 3584. [CrossRef]
21. Maier, H.T.; Ashraf, M.I.; Denecke, C.; Weiss, S.; Augustin, F.; Messner, F.; Vallant, N.; Böcklein, M.; Margreiter, C.; Göbel, G.; et al. Prediction of delayed graft function and long-term graft survival by serum and urinary neutrophil gelatinase-associated lipocalin during the early postoperative phase after kidney transplantation. *PLoS ONE* **2018**, *13*, e0189932. [CrossRef] [PubMed]
22. Ramirez-Sandoval, J.C.; Herrington, W.; Morales-Buenrostro, L.E. Neutrophil gelatinase-associated lipocalin in kidney transplantation: A review. *Transplant. Rev.* **2015**, *29*, 139–144. [CrossRef] [PubMed]
23. Li, Y.M.; Li, Y.; Yan, L.; Wang, H.; Wu, X.J.; Tang, J.T.; Wang, L.L.; Shi, Y.Y. Comparison of urine and blood NGAL for early prediction of delayed graft function in adult kidney transplant recipients: A meta-analysis of observational studies. *BMC Nephrol.* **2019**, *20*, 291. [CrossRef] [PubMed]
24. Sahraei, Z.; Mehdizadeh, M.; Salamzadeh, J.; Nafar, M.; Eshraghi, A. Association between Delayed Graft Function (DGF) Biomarkers and Long-term Outcomes after Living Donor Kidney Transplantation. *Rev. Recent Clin. Trials* **2018**, *13*, 312–318. [CrossRef]
25. Hu, X.; Su, M.; Lin, J.; Zhang, L.; Sun, W.; Zhang, J.; Tian, Y.; Qiu, W. Corin Is Downregulated in Renal Ischemia/Reperfusion Injury and Is Associated with Delayed Graft Function after Kidney Transplantation. *Dis. Markers* **2019**, *2019*, 9429323. [CrossRef]
26. Zmonarski, S.; Madziarska, K.; Banasik, M.; Mazanowska, O.; Magott-Procelewska, M.; Hap, K.; Krajewska, M. Expression of PBMC TLR4 in Renal Graft Recipients Who Experienced Delayed Graft Function Reflects Dynamic Balance Between Blood and Tissue Compartments and Helps Select a Problematic Patient. *Transplant. Proc.* **2018**, *50*, 1744–1749. [CrossRef]
27. Comai, G.; Baraldi, O.; Cuna, V.; Corradetti, V.; Angeletti, A.; Brunilda, S.; Capelli, I.; Cappuccilli, M.; LA Manna, G. Increase in Serum Amylase and Resistive Index after Kidney Transplant Are Biomarkers of Delayed Graft Function. *Vivo Athens Greece* **2018**, *32*, 397–402. [CrossRef]
28. Xu-Dubois, Y.-C.; Ahmadpoor, P.; Brocheriou, I.; Louis, K.; Snanoudj, N.A.; Rouvier, P.; Taupin, J.-L.; Corchia, A.; Galichon, P.; Barrou, B.; et al. Microvasculature partial endothelial mesenchymal transition in early posttransplant biopsy with acute tubular necrosis identifies poor recovery renal allografts. *Am. J. Transplant.* **2020**. [CrossRef]
29. Castellano, G.; Franzin, R.; Stasi, A.; Divella, C.; Sallustio, F.; Pontrelli, P.; Lucarelli, G.; Battaglia, M.; Staffieri, F.; Crovace, A.; et al. Complement Activation during Ischemia/Reperfusion Injury Induces Pericyte-to-Myofibroblast Transdifferentiation Regulating Peritubular Capillary Lumen Reduction Through pERK Signaling. *Front. Immunol.* **2018**, *9*, 1002. [CrossRef]
30. Castellano, G.; Franzin, R.; Sallustio, F.; Stasi, A.; Banelli, B.; Romani, M.; De Palma, G.; Lucarelli, G.; Divella, C.; Battaglia, M.; et al. Complement component C5a induces aberrant epigenetic modifications in renal tubular epithelial cells accelerating senescence by Wnt4/βcatenin signaling after ischemia/reperfusion injury. *Aging* **2019**, *11*, 4382–4406. [CrossRef]
31. Curci, C.; Castellano, G.; Stasi, A.; Divella, C.; Loverre, A.; Gigante, M.; Simone, S.; Cariello, M.; Montinaro, V.; Lucarelli, G.; et al. Endothelial-to-mesenchymal transition and renal fibrosis in ischaemia/reperfusion injury are mediated by complement anaphylatoxins and Akt pathway. *Nephrol. Dial. Transplant.* **2014**, *29*, 799–808. [CrossRef] [PubMed]
32. Lu, T.X.; Rothenberg, M.E. MicroRNA. *J. Allergy Clin. Immunol.* **2018**, *141*, 1202–1207. [CrossRef] [PubMed]
33. Gremmels, H.; de Jong, O.G.; Toorop, R.J.; Michielsen, L.; van Zuilen, A.D.; Vlassov, A.V.; Verhaar, M.C.; van Balkom, B.W.M. The Small RNA Repertoire of Small Extracellular Vesicles Isolated from Donor Kidney Preservation Fluid Provides a Source for Biomarker Discovery for Organ Quality and Posttransplantation Graft Function. *Transplant. Direct* **2019**, *5*, e484. [CrossRef] [PubMed]
34. Franco-Acevedo, A.; Melo, Z.; Echavarria, R. Diagnostic, Prognostic, and Therapeutic Value of Non-Coding RNA Expression Profiles in Renal Transplantation. *Diagnostics* **2020**, *10*, 60. [CrossRef] [PubMed]
35. Wilflingseder, J.; Reindl-Schwaighofer, R.; Sunzenauer, J.; Kainz, A.; Heinzel, A.; Mayer, B.; Oberbauer, R. MicroRNAs in kidney transplantation. *Nephrol. Dial. Transplant.* **2015**, *30*, 910–917. [CrossRef]
36. Trionfini, P.; Benigni, A.; Remuzzi, G. MicroRNAs in kidney physiology and disease. *Nat. Rev. Nephrol.* **2015**, *11*, 23–33. [CrossRef]

37. Su, M.; Hu, X.; Lin, J.; Zhang, L.; Sun, W.; Zhang, J.; Tian, Y.; Qiu, W. Identification of Candidate Genes Involved in Renal Ischemia/Reperfusion Injury. *DNA Cell Biol.* **2019**, *38*, 256–262. [CrossRef]
38. Cantaluppi, V.; Dellepiane, S.; Tamagnone, M.; Medica, D.; Figliolini, F.; Messina, M.; Manzione, A.M.; Gai, M.; Tognarelli, G.; Ranghino, A.; et al. Neutrophil Gelatinase Associated Lipocalin Is an Early and Accurate Biomarker of Graft Function and Tissue Regeneration in Kidney Transplantation from Extended Criteria Donors. *PLoS ONE* **2015**, *10*, e0129279. [CrossRef]
39. Bank, J.R.; Ruhaak, R.; Soonawala, D.; Mayboroda, O.; Romijn, F.P.; van Kooten, C.; Cobbaert, C.M.; de Fijter, J.W. Urinary TIMP-2 Predicts the Presence and Duration of Delayed Graft Function in Donation after Circulatory Death Kidney Transplant Recipients. *Transplantation* **2019**, *103*, 1014–1023. [CrossRef]
40. Van Niel, G.; D'Angelo, G.; Raposo, G. Shedding light on the cell biology of extracellular vesicles. *Nat. Rev. Mol. Cell Biol.* **2018**, *19*, 213–228. [CrossRef]
41. Karpman, D.; Ståhl, A.-L.; Arvidsson, I. Extracellular vesicles in renal disease. *Nat. Rev. Nephrol.* **2017**, *13*, 545–562. [CrossRef] [PubMed]
42. Quaglia, M.; Dellepiane, S.; Guglielmetti, G.; Merlotti, G.; Castellano, G.; Cantaluppi, V. Extracellular Vesicles as Mediators of Cellular Crosstalk between Immune System and Kidney Graft. *Front. Immunol.* **2020**, *11*, 74. [CrossRef] [PubMed]
43. Dursun, I.; Yel, S.; Unsur, E. Dynamics of circulating microparticles in chronic kidney disease and transplantation: Is it really reliable marker? *World J. Transplant.* **2015**, *5*, 267–275. [CrossRef] [PubMed]
44. Al-Massarani, G.; Vacher-Coponat, H.; Paul, P.; Widemann, A.; Arnaud, L.; Loundou, A.; Robert, S.; Berland, Y.; Dignat-George, F.; Camoin-Jau, L. Impact of immunosuppressive treatment on endothelial biomarkers after kidney transplantation. *Am. J. Transplant.* **2008**, *8*, 2360–2367. [CrossRef]
45. Al-Massarani, G.; Vacher-Coponat, H.; Paul, P.; Arnaud, L.; Loundou, A.; Robert, S.; Moal, V.; Berland, Y.; Dignat-George, F.; Camoin-Jau, L. Kidney transplantation decreases the level and procoagulant activity of circulating microparticles. *Am. J. Transplant.* **2009**, *9*, 550–557. [CrossRef]
46. Martins, S.R.; Alves, L.V.; Cardoso, C.N.; Silva, L.G.; Nunes, F.F.; de Lucas Júnior, F.M.; Silva, A.C.; Dusse, L.M.; Alpoim, P.N.; Mota, A.P. Cell-derived microparticles and von Willebrand factor in Brazilian renal transplant recipients. *Nephrol. Carlton* **2019**, *24*, 1304–1312. [CrossRef]
47. Alvarez, S.; Suazo, C.; Boltansky, A.; Ursu, M.; Carvajal, D.; Innocenti, G.; Vukusich, A.; Hurtado, M.; Villanueva, S.; Carreño, J.E.; et al. Urinary exosomes as a source of kidney dysfunction biomarker in renal transplantation. *Transplant. Proc.* **2013**, *45*, 3719–3723. [CrossRef]
48. Dimuccio, V.; Ranghino, A.; Praticò Barbato, L.; Fop, F.; Biancone, L.; Camussi, G.; Bussolati, B. Urinary CD133+ extracellular vesicles are decreased in kidney transplanted patients with slow graft function and vascular damage. *PLoS ONE* **2014**, *9*, e104490. [CrossRef]
49. Sonoda, H.; Yokota-Ikeda, N.; Oshikawa, S.; Kanno, Y.; Yoshinaga, K.; Uchida, K.; Ueda, Y.; Kimiya, K.; Uezono, S.; Ueda, A.; et al. Decreased abundance of urinary exosomal aquaporin-1 in renal ischemia-reperfusion injury. *Am. J. Physiol. Ren. Physiol.* **2009**, *297*, F1006–F1016. [CrossRef]
50. Asvapromtada, S.; Sonoda, H.; Kinouchi, M.; Oshikawa, S.; Takahashi, S.; Hoshino, Y.; Sinlapadeelerdkul, T.; Yokota-Ikeda, N.; Matsuzaki, T.; Ikeda, M. Characterization of urinary exosomal release of aquaporin-1 and -2 after renal ischemia-reperfusion in rats. *Am. J. Physiol. Ren. Physiol.* **2018**, *314*, F584–F601. [CrossRef]
51. Suthanthiran, M.; Schwartz, J.E.; Ding, R.; Abecassis, M.; Dadhania, D.; Samstein, B.; Knechtle, S.J.; Friedewald, J.; Becker, Y.T.; Sharma, V.K.; et al. Urinary-cell mRNA profile and acute cellular rejection in kidney allografts. *N. Engl. J. Med.* **2013**, *369*, 20–31. [CrossRef] [PubMed]
52. Christakoudi, S.; Runglall, M.; Mobillo, P.; Tsui, T.-L.; Duff, C.; Domingo-Vila, C.; Kamra, Y.; Delaney, F.; Montero, R.; Spiridou, A.; et al. Development of a multivariable gene-expression signature targeting T-cell-mediated rejection in peripheral blood of kidney transplant recipients validated in cross-sectional and longitudinal samples. *EBioMedicine* **2019**, *41*, 571–583. [CrossRef] [PubMed]
53. Zhang, W.; Yi, Z.; Keung, K.L.; Shang, H.; Wei, C.; Cravedi, P.; Sun, Z.; Xi, C.; Woytovich, C.; Farouk, S.; et al. A Peripheral Blood Gene Expression Signature to Diagnose Subclinical Acute Rejection. *J. Am. Soc. Nephrol.* **2019**, *30*, 1481–1494. [CrossRef] [PubMed]
54. Van Loon, E.; Gazut, S.; Yazdani, S.; Lerut, E.; de Loor, H.; Coemans, M.; Noël, L.-H.; Thorrez, L.; Van Lommel, L.; Schuit, F.; et al. Development and validation of a peripheral blood mRNA assay for the assessment of antibody-mediated kidney allograft rejection: A multicentre, prospective study. *EBioMedicine* **2019**, *46*, 463–472. [CrossRef] [PubMed]

55. Friedewald, J.J.; Kurian, S.M.; Heilman, R.L.; Whisenant, T.C.; Poggio, E.D.; Marsh, C.; Baliga, P.; Odim, J.; Brown, M.M.; Ikle, D.N.; et al. Development and clinical validity of a novel blood-based molecular biomarker for subclinical acute rejection following kidney transplant. *Am. J. Transplant.* **2019**, *19*, 98–109. [CrossRef] [PubMed]
56. Sigdel, T.; Nguyen, M.; Liberto, J.; Dobi, D.; Junger, H.; Vincenti, F.; Laszik, Z.; Sarwal, M.M. Assessment of 19 Genes and Validation of CRM Gene Panel for Quantitative Transcriptional Analysis of Molecular Rejection and Inflammation in Archival Kidney Transplant Biopsies. *Front. Med.* **2019**, *6*, 213. [CrossRef]
57. Roedder, S.; Sigdel, T.; Salomonis, N.; Hsieh, S.; Dai, H.; Bestard, O.; Metes, D.; Zeevi, A.; Gritsch, A.; Cheeseman, J.; et al. The kSORT assay to detect renal transplant patients at high risk for acute rejection: Results of the multicenter AART study. *PLoS Med.* **2014**, *11*, e1001759. [CrossRef]
58. Sis, B.; Jhangri, G.S.; Bunnag, S.; Allanach, K.; Kaplan, B.; Halloran, P.F. Endothelial gene expression in kidney transplants with alloantibody indicates antibody-mediated damage despite lack of C4d staining. *Am. J. Transplant.* **2009**, *9*, 2312–2323. [CrossRef]
59. Adam, B.A.; Smith, R.N.; Rosales, I.A.; Matsunami, M.; Afzali, B.; Oura, T.; Cosimi, A.B.; Kawai, T.; Colvin, R.B.; Mengel, M. Chronic Antibody-Mediated Rejection in Nonhuman Primate Renal Allografts: Validation of Human Histological and Molecular Phenotypes. *Am. J. Transplant.* **2017**, *17*, 2841–2850. [CrossRef]
60. Stites, E.; Renner, B.; Laskowski, J.; Le Quintrec, M.; You, Z.; Freed, B.; Cooper, J.; Jalal, D.; Thurman, J.M. Complement fragments are biomarkers of antibody-mediated endothelial injury. *Mol. Immunol.* **2020**, *118*, 142–152. [CrossRef]
61. Mueller, F.B.; Yang, H.; Lubetzky, M.; Verma, A.; Lee, J.R.; Dadhania, D.M.; Xiang, J.Z.; Salvatore, S.P.; Seshan, S.V.; Sharma, V.K.; et al. Landscape of innate immune system transcriptome and acute T cell-mediated rejection of human kidney allografts. *JCI Insight* **2019**, *4*. [CrossRef]
62. Hricik, D.E.; Nickerson, P.; Formica, R.N.; Poggio, E.D.; Rush, D.; Newell, K.A.; Goebel, J.; Gibson, I.W.; Fairchild, R.L.; Riggs, M.; et al. Multicenter validation of urinary CXCL9 as a risk-stratifying biomarker for kidney transplant injury. *Am. J. Transplant.* **2013**, *13*, 2634–2644. [CrossRef] [PubMed]
63. Rabant, M.; Amrouche, L.; Morin, L.; Bonifay, R.; Lebreton, X.; Aouni, L.; Benon, A.; Sauvaget, V.; Le Vaillant, L.; Aulagnon, F.; et al. Early Low Urinary CXCL9 and CXCL10 Might Predict Immunological Quiescence in Clinically and Histologically Stable Kidney Recipients. *Am. J. Transplant.* **2016**, *16*, 1868–1881. [CrossRef] [PubMed]
64. Faddoul, G.; Nadkarni, G.N.; Bridges, N.D.; Goebel, J.; Hricik, D.E.; Formica, R.; Menon, M.C.; Morrison, Y.; Murphy, B.; Newell, K.; et al. Analysis of Biomarkers within the Initial 2 Years Posttransplant and 5-Year Kidney Transplant Outcomes: Results from Clinical Trials in Organ Transplantation-17. *Transplantation* **2018**, *102*, 673–680. [CrossRef] [PubMed]
65. Mühlbacher, J.; Doberer, K.; Kozakowski, N.; Regele, H.; Camovic, S.; Haindl, S.; Bond, G.; Haslacher, H.; Eskandary, F.; Reeve, J.; et al. Non-invasive Chemokine Detection: Improved Prediction of Antibody-Mediated Rejection in Donor-Specific Antibody-Positive Renal Allograft Recipients. *Front. Med.* **2020**, *7*, 114. [CrossRef] [PubMed]
66. Rabant, M.; Amrouche, L.; Lebreton, X.; Aulagnon, F.; Benon, A.; Sauvaget, V.; Bonifay, R.; Morin, L.; Scemla, A.; Delville, M.; et al. Urinary C-X-C Motif Chemokine 10 Independently Improves the Noninvasive Diagnosis of Antibody-Mediated Kidney Allograft Rejection. *J. Am. Soc. Nephrol.* **2015**, *26*, 2840–2851. [CrossRef]
67. Bloom, R.D.; Bromberg, J.S.; Poggio, E.D.; Bunnapradist, S.; Langone, A.J.; Sood, P.; Matas, A.J.; Mehta, S.; Mannon, R.B.; Sharfuddin, A.; et al. Cell-Free DNA and Active Rejection in Kidney Allografts. *J. Am. Soc. Nephrol.* **2017**, *28*, 2221–2232. [CrossRef]
68. Huang, E.; Sethi, S.; Peng, A.; Najjar, R.; Mirocha, J.; Haas, M.; Vo, A.; Jordan, S.C. Early clinical experience using donor-derived cell-free DNA to detect rejection in kidney transplant recipients. *Am. J. Transplant.* **2019**, *19*, 1663–1670. [CrossRef]
69. Sigdel, T.K.; Archila, F.A.; Constantin, T.; Prins, S.A.; Liberto, J.; Damm, I.; Towfighi, P.; Navarro, S.; Kirkizlar, E.; Demko, Z.P.; et al. Optimizing Detection of Kidney Transplant Injury by Assessment of Donor-Derived Cell-Free DNA via Massively Multiplex PCR. *J. Clin. Med.* **2018**, *8*, 19. [CrossRef]

70. Oellerich, M.; Shipkova, M.; Asendorf, T.; Walson, P.D.; Schauerte, V.; Mettenmeyer, N.; Kabakchiev, M.; Hasche, G.; Gröne, H.-J.; Friede, T.; et al. Absolute quantification of donor-derived cell-free DNA as a marker of rejection and graft injury in kidney transplantation: Results from a prospective observational study. *Am. J. Transplant.* **2019**, *19*, 3087–3099. [CrossRef]
71. Jordan, S.C.; Bunnapradist, S.; Bromberg, J.S.; Langone, A.J.; Hiller, D.; Yee, J.P.; Sninsky, J.J.; Woodward, R.N.; Matas, A.J. Donor-derived Cell-free DNA Identifies Antibody-mediated Rejection in Donor Specific Antibody Positive Kidney Transplant Recipients. *Transplant. Direct* **2018**, *4*, e379. [CrossRef] [PubMed]
72. Sureshkumar, K.K.; Lyons, S.; Chopra, B. Letter to the Editors. Impact of kidney transplant type and previous transplant on baseline donor-derived cell free DNA. *Transpl. Int.* **2020**. [CrossRef]
73. Jordan, S.C.; Sawinsky, D.; Dholakia, S. Donor-derived cell-free DNA initiates De-Novo Donor Specific Antibody (DSA) responses. *Am. J. Transplant.* **2019**, *19*, 404–405.
74. Crespo, E.; Cravedi, P.; Martorell, J.; Luque, S.; Melilli, E.; Cruzado, J.M.; Jarque, M.; Meneghini, M.; Manonelles, A.; Donadei, C.; et al. Posttransplant peripheral blood donor-specific interferon-γ enzyme-linked immune spot assay differentiates risk of subclinical rejection and de novo donor-specific alloantibodies in kidney transplant recipients. *Kidney Int.* **2017**, *92*, 201–213. [CrossRef]
75. Dholakia, S.; De Vlaminck, I.; Khush, K.K. Adding Insult on Injury: Immunogenic Role for Donor-derived Cell-free DNA? *Transplantation* **2020**. [CrossRef] [PubMed]
76. Kim, K.; Moon, H.; Lee, Y.H.; Seo, J.-W.; Kim, Y.G.; Moon, J.-Y.; Kim, J.S.; Jeong, K.-H.; Lee, T.W.; Ihm, C.-G.; et al. Clinical relevance of cell-free mitochondrial DNA during the early postoperative period in kidney transplant recipients. *Sci. Rep.* **2019**, *9*, 18607. [CrossRef] [PubMed]
77. Karahan, G.E.; de Vaal, Y.J.H.; Krop, J.; Wehmeier, C.; Roelen, D.L.; Claas, F.H.J.; Heidt, S. A Memory B Cell Crossmatch Assay for Quantification of Donor-Specific Memory B Cells in the Peripheral Blood of HLA-Immunized Individuals. *Am. J. Transplant.* **2017**, *17*, 2617–2626. [CrossRef] [PubMed]
78. Pongpirul, W.; Chancharoenthana, W.; Pongpirul, K.; Leelahavanichkul, A.; Kittikowit, W.; Jutivorakool, K.; Nonthasoot, B.; Avihingsanon, Y.; Eiam-Ong, S.; Praditpornsilpa, K.; et al. B-cell activating factor, a predictor of antibody mediated rejection in kidney transplantation recipients. *Nephrol. Carlton* **2018**, *23*, 169–174. [CrossRef]
79. Hricik, D.E.; Augustine, J.; Nickerson, P.; Formica, R.N.; Poggio, E.D.; Rush, D.; Newell, K.A.; Goebel, J.; Gibson, I.W.; Fairchild, R.L.; et al. Interferon Gamma ELISPOT Testing as a Risk-Stratifying Biomarker for Kidney Transplant Injury: Results from the CTOT-01 Multicenter Study. *Am. J. Transplant.* **2015**, *15*, 3166–3173. [CrossRef]
80. Gorbacheva, V.; Fan, R.; Fairchild, R.L.; Baldwin, W.M.; Valujskikh, A. Memory CD4 T Cells Induce Antibody-Mediated Rejection of Renal Allografts. *J. Am. Soc. Nephrol.* **2016**, *27*, 3299–3307. [CrossRef]
81. Matz, M.; Fabritius, K.; Lorkowski, C.; Dürr, M.; Gaedeke, J.; Durek, P.; Grün, J.R.; Goestemeyer, A.; Bachmann, F.; Wu, K.; et al. Identification of T Cell-Mediated Vascular Rejection after Kidney Transplantation by the Combined Measurement of 5 Specific MicroRNAs in Blood. *Transplantation* **2016**, *100*, 898–907. [CrossRef] [PubMed]
82. Trailin, A.V.; Ostapenko, T.I.; Nykonenko, T.N.; Nesterenko, S.N.; Nykonenko, O.S. Peritransplant Soluble CD30 as a Risk Factor for Slow Kidney Allograft Function, Early Acute Rejection, Worse Long-Term Allograft Function, and Patients' Survival. *Dis. Markers* **2017**, *2017*, 9264904. [CrossRef] [PubMed]
83. Mirzakhani, M.; Shahbazi, M.; Akbari, R.; Dedinská, I.; Nemati, E.; Mohammadnia-Afrouzi, M. Soluble CD30, the Immune Response, and Acute Rejection in Human Kidney Transplantation: A Systematic Review and Meta-Analysis. *Front. Immunol.* **2020**, *11*, 295. [CrossRef] [PubMed]
84. Ashokkumar, C.; Shapiro, R.; Tan, H.; Ningappa, M.; Elinoff, B.; Fedorek, S.; Sun, Q.; Higgs, B.W.; Randhawa, P.; Humar, A.; et al. Allospecific CD154+ T-cytotoxic memory cells identify recipients experiencing acute cellular rejection after renal transplantation. *Transplantation* **2011**, *92*, 433–438. [CrossRef]
85. Verma, A.; Muthukumar, T.; Yang, H.; Lubetzky, M.; Cassidy, M.F.; Lee, J.R.; Dadhania, D.M.; Snopkowski, C.; Shankaranarayanan, D.; Salvatore, S.P.; et al. Urinary cell transcriptomics and acute rejection in human kidney allografts. *JCI Insight* **2020**, *5*. [CrossRef]
86. Lee, J.R.; Muthukumar, T.; Dadhania, D.; Ding, R.; Sharma, V.K.; Schwartz, J.E.; Suthanthiran, M. Urinary cell mRNA profiles predictive of human kidney allograft status. *Immunol. Rev.* **2014**, *258*, 218–240. [CrossRef]

87. O'Connell, P.J.; Zhang, W.; Menon, M.C.; Yi, Z.; Schröppel, B.; Gallon, L.; Luan, Y.; Rosales, I.A.; Ge, Y.; Losic, B.; et al. Biopsy transcriptome expression profiling to identify kidney transplants at risk of chronic injury: A multicentre, prospective study. *Lancet Lond. Engl.* **2016**, *388*, 983–993. [CrossRef]
88. Eikmans, M.; Gielis, E.M.; Ledeganck, K.J.; Yang, J.; Abramowicz, D.; Claas, F.F.J. Non-invasive Biomarkers of Acute Rejection in Kidney Transplantation: Novel Targets and Strategies. *Front. Med.* **2018**, *5*, 358. [CrossRef]
89. Jeon, H.J.; Lee, J.-G.; Kim, K.; Jang, J.Y.; Han, S.W.; Choi, J.; Ryu, J.-H.; Koo, T.Y.; Jeong, J.C.; Lee, J.W.; et al. Peripheral blood transcriptome analysis and development of classification model for diagnosing antibody-mediated rejection vs accommodation in ABO-incompatible kidney transplant. *Am. J. Transplant.* **2020**, *20*, 112–124. [CrossRef]
90. Marsh, C.L.; Kurian, S.M.; Rice, J.C.; Whisenant, T.C.; David, J.; Rose, S.; Schieve, C.; Lee, D.; Case, J.; Barrick, B.; et al. Application of TruGraf v1: A Novel Molecular Biomarker for Managing Kidney Transplant Recipients with Stable Renal Function. *Transplant. Proc.* **2019**, *51*, 722–728. [CrossRef]
91. Peddi, V.R.; Patel, P.S.; Schieve, C.; Rose, S.; First, M.R. Serial Peripheral Blood Gene Expression Profiling to Assess Immune Quiescence in Kidney Transplant Recipients with Stable Renal Function. *Ann. Transplant.* **2020**, *25*, e920839. [CrossRef]
92. Hruba, P.; Krejcik, Z.; Stranecky, V.; Maluskova, J.; Slatinska, J.; Gueler, F.; Gwinner, W.; Bräsen, J.H.; Wohlfahrtova, M.; Parikova, A.; et al. Molecular Patterns Discriminate Accommodation and Subclinical Antibody-mediated Rejection in Kidney Transplantation. *Transplantation* **2019**, *103*, 909–917. [CrossRef] [PubMed]
93. Halloran, P.F.; Reeve, J.; Akalin, E.; Aubert, O.; Bohmig, G.A.; Brennan, D.; Bromberg, J.; Einecke, G.; Eskandary, F.; Gosset, C.; et al. Real Time Central Assessment of Kidney Transplant Indication Biopsies by Microarrays: The INTERCOMEX Study. *Am. J. Transplant.* **2017**, *17*, 2851–2862. [CrossRef] [PubMed]
94. Barner, M.; DeKoning, J.; Kashi, Z.; Halloran, P. Recent Advancements in the Assessment of Renal Transplant Dysfunction with an Emphasis on Microarray Molecular Diagnostics. *Clin. Lab. Med.* **2018**, *38*, 623–635. [CrossRef]
95. Wu, H.; Malone, A.F.; Donnelly, E.L.; Kirita, Y.; Uchimura, K.; Ramakrishnan, S.M.; Gaut, J.P.; Humphreys, B.D. Single-Cell Transcriptomics of a Human Kidney Allograft Biopsy Specimen Defines a Diverse Inflammatory Response. *J. Am. Soc. Nephrol.* **2018**, *29*, 2069–2080. [CrossRef]
96. Stewart, B.J.; Clatworthy, M.R. Applying single-cell technologies to clinical pathology: Progress in nephropathology. *J. Pathol.* **2020**, *250*, 693–704. [CrossRef] [PubMed]
97. Franzin, R.; Stasi, A.; Fiorentino, M.; Stallone, G.; Cantaluppi, V.; Gesualdo, L.; Castellano, G. Inflammaging and Complement System: A Link between Acute Kidney Injury and Chronic Graft Damage. *Front. Immunol.* **2020**, *11*, 734. [CrossRef]
98. Bobka, S.; Ebert, N.; Koertvely, E.; Jacobi, J.; Wiesener, M.; Büttner-Herold, M.; Amann, K.; Daniel, C. Is Early Complement Activation in Renal Transplantation Associated with Later Graft Outcome? *Kidney Blood Press. Res.* **2018**, *43*, 1488–1504. [CrossRef]
99. Tower, C.M.; Reyes, M.; Nelson, K.; Leca, N.; Kieran, N.; Muczynski, K.; Jefferson, J.A.; Blosser, C.; Kukla, A.; Maurer, D.; et al. Plasma C4d+ Endothelial Microvesicles Increase in Acute Antibody-Mediated Rejection. *Transplantation* **2017**, *101*, 2235–2243. [CrossRef]
100. Wang, Z.; Yang, H.; Guo, M.; Han, Z.; Tao, J.; Chen, H.; Ge, Y.; Wang, K.; Tan, R.; Wei, J.-F.; et al. Impact of complement component 3/4/5 single nucleotide polymorphisms on renal transplant recipients with antibody-mediated rejection. *Oncotarget* **2017**, *8*, 94539–94553. [CrossRef]
101. Lazzeri, E.; Rotondi, M.; Mazzinghi, B.; Lasagni, L.; Buonamano, A.; Rosati, A.; Pradella, F.; Fossombroni, V.; La Villa, G.; Gacci, M.; et al. High CXCL10 expression in rejected kidneys and predictive role of pretransplant serum CXCL10 for acute rejection and chronic allograft nephropathy. *Transplantation* **2005**, *79*, 1215–1220. [CrossRef] [PubMed]
102. Rotondi, M.; Netti, G.S.; Lazzeri, E.; Stallone, G.; Bertoni, E.; Chiovato, L.; Grandaliano, G.; Gesualdo, L.; Salvadori, M.; Schena, F.P.; et al. High pretransplant serum levels of CXCL9 are associated with increased risk of acute rejection and graft failure in kidney graft recipients. *Transpl. Int.* **2010**, *23*, 465–475. [CrossRef] [PubMed]
103. Hirt-Minkowski, P.; De Serres, S.A.; Ho, J. Developing renal allograft surveillance strategies—Urinary biomarkers of cellular rejection. *Can. J. Kidney Health Dis.* **2015**, *2*, 28. [CrossRef] [PubMed]

104. Schiffer, L.; Wiehler, F.; Bräsen, J.H.; Gwinner, W.; Greite, R.; Kreimann, K.; Thorenz, A.; Derlin, K.; Teng, B.; Rong, S.; et al. Chemokine CXCL13 as a New Systemic Biomarker for B-Cell Involvement in Acute T Cell-Mediated Kidney Allograft Rejection. *Int. J. Mol. Sci.* **2019**, *20*, 2552. [CrossRef]
105. Katou, S.; Globke, B.; Morgul, M.H.; Vogel, T.; Struecker, B.; Otto, N.M.; Reutzel-Selke, A.; Marksteiner, M.; Brockmann, J.G.; Pascher, A.; et al. Urinary Biomarkers α-GST and π-GST for Evaluation and Monitoring in Living and Deceased Donor Kidney Grafts. *J. Clin. Med.* **2019**, *8*, 1899. [CrossRef] [PubMed]
106. Kim, S.-Y.; Kim, B.K.; Gwon, M.-R.; Seong, S.J.; Ohk, B.; Kang, W.Y.; Lee, H.W.; Jung, H.-Y.; Cho, J.-H.; Chung, B.H.; et al. Urinary metabolomic profiling for noninvasive diagnosis of acute T cell-mediated rejection after kidney transplantation. *J. Chromatogr. B* **2019**, *1118*, 157–163. [CrossRef] [PubMed]
107. Shen, J.; Zhou, Y.; Chen, Y.; Li, X.; Lei, W.; Ge, J.; Peng, W.; Wu, J.; Liu, G.; Yang, G.; et al. Dynamics of early post-operative plasma ddcf DNA levels in kidney transplantation: A single-center pilot study. *Transpl. Int.* **2019**, *32*, 184–192. [CrossRef]
108. Bloom, R.D. Using (cell-free) DNA to incriminate rejection as the cause of kidney allograft dysfunction: Do we have a verdict? *Am. J. Transplant.* **2019**, *19*, 1609–1610. [CrossRef]
109. Thongprayoon, C.; Vaitla, P.; Craici, I.M.; Leeaphorn, N.; Hansrivijit, P.; Salim, S.A.; Bathini, T.; Cabeza Rivera, F.H.; Cheungpasitporn, W. The Use of Donor-Derived Cell-Free DNA for Assessment of Allograft Rejection and Injury Status. *J. Clin. Med.* **2020**, *9*, 1480. [CrossRef]
110. Stites, E.; Kumar, D.; Olaitan, O.; Swanson, S.H.; Leca, N.; Weir, M.; Bromberg, J.; Melancon, J.; Agha, I.; Fattah, H.; et al. High levels of dd-cf DNA identify patients with TCMR 1A and borderline allograft rejection at elevated risk of graft injury. *Am. J. Transplant.* **2020**. [CrossRef]
111. Oweira, H.; Khajeh, E.; Mohammadi, S.; Ghamarnejad, O.; Daniel, V.; Schnitzler, P.; Golriz, M.; Mieth, M.; Morath, C.; Zeier, M.; et al. Pre-transplant CD200 and CD200R1 concentrations are associated with post-transplant events in kidney transplant recipients. *Med. Baltim.* **2019**, *98*, e17006. [CrossRef] [PubMed]
112. Lemerle, M.; Garnier, A.-S.; Planchais, M.; Brilland, B.; Subra, J.-F.; Blanchet, O.; Blanchard, S.; Croue, A.; Duveau, A.; Augusto, J.-F. CD45RC Expression of Circulating CD8(+) T Cells Predicts Acute Allograft Rejection: A Cohort Study of 128 Kidney Transplant Patients. *J. Clin. Med.* **2019**, *8*, 1147. [CrossRef] [PubMed]
113. Zhang, R. Donor-Specific Antibodies in Kidney Transplant Recipients. *Clin. J. Am. Soc. Nephrol.* **2018**, *13*, 182–192. [CrossRef] [PubMed]
114. Wehmeier, C.; Karahan, G.E.; Heidt, S. HLA-specific memory B-cell detection in kidney transplantation: Insights and future challenges. *Int. J. Immunogenet.* **2020**, *47*, 227–234. [CrossRef] [PubMed]
115. Zhang, X.; Reinsmoen, N.L. Impact and production of Non-HLA-specific antibodies in solid organ transplantation. *Int. J. Immunogenet.* **2020**, *47*, 235–242. [CrossRef]
116. Reindl-Schwaighofer, R.; Heinzel, A.; Gualdoni, G.A.; Mesnard., L.; Claas, F.H.J.; Oberbauer, R. Novel insights into non-HLA alloimmunity in kidney transplantation. *Transpl. Int.* **2020**, *33*, 5–17. [CrossRef]
117. Delville, M.; Lamarthée, B. Early Acute Microvascular Kidney Transplant Rejection in the Absence of Anti-HLA Antibodies Is Associated with Preformed IgG Antibodies against Diverse Glomerular Endothelial Cell Antigens. *J. Am. Soc. Nephrol.* **2019**, *30*, 692–709. [CrossRef]
118. Cardinal, H.; Dieudé, M.; Hébert, M.J. The Emerging Importance of Non-HLA Autoantibodies in Kidney Transplant Complications. *J. Am. Soc. Nephrol.* **2017**, *28*, 400–406. [CrossRef]
119. Dragun, D.; Catar, R.; Aurelie, P. Non-HLA antibodies against endothelial targets bridging allo-and autoimmunity. *Kidney Int.* **2016**, *90*, 280–288. [CrossRef]
120. Philogene, M.C.; Johnson, T.; Vaught, A.J.; Zakaria, S.; Fedarko., N. Antibodies against Angiotensin II Type 1 and Endothelin A Receptors: Relevance and pathogenicity. *Hum. Immunol.* **2019**, *80*, 561–567. [CrossRef]
121. Sas-Strózik, A.; Krajewska, M.; Banasik, M. The significance of angiotensin II type 1 receptor (AT1 receptor) in renal transplant injury. *Adv. Clin. Exp. Med.* **2020**, *29*, 629–633. [CrossRef] [PubMed]
122. Shinaeu, Y.; Hee, J.H.; Kyo, W.L.; Park, J.B.; Kim, S.; Huh, W.; Jang, H.R.; Kwon, G.Y.; Moon, H.H.; Kang, S. Pre-Transplant Angiotensin II Type 1 Receptor Antibodies and Anti-Endothelial Cell Antibodies Predict Graft Function and Allograft Rejection in a Low-Risk Kidney Transplantation Setting. *Ann. Lab. Med.* **2020**, *40*, 398–408. [CrossRef]
123. Pinelli, D.F.; Friedewald, J.J. Assessing the potential of angiotensin II type 1 receptor and donor specific anti-endothelial cell antibodies to predict long-term kidney graft outcome. *Hum. Immunol.* **2017**, *78*, 421–427. [CrossRef] [PubMed]

124. Philogene, M.C.; Zhou, S. Pre-transplant Screening for Non-HLA Antibodies: Who should be Tested? *Hum. Immunol.* **2018**, *79*, 195–202. [CrossRef] [PubMed]
125. Lim, M.A.; Palmer, M.; Trofe-Clark, J.; Bloom, R.D.; Jackson, A.; Philogene, M.C.; Kamoun, M. Histopathologic changes in anti-angiotensin II type 1 receptor antibody-positive kidney transplant recipients with acute rejection and no donor specific HLA antibodies. *Hum. Immunol.* **2017**, *78*, 350–356. [CrossRef] [PubMed]
126. Divanyan, T.; Acosta, E.; Patel, D.; Constantino, D.; Lopez-Soler, R.I. Anti-vimentin antibodies in transplant and disease. *Hum. Immunol.* **2019**, *80*, 602–607. [CrossRef]
127. Dieudé, M.; Cardinal, H.; Hébert, M.-J. Injury derived autoimmunity: Anti-perlecan/LG3 antibodies in transplantation. *Hum. Immunol.* **2019**, *80*, 608–613. [CrossRef]
128. Riesco, L.; Irure, J.; Rodrigo, E.; Guiral, S.; Ruiz, J.C.; Gómez, J.; Hoyos, M.L.; San Segundo, D. Anti-perlecan antibodies and acute humoral rejection in hypersensitized patients without forbidden HLA specificities after kidney transplantation. *Transpl. Immunol.* **2019**, *52*, 53–56. [CrossRef]
129. Padet, L.; Dieudé, M.; Karakeussian-Rimbaud, A.; Yang, B.; Turgeon, J.; Jean-Cailhier, F.; Cardinal, H.; Hébert, M.-J. New insights into immune mechanisms of antiperlecan/LG3 antibody production: Importance of T cells and innate B1 cells. *Am. J. Transplant.* **2019**, *19*, 699–712. [CrossRef]
130. Yang, B.; Dieudé, M.; Hamelin, K.; Hénault-Rondeau, M.; Patey, N.; Turgeon, J.; Lan, S.; Pomerleau, L.; Quesnel, M.; Peng, J.; et al. Anti-LG3 Antibodies Aggravate Renal Ischemia-Reperfusion Injury and Long-Term Renal Allograft Dysfunction. *Am. J. Transplant.* **2016**, *16*, 3416–3429. [CrossRef]
131. Jackson, A.M.; Sigdel, T.K.; Delville, M.; Hsieh, S.; Dai, H.; Bagnasco, S.; Montgomery, R.A.; Sarwal, M.M. Endothelial cell antibodies associated with novel targets and increased rejection. *J. Am. Soc. Nephrol.* **2015**, *26*, 1161–1171. [CrossRef] [PubMed]
132. Guo, X.; Hu, J.; Luo, W.; Luo, Q.; Guo, J.; Tian, F.; Ming, Y.; Zou, Y. Analysis of Sera of Recipients with Allograft Rejection Indicates that Keratin 1 Is the Target of Anti-Endothelial Antibodies. *Immunol. Res.* **2017**, *2017*, 8679841. [CrossRef] [PubMed]
133. Sánchez-Zapardiel, E.; Mancebo, E.; Díaz-Ordoñez, M.; de Jorge-Huerta, L.; Ruiz-Martínez, L.; Serrano, A.; Castro-Panete, M.J.; Utrero-Rico, A.; de Andrés, A.; Morales, J.M.; et al. Isolated de Novo Antiendothelial Cell Antibodies and Kidney Transplant Rejection. *Am. J. Kidney Dis.* **2016**, *68*, 933–943. [CrossRef] [PubMed]
134. Jackson, A.M.; Delville, M.; Lamarthée, B.; Anglicheau, D. Sensitization to endothelial cell antigens: Unraveling the cause or effect paradox. *Hum. Immunol.* **2019**, *80*, 614–620. [CrossRef]
135. Angaswamy, N.; Klein, C.; Tiriveedhi, V.; Gaut, J.; Anwar, S.; Rossi, A.; Phelan, D.; Wellen, J.R.; Shenoy, S.; Chapman, W.C.; et al. Immune responses to collagen-IV and fibronectin in renal transplant recipients with transplant glomerulopathy. *Am. J. Transplant.* **2014**, *14*, 685–693. [CrossRef]
136. Gunasekaran, M.; Vachharajani, N.; Gaut, J.P.; Maw, T.T.; Delos Santos, R.; Shenoy, S.; Chapman, W.C.; Wellen, J.; Mohanakumar, T. Development of immune response to tissue-restricted self-antigens in simultaneous kidney-pancreas transplant recipients with acute rejection. *Clin. Transplant.* **2017**, *31*, 8. [CrossRef]
137. Soma, O.; Hatakeyama, S.; Yoneyama, T.; Saito, M.; Sasaki, H.; Tobisawa, Y.; Noro, D.; Suzuki, Y.; Tanaka, M.; Nishimura, S.-I.; et al. Serum N-glycan profiling can predict biopsy-proven graft rejection after living kidney transplantation. *Clin. Exp. Nephrol.* **2020**, *24*, 174–184. [CrossRef]
138. Maehana, T.; Tanaka, T.; Kitamura, H.; Fukuzawa, N.; Ishida, H.; Harada, H.; Tanabe, K.; Masumori, N. Heat Shock Protein 90α Is a Potential Serological Biomarker of Acute Rejection after Renal Transplantation. *PLoS ONE* **2016**, *11*, e0162942. [CrossRef]
139. Barbas, A.S.; Lin, L.; McRae, M.; MacDonald, A.L.; Truong, T.; Yang, Y.; Brennan, T.V. Heparan sulfate is a plasma biomarker of acute cellular allograft rejection. *PLoS ONE* **2018**, *13*, e0200877. [CrossRef]
140. Kim, S.C.; Page, E.K.; Knechtle, S.J. Urine proteomics in kidney transplantation. *Transplant. Rev.* **2014**, *28*, 15–20. [CrossRef]
141. Perez, J.D.; Sakata, M.M.; Colucci, J.A.; Spinelli, G.A.; Felipe, C.R.; Carvalho, V.M.; Cardozo, K.H.M.; Medina-Pestana, J.O.; Tedesco-Silva, H.J.; Schor, N.; et al. Plasma proteomics for the assessment of acute renal transplant rejection. *Life Sci.* **2016**, *158*, 111–120. [CrossRef] [PubMed]
142. Zhang, H.; Huang, E.; Kahwaji, J.; Nast, C.C.; Li, P.; Mirocha, J.; Thomas, D.L.; Ge, S.; Vo, A.A.; Jordan, S.C.; et al. Plasma Exosomes from HLA-Sensitized Kidney Transplant Recipients Contain mRNA Transcripts Which Predict Development of Antibody-Mediated Rejection. *Transplantation* **2017**, *101*, 2419–2428. [CrossRef] [PubMed]

143. Qamri, Z.; Pelletier, R.; Foster, J.; Kumar, S.; Momani, H.; Ware, K.; Von Visger, J.; Satoskar, A.; Nadasdy, T.; Brodsky, S.V. Early posttransplant changes in circulating endothelial microparticles in patients with kidney transplantation. *Transpl. Immunol.* **2014**, *31*, 60–64. [CrossRef] [PubMed]
144. Sigdel, T.K.; Ng, Y.W.; Lee, S.; Nicora, C.D.; Qian, W.-J.; Smith, R.D.; Camp, D.G., 2nd; Sarwal, M.M. Perturbations in the urinary exosome in transplant rejection. *Front. Med.* **2014**, *1*, 57. [CrossRef]
145. Lim, J.-H.; Lee, C.-H.; Kim, K.Y.; Jung, H.-Y.; Choi, J.-Y.; Cho, J.-H.; Park, S.-H.; Kim, Y.-L.; Baek, M.-C.; Park, J.B.; et al. Novel urinary exosomal biomarkers of acute T cell-mediated rejection in kidney transplant recipients: A cross-sectional study. *PLoS ONE* **2018**, *13*, e0204204. [CrossRef]
146. Park, J.; Lin, H.-Y.; Assaker, J.P.; Jeong, S.; Huang, C.-H.; Kurdi, A.; Lee, K.; Fraser, K.; Min, C.; Eskandari, S.; et al. Integrated Kidney Exosome Analysis for the Detection of Kidney Transplant Rejection. *ACS Nano* **2017**, *11*, 11041–11046. [CrossRef]
147. Yang, C.; Qi, R.; Yang, B. Pathogenesis of Chronic Allograft Dysfunction Progress to Renal Fibrosis. *Adv. Exp. Med. Biol.* **2019**, *1165*, 101–116. [CrossRef]
148. Sellarés, J.; de Freitas, D.G.; Mengel, M.; Reeve, J.; Einecke, G.; Sis, B.; Hidalgo, L.G.; Famulski, K.; Matas, A.; Halloran, P.F. Understanding the causes of kidney transplant failure: The dominant role of antibody-mediated rejection and nonadherence. *Am. J. Transplant.* **2012**, *12*, 388–399. [CrossRef]
149. Castellano, G.; Intini, A.; Stasi, A.; Divella, C.; Gigante, M.; Pontrelli, P.; Franzin, R.; Accetturo, M.; Zito, A.; Fiorentino, M.; et al. Complement Modulation of Anti-Aging Factor Klotho in Ischemia/Reperfusion Injury and Delayed Graft Function. *Am. J. Transplant.* **2016**, *16*, 325–333. [CrossRef]
150. Humphreys, B.D. Mechanisms of Renal Fibrosis. *Annu. Rev. Physiol.* **2018**, *80*, 309–326. [CrossRef]
151. Yiu, W.H.; Li, R.X.; Wong, D.W.L.; Wu, H.J.; Chan, K.W.; Chan, L.Y.Y.; Leung, J.C.K.; Lai, K.N.; Sacks, S.H.; Zhou, W.; et al. Complement C5a inhibition moderates lipid metabolism and reduces tubulointerstitial fibrosis in diabetic nephropathy. *Nephrol. Dial. Transplant.* **2018**, *33*, 1323–1332. [CrossRef] [PubMed]
152. Tang, Z.; Lu, B.; Hatch, E.; Sacks, S.H.; Sheerin, N.S. C3a mediates epithelial-to-mesenchymal transition in proteinuric nephropathy. *J. Am. Soc. Nephrol.* **2009**, *20*, 593–603. [CrossRef] [PubMed]
153. Xavier, S.; Sahu, R.K.; Landes, S.G.; Yu, J.; Taylor, R.P.; Ayyadevara, S.; Megyesi, J.; Stallcup, W.B.; Duffield, J.S.; Reis, E.S.; et al. Pericytes and immune cells contribute to complement activation in tubulointerstitial fibrosis. *Am. J. Physiol. Ren. Physiol.* **2017**, *312*, F516–F532. [CrossRef]
154. Modena, B.D.; Kurian, S.M.; Gaber, L.W.; Waalen, J.; Su, A.I.; Gelbart, T.; Mondala, T.S.; Head, S.R.; Papp, S.; Heilman, R.; et al. Gene Expression in Biopsies of Acute Rejection and Interstitial Fibrosis/Tubular Atrophy Reveals Highly Shared Mechanisms That Correlate with Worse Long-Term Outcomes. *Am. J. Transplant.* **2016**, *16*, 1982–1998. [CrossRef] [PubMed]
155. Mas, V.; Maluf, D.; Archer, K.; Yanek, K.; Mas, L.; King, A.; Gibney, E.; Massey, D.; Cotterell, A.; Fisher, R.; et al. Establishing the molecular pathways involved in chronic allograft nephropathy for testing new noninvasive diagnostic markers. *Transplantation* **2007**, *83*, 448–457. [CrossRef] [PubMed]
156. Li, L.; Greene, I.; Readhead, B.; Menon, M.C.; Kidd, B.A.; Uzilov, A.V.; Wei, C.; Philippe, N.; Schroppel, B.; He, J.C.; et al. Novel Therapeutics Identification for Fibrosis in Renal Allograft Using Integrative Informatics Approach. *Sci. Rep.* **2017**, *7*, 39487. [CrossRef]
157. Zununi Vahed, S.; Omidi, Y.; Ardalan, M.; Samadi, N. Dysregulation of urinary miR-21 and miR-200b associated with interstitial fibrosis and tubular atrophy (IFTA) in renal transplant recipients. *Clin. Biochem.* **2017**, *50*, 32–39. [CrossRef]
158. Zununi Vahed, S.; Poursadegh Zonouzi, A.; Mahmoodpoor, F.; Samadi, N.; Ardalan, M.; Omidi, Y. Circulating miR-150, miR-192, miR-200b, and miR-423-3p as Non-invasive Biomarkers of Chronic Allograft Dysfunction. *Arch. Med. Res.* **2017**, *48*, 96–104. [CrossRef]
159. Zununi Vahed, S.; Poursadegh Zonouzi, A.; Ghanbarian, H.; Ghojazadeh, M.; Samadi, N.; Omidi, Y.; Ardalan, M. Differential expression of circulating miR-21, miR-142-3p and miR-155 in renal transplant recipients with impaired graft function. *Int. Urol. Nephrol.* **2017**, *49*, 1681–1689. [CrossRef]
160. Matz, M.; Heinrich, F.; Lorkowski, C.; Wu, K.; Klotsche, J.; Zhang, Q.; Lachmann, N.; Durek, P.; Budde, K.; Mashreghi, M.-F. MicroRNA regulation in blood cells of renal transplanted patients with interstitial fibrosis/tubular atrophy and antibody-mediated rejection. *PLoS ONE* **2018**, *13*, e0201925. [CrossRef]
161. Granata, S.; Benedetti, C.; Gambaro, G.; Zaza, G. Kidney allograft fibrosis: What we learned from latest translational research studies. *J. Nephrol.* **2020**. [CrossRef] [PubMed]

162. Matas, A.J.; Helgeson, E.S.; Gaston, R.; Cosio, F.; Mannon, R.; Kasiske, B.L.; Hunsicker, L.; Gourishankar, S.; Rush, D.; Michael Cecka, J.; et al. Inflammation in areas of fibrosis: The DeKAF prospective cohort. *Am. J. Transplant.* **2020**. [CrossRef] [PubMed]
163. Maluf, D.G.; Dumur, C.I.; Suh, J.L.; Scian, M.J.; King, A.L.; Cathro, H.; Lee, J.K.; Gehrau, R.C.; Brayman, K.L.; Gallon, L.; et al. The urine microRNA profile may help monitor post-transplant renal graft function. *Kidney Int.* **2014**, *85*, 439–449. [CrossRef] [PubMed]
164. Bontha, S.V.; Maluf, D.G.; Archer, K.J.; Dumur, C.I.; Dozmorov, M.G.; King, A.L.; Akalin, E.; Mueller, T.F.; Gallon, L.; Mas, V.R. Effects of DNA Methylation on Progression to Interstitial Fibrosis and Tubular Atrophy in Renal Allograft Biopsies: A Multi-Omics Approach. *Am. J. Transplant.* **2017**, *17*, 3060–3075. [CrossRef] [PubMed]
165. Kalluri, R.; Weinberg, R.A. The basics of epithelial-mesenchymal transition. *J. Clin. Investig.* **2009**, *119*, 1420–1428. [CrossRef] [PubMed]
166. Srivastava, S.M.; Hedayat, A.F.; Kanasaki, K.; Goodwin, G.E. MicroRNA Crosstalk Influences Epithelial-to-Mesenchymal, Endothelial-to-Mesenchymal, and Macrophage-to-Mesenchymal Transitions in the Kidney. *Front. Pharmacol.* **2019**, *10*, 904. [CrossRef]
167. Alfieri, C.; Regalia, A.; Moroni, G.; Cresseri, D.; Zanoni, F.; Ikehata, M.; Simonini, P.; Rastaldi, M.P.; Tripepi, G.; Zoccali, C.; et al. Novel markers of graft outcome in a cohort of kidney transplanted patients: A cohort observational study. *J. Nephrol.* **2019**, *32*, 139–150. [CrossRef]
168. Zhou, J.; Cheng, H.; Wang, Z.; Chen, H.; Suo, C.; Zhang, H.; Zhang, J.; Yang, Y.; Geng, L.; Gu, M.; et al. Bortezomib attenuates renal interstitial fibrosis in kidney transplantation via regulating the EMT induced by TNF-α-Smurf1-Akt-mTOR-P70S6K pathway. *J. Cell. Mol. Med.* **2019**, *23*, 5390–5402. [CrossRef]
169. Hazzan, M.; Hertig, A.; Buob, D.; Copin, M.-C.; Noël, C.; Rondeau, E.; XuDubois, Y.C. Epithelial-to-mesenchymal transition predicts cyclosporine nephrotoxicity in renal transplant recipients. *J. Am. Soc. Nephrol.* **2011**, *22*, 1375–1381. [CrossRef]
170. Sosa Peña, M.D.P.; Lopez-Soler, R.; Melendez, J.A. Senescence in chronic allograft nephropathy. *Am. J. Physiol. Ren. Physiol.* **2018**, *315*, F880–F889. [CrossRef]
171. Mezni, I.; Galichon, P.; Bacha, M.M.; XuDubois, Y.C.; Sfar, I.; Buob, D.; Benbouzid, S.; Goucha, R.; Gorgi, Y.; Abderrhaim, E.; et al. Urinary mRNA analysis of biomarkers to epithelial mesenchymal transition of renal allograft. *Nephrol. Ther.* **2018**, *14*, 153–161. [CrossRef] [PubMed]
172. Galichon, P.; XuDubois, Y.C.; Buob, D.; Tinel, C.; Anglicheau, D.; Benbouzid, S.; Dahan, K.; Ouali, N.; Hertig, A.; Brocheriou, I.; et al. Urinary transcriptomics reveals patterns associated with subclinical injury of the renal allograft. *Biomark. Med.* **2018**, *12*, 427–438. [CrossRef] [PubMed]
173. Xu-Dubois, Y.-C.; Peltier, J.; Brocheriou, I.; Suberbielle-Boissel, C.; Djamali, A.; Reese, S.; Mooney, N.; Keuylian, Z.; Lion, J.; Ouali, N.; et al. Markers of Endothelial-to-Mesenchymal Transition: Evidence for Antibody-Endothelium Interaction during Antibody-Mediated Rejection in Kidney Recipients. *J. Am. Soc. Nephrol.* **2016**, *27*, 324–332. [CrossRef]
174. Wang, Z.; Han, Z.; Tao, J.; Wang, J.; Liu, X.; Zhou, W.; Xu, Z.; Zhao, C.; Wang, Z.; Tan, R.; et al. Role of endothelial-to-mesenchymal transition induced by TGF-β1 in transplant kidney interstitial fibrosis. *J. Cell. Mol. Med.* **2017**, *21*, 2359–2369. [CrossRef]
175. Glover, E.K.; Jordan, N.; Sheerin, N.S.; Ali, S. Regulation of Endothelial-to-Mesenchymal Transition by MicroRNAs in Chronic Allograft Dysfunction. *Transplantation* **2019**, *103*, e64–e73. [CrossRef] [PubMed]
176. Fernando, M.; Peake, P.W.; Endre, Z.H. Biomarkers of calcineurin inhibitor nephrotoxicity in transplantation. *Biomark. Med.* **2014**, *8*, 1247–1262. [CrossRef] [PubMed]
177. Xia, T.; Fu, S.; Wang, Q.; Wen, Y.; Chan, S.-A.; Zhu, S.; Gao, S.; Tao, X.; Zhang, F.; Chen, W. Targeted metabolomic analysis of 33 amino acids and biogenic amines in human urine by ion-pairing HPLC-MS/MS: Biomarkers for tacrolimus nephrotoxicity after renal transplantation. *Biomed. Chromatogr. BMC* **2018**, *32*, e4198. [CrossRef] [PubMed]
178. Gacka, E.; Życzkowski, M.; Bogacki, R.; Paradysz, A.; Hyla-Klekot, L. The Usefulness of Determining Neutrophil Gelatinase-Associated Lipocalin Concentration Excreted in the Urine in the Evaluation of Cyclosporine A Nephrotoxicity in Children with Nephrotic Syndrome. *Dis. Markers* **2016**, *2016*, 6872149. [CrossRef]
179. Wu, Z.; Xu, Q.; Qiu, X.; Xu, L.; Jiao, Z.; Zhang, M.; Zhong, M. FKBP1A rs6041749 polymorphism is associated with allograft function in renal transplant patients. *Eur. J. Clin. Pharmacol.* **2019**, *75*, 33–40. [CrossRef]

180. Carlos, C.P.; Sonehara, N.M.; Oliani, S.M.; Burdmann, E.A. Predictive usefulness of urinary biomarkers for the identification of cyclosporine. *PLoS ONE* **2014**, *9*, e103660. [CrossRef]
181. Cui, Y.; Huang, Q.; Auman, J.T.; Knight, B.; Jin, X.; Blanchard, K.T.; Chou, J.; Jayadev, S.; Paules, R.S. Genomic-derived markers for early detection of calcineurin inhibitor immunosuppressant-mediated nephrotoxicity. *Toxicol. Sci.* **2011**, *124*, 23–34. [CrossRef] [PubMed]
182. Masutani, K. Viral infections directly involved in kidney allograft function. *Nephrol. Carlton* **2018**, *23* (Suppl. 2), 31–37. [CrossRef]
183. Kim, M.H.; Lee, Y.H.; Seo, J.-W.; Moon, H.; Kim, J.S.; Kim, Y.G.; Jeong, K.-H.; Moon, J.-Y.; Lee, T.W.; Ihm, C.-G.; et al. Urinary exosomal viral microRNA as a marker of BK virus nephropathy in kidney transplant recipients. *PLoS ONE* **2017**, *12*, e0190068. [CrossRef] [PubMed]
184. Ho, J.; Schaub, S.; Wiebe, C.; Gao, A.; Wehmeier, C.; Koller, M.T.; Hirsch, H.H.; Hopfer, H.; Nickerson, P.; Hirt-Minkowski, P. Urinary CXCL10 Chemokine Is Associated with Alloimmune and Virus Compartment-Specific Renal Allograft Inflammation. *Transplantation* **2018**, *102*, 521–529. [CrossRef] [PubMed]
185. Dvir, R.; Paloschi, V.; Canducci, F.; Dell'Antonio, G.; Racca, S.; Caldara, R.; Pantaleo, G.; Clementi, M.; Secchi, A. IL28B rs12979860 genotype as a predictor marker of progression to BKVirus Associated nephropathy, after kidney transplantation. *Sci. Rep.* **2017**, *7*, 6746. [CrossRef] [PubMed]
186. Pan, L.; Lyu, Z.; Adam, B.; Zeng, G.; Wang, Z.; Huang, Y.; Abedin, Z.; Randhawa, P. Polyomavirus BK Nephropathy-Associated Transcriptomic Signatures: A Critical Reevaluation. *Transplant. Direct* **2018**, *4*, e339. [CrossRef]
187. Verhoeven, J.G.H.P.; Boer, K.; Van Schaik, R.H.N.; Manintveld, O.C.; Huibers, M.M.H.; Baan, C.C.; Hesselink, D.A. Liquid Biopsies to Monitor Solid Organ Transplant Function: A Review of New Biomarkers. *Ther. Drug Monit.* **2018**, *40*, 515–525. [CrossRef]
188. Peeters, L.E.J.; Andrews, L.M.; Hesselink, D.A.; de Winter, B.C.M.; van Gelder, T. Personalized immunosuppression in elderly renal transplant recipients. *Pharmacol. Res.* **2018**, *130*, 303–307. [CrossRef]
189. Newell, K.A.; Adams, A.B.; Turka, L.A. Biomarkers of operational tolerance following kidney transplantation—The immune tolerance network studies of spontaneously tolerant kidney transplant recipients. *Hum. Immunol.* **2018**, *79*, 380–387. [CrossRef]
190. Massart, A.; Ghisdal, L.; Abramowicz, M.; Abramowicz, D. Operational tolerance in kidney transplantation and associated biomarkers. *Clin. Exp. Immunol.* **2017**, *189*, 138–157. [CrossRef]
191. Newell, K.A.; Asare, A.; Kirk, A.D.; Gisler, T.D.; Bourcier, K.; Suthanthiran, M.; Burlingham, W.J.; Marks, W.H.; Sanz, I.; Lechler, R.I.; et al. Identification of a B cell signature associated with renal transplant tolerance in humans. *J. Clin. Investig.* **2010**, *120*, 1836–1847. [CrossRef] [PubMed]
192. Danger, R.; Chesneau, M.; Paul, C.; Guérif, P.; Durand, M.; Newell, K.A.; Kanaparthi, S.; Turka, L.A.; Soulillou, J.-P.; Houlgatte, R.; et al. A composite score associated with spontaneous operational tolerance in kidney transplant recipients. *Kidney Int.* **2017**, *91*, 1473–1481. [CrossRef] [PubMed]
193. Kurian, S.M.; Whisenant, T.C.; Mathew, J.M.; Miller, J.; Leventhal, J.R. Transcriptomic studies in tolerance: Lessons learned and the path forward. *Hum. Immunol.* **2018**, *79*, 395–401. [CrossRef] [PubMed]
194. Girmanova, E.; Hruba, P.; Viklicky, O. Circulating biomarkers of tolerance. *Transplant. Rev.* **2015**, *29*, 68–72. [CrossRef] [PubMed]
195. Bontha, S.V.; Fernandez-Piñeros, A.; Maluf, D.G.; Mas, V.R. Messengers of tolerance. *Hum. Immunol.* **2018**, *79*, 362–372. [CrossRef]
196. Niel, O.; Bastard, P. Artificial Intelligence in Nephrology: Core Concepts, Clinical Applications, and Perspectives. *Am. J. Kidney Dis.* **2019**, *74*, 803–810. [CrossRef]
197. Briganti, G.; Le Moine, O. Artificial Intelligence in Medicine: Today and Tomorrow. *Front. Med.* **2020**, *7*, 27. [CrossRef]
198. Hummel, A.D.; Maciel, R.F.; Sousa, F.S.; Cohrs, F.M.; Falcão, A.E.J.; Teixeira, F.; Baptista, R.; Mancini, F.; da Costa, T.M.; Alves, D.; et al. Artificial intelligence techniques: Predicting necessity for biopsy in renal transplant recipients suspected of acute cellular rejection or nephrotoxicity. *Transplant. Proc.* **2011**, *43*, 1343–1344. [CrossRef]

199. Niel, O.; Bastard, P. Artificial intelligence improves estimation of tacrolimus area under the concentration over time curve in renal transplant recipients. *Transpl. Int.* **2018**, *31*, 940–941. [CrossRef]
200. Aubert, O.; Higgins, S.; Bouatou, Y.; Yoo, D.; Raynaud, M.; Viglietti, D.; Rabant, M.; Hidalgo, L.; Glotz, D.; Legendre, C.; et al. Archetype Analysis Identifies Distinct Profiles in Renal Transplant Recipients with Transplant Glomerulopathy Associated with Allograft Survival. *J. Am. Soc. Nephrol.* **2019**, *30*, 625–639. [CrossRef]

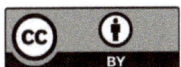

© 2020 by the authors. Licensee MDPI, Basel, Switzerland. This article is an open access article distributed under the terms and conditions of the Creative Commons Attribution (CC BY) license (http://creativecommons.org/licenses/by/4.0/).

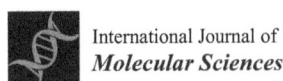 International Journal of
Molecular Sciences

Article

Proteomics-Based Machine Learning Approach as an Alternative to Conventional Biomarkers for Differential Diagnosis of Chronic Kidney Diseases

Yury E. Glazyrin [1,2,*], Dmitry V. Veprintsev [2], Irina A. Ler [3], Maria L. Rossovskaya [3], Svetlana A. Varygina [3], Sofia L. Glizer [3,4], Tatiana N. Zamay [1], Marina M. Petrova [4], Zoran Minic [5], Maxim V. Berezovski [5] and Anna S. Kichkailo [1,2]

1. Laboratory for Biomolecular and Medical Technologies, Krasnoyarsk State Medical University Named after Prof. V.F. Voyno-Yasenetsky, 660022 Krasnoyarsk, Russia; tzamay@yandex.ru (T.N.Z.); annazamay@yandex.ru (A.S.K.)
2. Laboratory for Digital Controlled Drugs and Theranostics, Federal Research Center "Krasnoyarsk Science Center of the Siberian Branch of the Russian Academy of Science", 660036 Krasnoyarsk, Russia; d_veprintsev@mail.ru
3. Department of Nephrology, Krasnoyarsk Interdistrict Clinical Hospital of Emergency Medical Care Named after N.S. Karpovich, 660062 Krasnoyarsk, Russia; irina-ler@bk.ru (I.A.L.); mross@mail.ru (M.L.R.); alfasv-ja@list.ru (S.A.V.); sofiaglizer@mail.ru (S.L.G.)
4. Faculty of Medicine, Krasnoyarsk State Medical University Named after Prof. V.F. Voyno-Yasenetsky, 660022 Krasnoyarsk, Russia; stk99@yandex.ru
5. Department of Chemistry and Biomolecular Sciences, University of Ottawa, Ottawa, ON K1N6N5, Canada; zminic@uottawa.ca (Z.M.); Maxim.Berezovski@uottawa.ca (M.V.B.)
* Correspondence: yury.glazyrin@gmail.com

Received: 17 June 2020; Accepted: 6 July 2020; Published: 7 July 2020

Abstract: Diabetic nephropathy, hypertension, and glomerulonephritis are the most common causes of chronic kidney diseases (CKD). Since CKD of various origins may not become apparent until kidney function is significantly impaired, a differential diagnosis and an appropriate treatment are needed at the very early stages. Conventional biomarkers may not have sufficient separation capabilities, while a full-proteomic approach may be used for these purposes. In the current study, several machine learning algorithms were examined for the differential diagnosis of CKD of three origins. The tested dataset was based on whole proteomic data obtained after the mass spectrometric analysis of plasma and urine samples of 34 CKD patients and the use of label-free quantification approach. The k-nearest-neighbors algorithm showed the possibility of separation of a healthy group from renal patients in general by proteomics data of plasma with high confidence (97.8%). This algorithm has also be proven to be the best of the three tested for distinguishing the groups of patients with diabetic nephropathy and glomerulonephritis according to proteomics data of plasma (96.3% of correct decisions). The group of hypertensive nephropathy could not be reliably separated according to plasma data, whereas analysis of entire proteomics data of urine did not allow differentiating the three diseases. Nevertheless, the group of hypertensive nephropathy was reliably separated from all other renal patients using the k-nearest-neighbors classifier "one against all" with 100% of accuracy by urine proteome data. The tested algorithms show good abilities to differentiate the various groups across proteomic data sets, which may help to avoid invasive intervention for the verification of the glomerulonephritis subtypes, as well as to differentiate hypertensive and diabetic nephropathy in the early stages based not on individual biomarkers, but on the whole proteomic composition of urine and blood.

Keywords: chronic kidney disease; machine learning; differential diagnosis; proteomics; mass spectrometry; label-free quantification

1. Introduction

Chronic kidney disease (CKD) is a supra-nosological concept that unites all patients with signs of kidney damage and/or a decrease in their function [1]. CKD is one of the major health problems with high mortality, because it causes irreversible changes in renal failure. No obvious clinical symptoms appear in early stage disease until severe damage has occurred [2]. Therefore, the need for early diagnosis of CKD is obvious. Diseases leading to CKD can be divided into two groups: (1) processes localized directly in the kidneys and urinary tract (glomerulonephritis, pyelonephritis, etc.), and (2) diseases in which the kidneys are target organs (diabetes, hypertensive disease, systemic diseases, etc.). Diagnosis of the disease causing the damage is paramount in all cases of the CKD presence [3–5]. The most common causes of CKD are diabetic nephropathy, hypertension, and glomerulonephritis [6]. Clinical manifestations, serum creatinine (Scr), and renal histopathology are commonly used to diagnose CKD and determine its different stages. The role of Scr is very limited [2]. Although kidney biopsy for histopathology may be an invasive and painful procedure, it is considered as the gold standard for the diagnosis of renal disease [7]. Bleeding and other surgical complications may follow this procedure. To reduce these risks, it could be safer to use alternative techniques.

The study of proteomic composition of urine and other human bio-fluids is very promising for the diagnosis of different kidney pathologies and for understanding the mechanisms of their occurrence. Proteinuria may reflect abnormal plasma protein loss, as a result of: (a) an increase in glomerular permeability for macromolecular proteins (glomerular proteinuria), (b) incomplete tubular reabsorption of low molecular weight proteins (tubular proteinuria), (c) abnormal loss of proteins of renal origin and urinary tract. Thus, the analysis of the urine proteome potentially allows us to speak about the localization of nephron damage, which greatly facilitates the differential diagnosis [8,9]. Research is currently underway, both in the search for specific proteins found in CKD [10–14] and attempts to highlight individual proteins that would become markers of specific diseases that cause CKD [15,16].

Often, information on changes in the expression level of a single protein is not enough to obtain sufficient accuracy and the sensitivity required for a clinical diagnostic system, and it is necessary to apply several indicators simultaneously. Thus, the use of a panel of 28 urinal proteins has shown the ability to differentiate Immunoglobulin-A nephropathy and primary membranous nephropathy with a sensitivity of 77% and specificity of 100% [17]. The sets of differently expressed urinal proteins were used for the differential diagnosis of lupus nephritis, primary membranous nephropathy, diabetic nephropathy, and focal segmental glomerulosclerosis. The sensitivity of differential diagnosis remained at 70% when using a set of 5 proteins, but the accuracy fell below 50% when using a set of less than 20 proteins [18]. It shows that these indicators are still insufficient for the effective differentiation of CKDs.

However, the most versatile and universal approach for differential diagnosis should consider the full quantitative information about a large number of proteins contained in patient's fluids. Multicomponent proteomics data derived from mass spectrometric analysis of a non-diagnosed patient's sample can be processed in comparison with similar data sets obtained from people with known diagnoses, to assign a new patient to a particular group. For this purpose the mathematical models of machine learning, which take into account the interactions of a large amount of data in a multidimensional space, can be used. Such an approach may become a new concept of an effective and universal test system for both early diagnosis of CKD and post diagnostic differentiation of renal diseases of different origin.

Recent methods of large data sets processing are often based on the principle of "black box", where input data are transformed into decision factors without any additional knowledge of internal working. Mathematical instruments, such as machine learning and data analysis, are increasingly being used in medicine [19,20]. Machine learning is a branch of the data science that trains computers to perform tasks by observing patterns in large datasets and using them to derive rules or algorithms that optimize task performance [21]. It is used for computer-aided diagnosis of acute neurological events [22] and retinal disease [23]. These studies were mainly based on general clinical indicators, whereas the application of the wide-scale method of quantitative proteomics based on a comparison of relative expressions of a large number of proteins can show much greater efficiency.

In this paper, we introduce a new approach to the differential diagnosis of CKDs of different origins, such as diabetic nephropathy, chronic glomerulonephritis and hypertensive nephropathy, which is based on large proteomics data sets obtained by mass spectrometry of blood plasma and urine, by means of several models of machine learning. The tested algorithms showed good abilities to differentiate the various groups of the tested renal patients according to the proteomic data.

2. Results

Plasma and urine samples were collected from 15 patients with diabetic nephropathy (group D), from 14 patients with glomerulonephritis (group G), from 5 patients with hypertensive nephropathy (group H), and from 14 healthy volunteers (group N). Table 1 summarizes the principal characteristics of the CKD patients.

Table 1. Principal characteristics of the chronic kidney diseases (CKD) patients.

Variable	Group D	Group G	Group H
Sex, n (%)			
Male	6 (40)	8 (57)	2 (40)
Female	9 (60)	6 (43)	3 (60)
Age, mean ± SD (years)	62.11 ± 17.91	48.46 ± 16.83	60.6 ± 14.15
Stage of renal disease, n (%)			
Stage 1	6 (40)	7 (50)	0 (0)
Stage 2 + 3	7 (46.7)	2 (14.3)	0 (0)
Stage 4 + 5	2 (13.3)	5 (35.7)	5 (100)
Level of proteinuria			
Below 30 mg/l, n (%)	0 (0)	0 (0)	0 (0)
30 - 300 mg/l, n (%)	5 (33.4)	5 (35.7)	1 (20)
Above 300 mg/l, n (%)	10 (66.6)	9 (64.3)	4 (80)
Presence of hypertension, n (%)	8 (53)	10 (71.4)	5 (100)
eGFR, mean ± SD (mL/min)	39.56 ± 15.27	68.38 ± 48.36	14.8 ± 7.19
Biopsy tested patients, n (%)	0 (0)	2 (14.3)	0 (0)
Type of glomerulonephritis			
Chronic glomerulonephritis, n (%)		10 (71.4)	
Nephrotic syndrome, n (%)		4 (28.6)	

Abbreviations: SD, standard deviation; eGFR, estimated glomerular filtration rate.

The plasma samples were depleted from albumin and immunoglobulin, the urine samples were concentrated by filter columns. All protein samples were prepared for mass spectrometry in duplicates and each duplicate was analyzed twice. These technical replicates were marked as A and B. The total set of plasma probes contained 190 samples (group G—56, group D—58, group H—20, and group N—56). The number of urine samples derived from patients was 97 (group G—40, group D—41, and group H—16); urine from healthy people was not taken due to low normal protein concentrations. The samples were not divided into fractions to limit the resulted data set for the convenience of bioinformatic processing. Two sets of quantitative proteomics data from blood and urine samples (Table S1) were obtained. No specific differences on proteome profiles between different patients groups expressed in the distribution of individual proteins were found by conventional statistical methods. Thus, machine learning algorithms, taking into account the overall contribution of the proteomic composition of the samples, were applied. The data were independently tested in two ways. At first, we distinguished the total CKD patients from the healthy individuals, and then we differentiated three groups of patients from each other without comparison with healthy control.

2.1. Separation of CKD Patients from the Healthy Individuals by Plasma Proteome

A total of 246 proteins were identified and quantified by label-free quantification (LFQ) from the plasma probes, and 184 of them were considered as relevant after the quality filtration. Then, the differences in plasma proteome of CKD patients and healthy individuals were estimated by principal component analysis (PCA). After the consistency check and averaging of the replicates, the dataset was reduced to 90 samples (group G—27, group D—28, group H—9, and group N—26) and label-free quantification (LFQ) values of 184 proteins were converted to the 17 principal components providing the cumulative variance of 70%.

The KNeighbors machine learning model (kNN) with the Euclidean distance was used for the separation of the total set of CKD patients (groups G, D, H) from the healthy individuals (group N). The best number of neighbors was found as 3. The mean proportion of correct classifier responses was 97.8%. Thus, the total CKD patients were differentiated from the healthy individuals using proteomics data of plasma with high confidence.

2.2. Differentiation of the Three Groups of Renal Patients by Plasma Proteome

The possibility of differentiation of various types of CKD with similar symptoms by proteomics data was tested. At this step, the control samples obtained from healthy people (group N) were discarded and 134 CKD patient's samples were taken; 175 proteins in 131 samples were left after the quality control check.

The PCA analysis showed that 14 principal components were necessary for 70% of cumulative variance, and 64 averaged results were obtained after the consistency check. Three models of machine learning were tested: KNeighbors, logistic regression, and support vector machine (SVM). The optimal hyper parameters were found: number of neighbors (n_neighbors = 1) for KNeighbors, constant of regularization (C = 1) for logistic regression, kernel (kernel = 'rbf') and gamma (gamma = 0.5) for SVM. The mean proportions of correct classifier responses were 87.5%, 84.3%, 82.8%, respectively. Based on this cross-validation quality assessment, the KNeighbors classifier was chosen as the best for further calculations. A number of errors of the nearest-neighbors algorithm were found for each class for the entire set. Class D had 2 errors from 28 (7.1%), class G had 2 errors from 27 (7.4%), and class H had 4 errors from 9 (44.4%). Thus, this algorithm works well for differential separation of group D from group G, but does not allow distinguishing class H.

Finally, the class H samples were excluded from the analysis and 55 samples were left in the set. The nearest-neighbor algorithm gave only two errors for this set (the proportions of correct decisions were 96.3% for class G and 96.4% for class D). Thus, this algorithm showed good results for the use in a medical test system that can separate glomerulonephritis from diabetic nephropathy based on plasma proteome.

2.3. Differential Diagnosis Based on Urine Proteome and Separation of Group H from the Total Patients

A total of 409 proteins were identified and quantified by LFQ, and 241 proteins in 96 samples left after the quality control.

We found 13 principal components to be optimal after the PCA. The consistency check and averaging resulted in 47 samples (group G—19, group D—20, and group H—8). Four machine learning models were tested. A decision tree was added to the three algorithms mentioned above. None of the tested algorithms with optimized hyper parameters showed high proportion of correct decisions. It was lower than 80% overall, thus showing no evident possibility to differentiate the three tested groups on the basis of urine proteome data, and allowing us to conclude that the urine proteome in comparison with plasma proteome has much less differences in the tested groups of patients.

The capabilities of "one against all" models for the separation of classes were tested. It was found that the classifier 1-nn (nearest-neighbor algorithm) gives an accuracy equal to 100% for class H by the entire set of urine proteomics data. It correctly defined all the samples of class H and had no false definitions. Thus, this model showed good capability to separate patients of group H (hypertensive nephropathy) from the remaining groups of renal patients.

3. Discussion

Focused on efficient processing of proteomics data, this work had two goals: 1) development of the concept of a non-invasive early-stage test system for general kidney malfunctions, and 2) the differentiation by origin of previously diagnosed renal diseases with similar symptoms. For these, using our data set, we first tried to distinguish the total group of CKD patients from the healthy group, and then to differentiate the three groups of patients from each other.

At the first step, it was important to find out whether the common differences in plasma proteome appear in patients with renal disease and in healthy people. This task was not particularly difficult. It turned out that KNeighbors machine learning model (kNN) is able to differentiate CKD patients from healthy individuals with high confidence (97.8% of correct classifier responses).

Glomerular filtration rate (GFR) remains for today the most operating marker of kidney malfunction, which is usually estimated taking into account endogenous filtration markers like serum creatinine and cystatin C [24], but the accuracy of their measuring is still under consideration [25]. It shows that new proteomic biomarkers may facilitate more accurate and earlier detection of renal pathologies [26]. Machine learning has been successfully applied to proteomics data for classification of samples and identification of biomarkers, and can be used across a wide range of diseases [27]. Thus, the high accuracy in separating a group of renal patients from healthy ones that we demonstrated by processing of plasma proteome data using machine learning proved to be effective for the introduction of this approach into clinical diagnosis.

The second goal of our research was to examine the ability of complex differentiation of various CKDs by plasma proteome data. It is difficult to predict in advance the most efficient processing algorithm for analyzing multidimensional data, thus we tested three models. The KNeighbors classifier (Model 1) was chosen as the most effective after comparing with the logistic regression and support vector machine (SVM), because of the best proportion of correct classifier responses (87.5%). After the less represented group of hypertensive patients was excluded, the proportion of correct decisions increased above 96%, thus showing a high ability to separate diabetic patients with indirect kidney damage from patients with autoimmune-caused internal kidney degradation (glomerulonephritis).

Diseases of different origins, which are not only related to kidneys but expressed in symptoms of kidney degradation, may appear in plasma proteomic composition. According to our results, diabetic nephropathy has a specific proteomic signature in blood which is independent of renal degradation. The distinct changes in the expression of individual proteins, such as monocyte chemoattractant protein-1 (MCP-1) and transforming growth factor-β1 (TGF-β1) [28], or even in panels of several proteins [29] noted previously as predicting the rate of renal function decline in diabetes, may also be accompanied by other more complex changes in the plasma proteome. On the other hand, the hypertonic signature of renal degradation with the damage of the tubules and the interstitium was not expressed in specific changes in the blood proteome, according to our data. Therefore, the proposed approach can be recommended for further development as a medical test system based on plasma proteome that can separate glomerulonephritis from other CKD patients, e.g., diabetics.

Urine sampling is even easier compared to venous blood collection and the sample preparation procedure eliminates the extra step of plasma depletion from major proteins. We tried to use both bio-fluids to obtain the proteomics data and compared them to find the most suitable way for differential diagnosis of the three types of kidney diseases. Urine samples obtained from healthy people were not used in this study, due to much lower protein concentrations compared with renal patients.

As well as for the plasma proteome, we tested kNN, SVM, and logistic regression as means for distinguishing the urine proteome datasets. In addition, the decision tree algorithm has been added to the comparison. However, as a result, none of the tested models gave the proportion of correct decisions above the level of 80%, thus showing no clear ability to differentiate simultaneously the three tested groups based on urine proteome data.

The additional "one against all" model showed the best results in the separation of only one tested group of patients. The classifier 1-nn (nearest-neighbor algorithm, Model 2) gives an accuracy of 100% for class H, showing no false definitions across the entire data set. Processing of urine proteome by machine learning showed the ability of distinguishing hypertensive nephropathy from other renal diseases. Since, here, we used a sample set that is not very representative (only 5 hypertensive patients), this approach should be recommended for further testing on larger groups.

Diabetic nephropathy and proliferative forms of glomerulonephritis have a similar histological picture of diffuse glomerulosclerosis, tubulointerstitial fibrosis, and atrophy, and also variable degrees of hyaline arteriolosclerosis and arterial sclerosis. In hypertensive nephropathy, primary pathological changes in afferent arterioles lead to ischemic damage to the glomerular apparatus [30]. Thus, the degradation of various kidney structures can result in a difference in the transmitted proteins that enter the urine of hypertensive patients. Proteinuria of the same origin, associated with glomerular defects probably did not have specific features depending on the genesis of renal degradation, and therefore diabetes and glomerulonephritis did not appear in urinal protein variations according to our study.

To test the differences in pathological renal filtration in the context of protein size, we compared molecular masses of the proteins found in the urine of patients from the three CKD groups. No distinct specificity for a particular disease was found in our case, as shown in Figure 1. Thus, the differences in the total proteome, which can be traced by machine learning, do not concern the molecular masses and sizes of proteins and are manifested in other complex features.

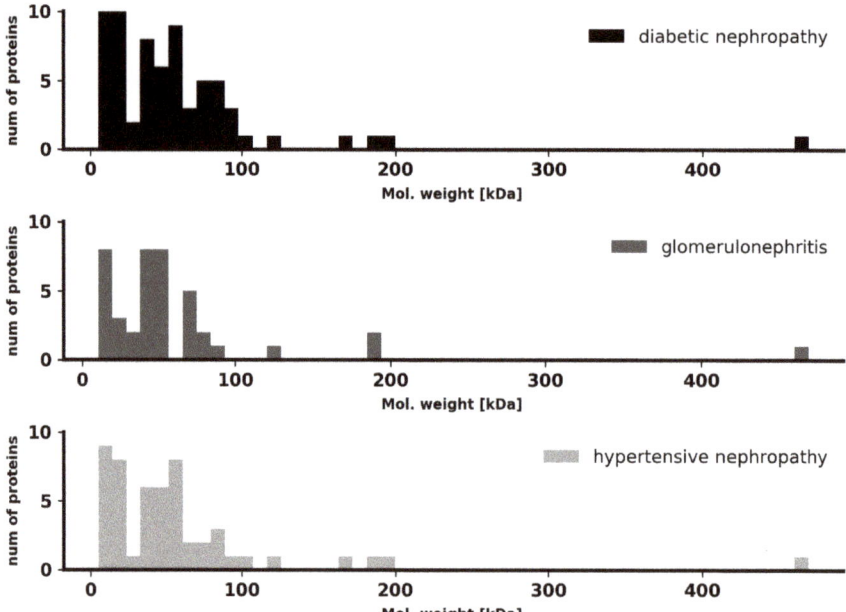

Figure 1. Distribution of urine proteins by molecular weight in the three studied groups of patients.

In this study, we conclude that the urine proteome, compared with the plasma proteome, has much less differences in our tested groups. As a result, urine is not quite suited for universal differential diagnosis in this analytical way, but this approach may remain useful in some cases, for example, to isolate patients with hypertensive nephropathy.

In addition, it is possible to use a two-stage approach to the differential diagnosis of CKD (Figure 2), including a combination of primary proteomic analysis of urine to cut off the hypertensive origin of the disease (using Model 2), followed by proteomic analysis of blood plasma to separate diabetic nephropathy and glomerulonephritis (using Model 1).

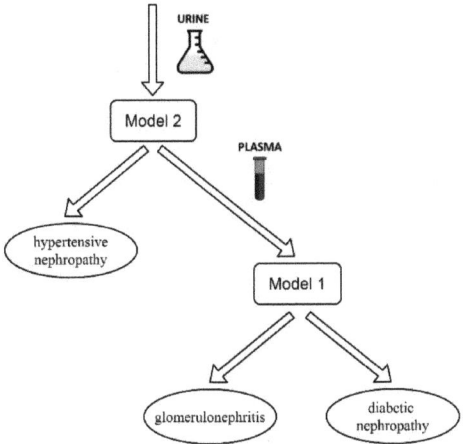

Figure 2. Scheme of two-stage differential diagnosis of chronic kidney disease using proteomic data of urine and plasma.

While the application of the presented strategy can be limited for the hypertensive nephropathy due to the fact that its diagnosis is mostly clinical and proteinuria is absent in most of the cases, for correctly diagnosed diabetic nephropathy, a specific therapy aimed at correcting sugar levels can be more actively applied. Treatment strategies for glomerulonephritis include immunosuppression with glucocorticosteroids and cytostatics, associated with the risk of serious infectious complications. The similar therapy for patients with diabetes can be dangerous, since they have a higher risk of purulent complications. Generally, differential diagnosis between glomerulonephritis and diabetic nephropathy should be carried out on the basis of kidney biopsy. However, several complicating points exist: (1) kidney biopsy is not always unambiguous, (2) this is an invasive method, (3) kidney biopsy should be performed in a specialized center, (4) to assess the dynamics of the process, a second study is required, which in the case of kidney biopsy is associated with repeated invasive intervention, and (5) the patient may refuse an invasive procedure. In this work, we studied the phenotypes expressed in the proteomes that distinguish the presented groups. All associated pathologies, including diabetes, should be undoubtedly reflected in the phenotypic proteomes, which we examined by choosing groups in this way (with and without diabetes) and dividing them using a machine learning approach.

4. Materials and Methods

4.1. Patients

A total of 34 CKD patients participated in the study (Table 1). Diagnosis of diabetic nephropathy patients was made clinically by the presence of diabetes; most patients had hypertension. Hypertensive nephropathy was diagnosed clinically by the presence of hypertension without presence of diabetes; no biopsy was performed in these groups. A group of glomerulonephritis patients were diagnosed by biopsy. All participants signed an informed consent. The study was approved by the Ethical Committee of the Krasnoyarsk State Medical University named after Professor V.F. Voyno-Yasenetsky (ethical code 88/2019 of 27 February 2019).

4.2. Sample Preparation

The plasma samples were depleted from albumin and immunoglobulin using ProteoPrep depletion columns (Sigma-Aldrich, St. Louis, MO, USA) according to the manufacturer's protocol. Proteins from the urine samples were concentrated with Amicon Ultra-4 3 kDa centrifugal filter columns (Merck Millipore, County Cork, Ireland). The protein concentrations were determined by UV-1280 spectrophotometer (Shimadzu, Kyoto, Japan) and samples with 4 µg of protein were taken for mass spectrometry. The proteins were reduced by dithiothreitol, alkylated by iodoacetamide, and digested by trypsin according to the manufacturer's protocols (Thermo Scientific, Waltham, MA, USA). The samples were desalted by 10 µL C18 pipette tips from the same manufacturer in accordance with its protocol and dried before analysis.

4.3. Liquid Chromatography and Mass Spectrometry

The samples were dissolved in phase "A" (0.1% of formic acid) and 2 µg of each sample were injected into the Dionex UltiMate 3000 RSLC nano liquid chromatographer (Thermo Scientific, USA) with Acclaim RSLC PepMap C18 separation column (15 cm length, 75 µm inner diameter, 2 µm particles). The solvent gradient was increased from 0% to 40% of phase "B" (0.1% of formic acid in 80% acetonitrile) for 90 min, maintaining a constant flow rate of 200 nL/min. The Orbitrap Fusion mass spectrometer (Thermo Scientific, USA) was operated in data-dependent mode with scans of parent and fragment ions changing in cycle of 4 s. Full scans were made at a resolution of 60,000 by the Orbitrap mass detector, and fragments generated by high energy collision dissociation (HCD) were registered by ion trap at normal rate.

4.4. Protein Search and Label-Free Quantification

The raw data files were processed by MaxQuant 1.6 software (Max Planck Institute for Biochemistry, Martinsried, Germany) [31]. Label-free quantification (LFQ) parameter was enabled. Unique and razor peptides were chosen for protein quantification. Carbamidomethylation of cysteine was set as a fixed modification, and oxidation of methionine and N-term acetylation were set as variable modifications. Protein search was performed against an actual SwissProt protein database with the human taxonomy restriction. The Orbitrap instrument was chosen and mass tolerance of 20 ppm was set for the first search and 4.5 ppm was set for the main search. Protein false discovery rate (FDR) of 0.01 was set. The obtained values of LFQ intensities (Table S1) were considered as relative indicators of protein expressions over the sample groups.

4.5. Data Analysis

All LFQ data analysis was performed using Anaconda Python 3 with Pandas and Scikit-learn libraries. Two steps of data filtration were made. Non-widespread proteins and low quality samples were excluded from the further analysis. Proteins detected in less than 5 samples and samples in which less than 50 proteins were found were not taken into account. Then, the LFQ normalization procedure was performed as follows: protein LFQ level for each sample was divided to the maximum of LFQ level of the certain protein among all the samples, giving the quantitative values to the range from 0 to 1. Then principal component analysis (PCA) was applied to reduce the data dimensions. We switched to a lower number of features expressed in projections of multiple protein LFQ values to the vectors of principal components. The next step was performed to check the consistency of the samples using data from the pairs of technical replicates. A closest Euclidean neighbor in the space of the principal components was found for each sample. The replicated samples were considered as consistent if a closest neighbor for replicate A was the corresponding replicate B and vice versa. The coordinates in the space of principal components for these replicates were averaged and they were considered as one sample. Samples that were not verified by this method were excluded.

Machine learning algorithms KNeighbors (kNN), logistic regression, support vector machine (SVM) and decision tree were used at the final step of the data analysis. In order to find optimal model hyper parameters, a grid search was used. As the number of experimental samples was not large enough, we did not use the separation of the dataset into training and test sets. We could not select a test set for the final quality verification of the models, since in this case the evaluation of the quality of the trained model would be very unstable, due to the randomness of the division of training and test sets, when marginal measurements may fall into the test set. Instead, we used the leave-one-out cross-validation on the whole dataset to control the model quality.

Accordingly, we excluded each sample from the entire set, trained the model on the remaining set, and then checked it on this extracted sample.

Then, we used mean accuracy metrics, i.e., the average proportion of correct answers to estimate the quality. This metrics seems to be adequate, because the class imbalance is insignificant (the ratio of class sizes does not exceed 3.2).

These procedures allowed us to use all available data as efficiently as possible and to avoid randomness in choosing a test sample.

5. Conclusions

The machine learning algorithms show good abilities to differentiate various groups across large data sets. Full proteomics data obtained by mass spectrometry can be very useful for this approach to medical diagnosis. These data contain general information about changes in normal body processes in those cases when common diagnostic approaches using single biomarkers or even panels of biomarkers do not work well enough. With the testing machine learning models on proteomics data obtained from the plasma and urine of patients of three types of CKD, the best results were obtained using the nearest-neighbor algorithm. In this case, according to the proteomics data of plasma, the two groups of patients with diabetic nephropathy and glomerulonephritis are well separated from the group of healthy people. On the other hand, a less presented group of patients with hypertensive nephropathy is better isolated from groups of patients of the two other CKD types by the "one against all" method based on the urine proteome data set.

The further development of the approach presented here may help to avoid invasive intervention and contraindicated intervention in some cases for the verification of the glomerulonephritis subtypes, which is currently performed only by kidney biopsy and microscopic morphological confirmation. The diagnosis of hypertensive and diabetic nephropathy at an early stage also remains relevant and the capabilities of machine learning methods based on proteomics data may be useful for this purpose.

Supplementary Materials: The following are available online at http://www.mdpi.com/1422-0067/21/13/4802/s1, Table S1. Plasma and urine proteins LFQ values.

Author Contributions: Conceptualization, methodology, mass spectrometry, software calculations, writing—original draft preparation, Y.E.G. and D.V.V.; blood and urine samples collection and preparation, medical investigations, I.A.L., M.L.R., S.A.V., and S.L.G.; medical investigations, writing—review and editing, T.N.Z. and M.M.P.; mass spectrometry experiments, Z.M.; supervision, review, and editing of the final version of the manuscript, M.V.B. and A.S.K. All authors have read and agreed to the published version of the manuscript.

Funding: This research received no external funding.

Acknowledgments: The authors sincerely thank Ivan Denisov for help in preparing the manuscript.

Conflicts of Interest: The authors declare no conflict of interest.

Abbreviations

CKD	Chronic kidney disease
Scr	Serum creatinine
D	Diabetic nephropathy group
G	Glomerulonephritis group
H	Hypertonic nephropathy group
N	Healthy volunteers group
SD	Standard deviation
PCA	Principal components analysis
LFQ	Label-free quantification
kNN	K nearest neighbors algorithm
SVM	Support vector machine
MCP-1	Monocyte chemoattractant protein-1
TGF-β1	Transforming growth factor-β1
eGFR	Estimated glomerular filtration rate
FDR	False discovery rate

References

1. Levey, A.S.; Eckardt, K.-U.; Tsukamoto, Y.; Levin, A.; Coresh, J.; Rossert, J.; Zeeuw, D.D.E.; Hostetter, T.H.; Lameire, N.; Eknoyan, G. Definition and classification of chronic kidney disease: A position statement from Kidney Disease: Improving Global Outcomes (KDIGO). *Kidney Int.* **2005**, *67*, 2089–2100. [CrossRef]
2. Wang, Y.-N.; Ma, S.-X.; Chen, Y.-Y.; Chen, L.; Liu, B.-L.; Liu, Q.-Q.; Zhao, Y.-Y. Chronic kidney disease: Biomarker diagnosis to therapeutic targets. *Clin. Chim. Acta* **2019**, *499*, 54–63. [CrossRef] [PubMed]
3. Lamb, E.J.; MacKenzie, F.; Stevens, P.E. How should proteinuria be detected and measured? *Ann. Clin. Biochem.* **2009**, *46*, 205–217. [CrossRef] [PubMed]
4. Uchida, S. Differential diagnosis of chronic kidney disease (CKD): By primary diseases. *Jpn. Med. Assoc. J.* **2011**, *54*, 22–26.
5. Vassalotti, J.A.; Centor, R.; Turner, B.J.; Greer, R.C.; Choi, M.; Sequist, T.D. Practical Approach to Detection and Management of Chronic Kidney Disease for the Primary Care Clinician. *Am. J. Med.* **2016**, *129*, 153–162. [CrossRef] [PubMed]
6. Alebiosu, C.O.; Ayodele, O.E. The global burden of chronic kidney disease and the way forward. *Ethn. Dis.* **2005**, *15*, 418–423.
7. Cunningham, A.; Benediktsson, H.; Muruve, D.A.; Hildebrand, A.M.; Ravani, P. Trends in Biopsy-Based Diagnosis of Kidney Disease: A Population Study. *Can. J. Kidney Health Dis.* **2018**, *5*, 205435811879969. [CrossRef]
8. McMahon, G.M.; Waikar, S.S. Biomarkers in Nephrology: Core Curriculum 2013. *Am. J. Kidney Dis.* **2013**, *62*, 165–178. [CrossRef]
9. Bergón, E.; Granados, R.; Fernández-Segoviano, P.; Miravalles, E.; Bergón, M. Classification of Renal Proteinuria: A Simple Algorithm. *Clin. Chem. Lab. Med.* **2002**, *40*, 1143–1150. [CrossRef]
10. Mischak, H.; Delles, C.; Vlahou, A.; Vanholder, R. Proteomic biomarkers in kidney disease: Issues in development and implementation. *Nat. Rev. Nephrol.* **2015**, *11*, 221–232. [CrossRef] [PubMed]
11. Dakna, M.; Harris, K.; Kalousis, A.; Carpentier, S.; Kolch, W.; Schanstra, J.P.; Haubitz, M.; Vlahou, A.; Mischak, H.; Girolami, M. Addressing the Challenge of Defining Valid Proteomic Biomarkers and Classifiers. *BMC Bioinform.* **2010**, *11*, 594. [CrossRef] [PubMed]
12. Good, D.M.; Zürbig, P.; Argilés, À.; Bauer, H.W.; Behrens, G.; Coon, J.J.; Dakna, M.; Decramer, S.; Delles, C.; Dominiczak, A.F.; et al. Naturally Occurring Human Urinary Peptides for Use in Diagnosis of Chronic Kidney Disease. *Mol. Cell. Proteom.* **2010**, *9*, 2424–2437. [CrossRef] [PubMed]
13. Schanstra, J.P.; Zürbig, P.; Alkhalaf, A.; Argiles, A.; Bakker, S.J.L.; Beige, J.; Bilo, H.J.G.; Chatzikyrkou, C.; Dakna, M.; Dawson, J.; et al. Diagnosis and Prediction of CKD Progression by Assessment of Urinary Peptides. *J. Am. Soc. Nephrol.* **2015**, *26*, 1999–2010. [CrossRef] [PubMed]

14. Pontillo, C.; Jacobs, L.; Staessen, J.A.; Schanstra, J.P.; Rossing, P.; Heerspink, H.J.L.; Siwy, J.; Mullen, W.; Vlahou, A.; Mischak, H.; et al. A urinary proteome-based classifier for the early detection of decline in glomerular filtration. *Nephrol. Dial. Transplant.* **2017**, *32*, 1510–1516. [PubMed]
15. Argyropoulos, C.P.; Chen, S.S.; Ng, Y.-H.; Roumelioti, M.-E.; Shaffi, K.; Singh, P.P.; Tzamaloukas, A.H. Rediscovering Beta-2 Microglobulin As a Biomarker across the Spectrum of Kidney Diseases. *Front. Med.* **2017**, *4*, 73. [CrossRef]
16. Wu, J.; Chen, Y.; Gu, W. Urinary proteomics as a novel tool for biomarker discovery in kidney diseases. *J. Zhejiang Univ. Sci. B* **2010**, *11*, 227–237. [CrossRef]
17. Haubitz, M.; Wittke, S.; Weissinger, E.M.; Walden, M.; Rupprecht, H.D.; Floege, J.; Haller, H.; Mischak, H. Urine protein patterns can serve as diagnostic tools in patients with IgA nephropathy. *Kidney Int.* **2005**, *67*, 2313–2320. [CrossRef]
18. Varghese, S.A.; Powell, T.B.; Budisavljevic, M.N.; Oates, J.C.; Raymond, J.R.; Almeida, J.S.; Arthur, J.M. Urine Biomarkers Predict the Cause of Glomerular Disease. *J. Am. Soc. Nephrol.* **2007**, *18*, 913–922. [CrossRef]
19. Sajda, P. Machine Learning for Detection and Diagnosis of Disease. *Annu. Rev. Biomed. Eng.* **2006**, *8*, 537–565. [CrossRef]
20. Sun, D. Development of New Diagnostic Techniques—Machine Learning. In *Substance and Non-substance Addiction*; Zhang, X., Shi, J., Tao, R., Eds.; Springer: Singapore, 2017; Volume 1010, pp. 203–215.
21. Lynch, C.J.; Liston, C. New machine-learning technologies for computer-aided diagnosis. *Nat. Med.* **2018**, *24*, 1304–1305. [CrossRef]
22. Titano, J.J.; Badgeley, M.; Schefflein, J.; Pain, M.; Su, A.; Cai, M.; Swinburne, N.; Zech, J.; Kim, J.; Bederson, J.; et al. Automated deep-neural-network surveillance of cranial images for acute neurologic events. *Nat. Med.* **2018**, *24*, 1337–1341. [CrossRef] [PubMed]
23. De Fauw, J.; Ledsam, J.R.; Romera-Paredes, B.; Nikolov, S.; Tomasev, N.; Blackwell, S.; Askham, H.; Glorot, X.; O'Donoghue, B.; Visentin, D.; et al. Clinically applicable deep learning for diagnosis and referral in retinal disease. *Nat. Med.* **2018**, *24*, 1342–1350. [CrossRef] [PubMed]
24. Lopez-Giacoman, S. Biomarkers in chronic kidney disease, from kidney function to kidney damage. *World J. Nephrol.* **2015**, *4*, 57–73. [CrossRef] [PubMed]
25. MacIsaac, R.J.; Tsalamandris, C.; Thomas, M.C.; Premaratne, E.; Panagiotopoulos, S.; Smith, T.J.; Poon, A.; Jenkins, M.A.; Ratnaike, S.I.; Power, D.A.; et al. The accuracy of cystatin C and commonly used creatinine-based methods for detecting moderate and mild chronic kidney disease in diabetes. *Diabet. Med.* **2007**, *24*, 443–448. [CrossRef] [PubMed]
26. Rysz, J.; Gluba-Brzózka, A.; Franczyk, B.; Jabłonowski, Z.; Ciałkowska-Rysz, A. Novel Biomarkers in the Diagnosis of Chronic Kidney Disease and the Prediction of Its Outcome. *Int. J. Mol. Sci.* **2017**, *18*, 1702. [CrossRef]
27. Swan, A.L.; Mobasheri, A.; Allaway, D.; Liddell, S.; Bacardit, J. Application of Machine Learning to Proteomics Data: Classification and Biomarker Identification in Postgenomics Biology. *OMICS J. Integr. Biol.* **2013**, *17*, 595–610. [CrossRef]
28. Verhave, J.C.; Bouchard, J.; Goupil, R.; Pichette, V.; Brachemi, S.; Madore, F.; Troyanov, S. Clinical value of inflammatory urinary biomarkers in overt diabetic nephropathy: A prospective study. *Diabetes Res. Clin. Pract.* **2013**, *101*, 333–340. [CrossRef] [PubMed]
29. Pena, M.J.; Heinzel, A.; Heinze, G.; Alkhalaf, A.; Bakker, S.J.L.; Nguyen, T.Q.; Goldschmeding, R.; Bilo, H.J.G.; Perco, P.; Mayer, B.; et al. A Panel of Novel Biomarkers Representing Different Disease Pathways Improves Prediction of Renal Function Decline in Type 2 Diabetes. *PLoS ONE* **2015**, *10*, e0120995. [CrossRef]
30. Alsaad, K.O.; Herzenberg, A.M. Distinguishing diabetic nephropathy from other causes of glomerulosclerosis: An update. *J. Clin. Pathol.* **2007**, *60*, 18–26. [CrossRef]
31. Cox, J.; Mann, M. MaxQuant enables high peptide identification rates, individualized p.p.b.-range mass accuracies and proteome-wide protein quantification. *Nat. Biotechnol.* **2008**, *26*, 1367–1372. [CrossRef]

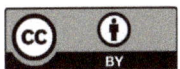

© 2020 by the authors. Licensee MDPI, Basel, Switzerland. This article is an open access article distributed under the terms and conditions of the Creative Commons Attribution (CC BY) license (http://creativecommons.org/licenses/by/4.0/).

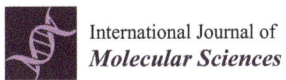

Article

Differential Urinary Proteome Analysis for Predicting Prognosis in Type 2 Diabetes Patients with and without Renal Dysfunction

Hee-Sung Ahn [1,†], Jong Ho Kim [2,†], Hwangkyo Jeong [3], Jiyoung Yu [1], Jeonghun Yeom [4], Sang Heon Song [2], Sang Soo Kim [2], In Joo Kim [2,*] and Kyunggon Kim [1,3,5,6,*]

1. Asan Institute for Life Sciences, Asan Medical Center, Seoul 05505, Korea; zaulim3@gmail.com (H.-S.A.); yujiyoung202@gmail.com (J.Y.)
2. Department of Internal Medicine and Biomedical Research Institute, Pusan National University Hospital, Busan 49241, Korea; bedaya@hanmail.net (J.H.K.); shsong0209@gmail.com (S.H.S.); drsskim7@gmail.com (S.S.K.)
3. Department of Biomedical Sciences, University of Ulsan College of Medicine, Seoul 05505, Korea; hkyo723@naver.com
4. Convergence Medicine Research Center, Asan Institute for Life Sciences, Seoul 05505, Korea; nature8309@gmail.com
5. Clinical Proteomics Core Laboratory, Convergence Medicine Research Center, Asan Medical Center, Seoul 05505, Korea
6. Bio-Medical Institute of Technology, Asan Medical Center, Seoul 05505, Korea
* Correspondence: injkim@pusan.ac.kr (I.J.K.); kkkon1@amc.seoul.kr (K.K.); Tel.: +82-51-240-7224 (I.J.K.); +82-2-1688-7575 (K.K.)
† These authors contributed equally to this work.

Received: 3 April 2020; Accepted: 12 June 2020; Published: 14 June 2020

Abstract: Renal dysfunction, a major complication of type 2 diabetes, can be predicted from estimated glomerular filtration rate (eGFR) and protein markers such as albumin concentration. Urinary protein biomarkers may be used to monitor or predict patient status. Urine samples were selected from patients enrolled in the retrospective diabetic kidney disease (DKD) study, including 35 with good and 19 with poor prognosis. After removal of albumin and immunoglobulin, the remaining proteins were reduced, alkylated, digested, and analyzed qualitatively and quantitatively with a nano LC-MS platform. Each protein was identified, and its concentration normalized to that of creatinine. A prognostic model of DKD was formulated based on the adjusted quantities of each protein in the two groups. Of 1296 proteins identified in the 54 urine samples, 66 were differentially abundant in the two groups (area under the curve (AUC): p-value < 0.05), but none showed significantly better performance than albumin. To improve the predictive power by multivariate analysis, five proteins (ACP2, CTSA, GM2A, MUC1, and SPARCL1) were selected as significant by an AUC-based random forest method. The application of two classifiers—support vector machine and random forest—showed that the multivariate model performed better than univariate analysis of mucin-1 (AUC: 0.935 vs. 0.791) and albumin (AUC: 1.0 vs. 0.722). The urinary proteome can reflect kidney function directly and can predict the prognosis of patients with chronic kidney dysfunction. Classification based on five urinary proteins may better predict the prognosis of DKD patients than urinary albumin concentration or eGFR.

Keywords: urine; diabetic kidney disease; kidney function; proteomics; mass spectrometry; statistical clinical model; machine learning

1. Introduction

About 30% of people with diabetes develop diabetic kidney disease (DKD), and the spread of diabetes is increasing worldwide [1,2]. Complications of type 2 diabetes (T2D) mainly cause end-stage renal disease, which is related to high heart disease incidence and mortality [2,3]. Early detection and screening of patients at risk for DKD is important, which may reduce the global burden of T2D.

Because the kidneys filter waste from blood and discharge it as urine, urine can directly reflect kidney function. Unlike plasma, urine can be easily collected non-invasively, with proteins in urine being stable and not vulnerable to sudden degradation [4]. Albuminuria and estimated glomerular filtration rate (eGFR), have been generally used to assess kidney function [2,5]. However, albuminuria is only evaluated after glomerular damage has occurred, and sometimes kidney disease develops before the outbreak of albuminuria [6,7]. Better markers are required to help delay progression to DKD.

Multiple-biomarker approaches based on proteomics, including urinary proteomics, may overcome the limitations of markers diagnostic for DKD [4,8]. This study was designed to identify a urinary multi-protein panel that could predict progression to DKD in patients with T2D.

2. Results

2.1. Baseline Characteristics of Clinical Samples Used in the Study

Table 1 summarizes the baseline characteristics of patients in the poor and good prognosis groups. All factors did not differ significantly in the two groups, including sex, age, body mass index (BMI), duration of follow-up, systolic blood pressure (SBP), glycated hemoglobin concentration (HbA1c), lipid profile, percent with diabetic retinopathy, and the percentages treated with RAS inhibitors, anti-hypertensive agents, and lipid-lowering agents (Bonferroni corrected p-value > 0.05/17 = 0.0029; Table S1).

Table 1. Baseline characteristics of the patients with type 2 diabetes (T2D) with and without renal outcomes.

Variable	With Renal Outcome	Without Renal Outcome
Sex, n (%)		
Male	8 (42.1)	11 (31.4)
Female	11 (57.9)	24 (68.6)
Age at diagnosis of diabetic kidney disease, mean ± SD (years)	54.58 ± 11.66	58.66 ± 9.19
BMI, mean ± SD (kg/m^2)	22.64 ± 3.46	23.81 ± 3.00
Duration of follow-up, mean ± SD (years)	4.80 ± 1.96	4.73 ± 1.94
SBP, mean ± SD (mmHg)	126.58 ± 15.70	125.97 ± 12.07
LDL cholesterol, mean ± SD (mg/dL)	104.89 ± 41.00	99.83 ± 32.32
HDL cholesterol, mean ± SD (mg/dL)	48.42 ± 7.50	52.51 ± 11.51
Triglycerides, mean ± SD (mg/dL)	145.74 ± 99.80	154.57 ± 128.88
eGFR after 1 years, mean ± SD (mL/min/1.73 m^2)	91.52 ± 17.57	88.33 ± 15.46
HbA1c, mean ± SD (%)	8.34 ± 2.09	7.16 ± 1.36
ACR, mean ± SD (mg/g)	213.66 ± 446.75	126.11 ± 419.70
NAPCR, mean ± SD (mg/g)	178.18 ± 209.30	154.76 ± 299.68
PCR, mean ± SD (mg/g)	391.84 ± 652.79	280.87 ± 711.04
Diabetic retinopathy, n (%)	9 (47.37)	11 (31.43)
RAS inhibitor, n (%)	6 (31.58)	15 (42.86)
Anti-hypertensive agent, n (%)	5 (26.32)	12 (34.29)
Lipid-lowering agent, n (%)	10 (52.63)	20 (57.14)

Abbreviations: BMI, body mass index; SBP, systolic blood pressure; LDL, low-density lipoprotein; HDL, high-density lipoprotein; eGFR, estimated glomerular filtration rate; HbA1c, glycated hemoglobin; ACR, urine albumin-to-creatinine ratio; NAPCR, urine nonalbumin protein-to-creatinine ratio; PCR, urine protein-to-creatinine ratio.

2.2. Urinary Proteome Analysis for Identification and Label-Free Quantitation

The workflow of data processes contained identified and quantified urinary proteins indicative of disease status, as well as significant proteins to build the clinical models (Figure 1A). Liquid chromatography–mass spectrometry (LC-MS) analysis of the 54 urine samples identified 1296 proteins (Table S2). Of these proteins, 1244 were quantified, and their quantities were adjusted relative to the concentration of creatinine [9,10]. Sample-to-sample variation was subsequently fixed by the amount of proteins, leading to the selection of six endogenous normalization proteins that showed stable abundance in all LC-MS analyses. A boxplot of protein abundances in the 54 samples, composed of 35 patients in good-prognostic group (GPG) and 19 patients in poor-prognostic group (PPG), is depicted in Figure 1B. The normalized abundance of 68 proteins significantly correlated with their immunoassay [11] determined concentrations in urine, with a Pearson's coefficient of 0.502 (permutation p-value < 0.001; Figure 1C).

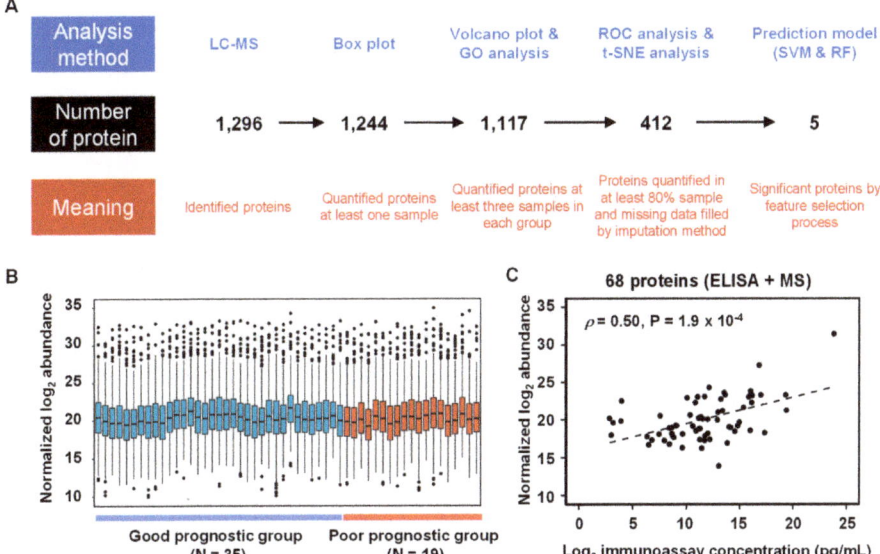

Figure 1. (**A**) Analysis workflow of urinary proteins in the 54 diabetic kidney disease (DKD) patients. The analysis method is written in the upper part, the number of proteins in the middle, and the meaning of the protein in the bottom part. (**B**) Boxplots of normalized urinary protein abundances in the 54 samples (35 patients in good-prognostic group and 19 patients in poor-prognostic group) measured by LC-MS analysis. (**C**) Scatter plot of 68 urine proteins between normalized log2 abundance and log2 immunoassays concentration (Pearson correlation coefficient (ρ): 0.5 and p-value: 1.9×10^{-4}).

2.3. Functional Annotation of Differential Protein Expression in the PPG and GPG Groups

To find the differential abundant proteins (DAPs) from among the 1117 proteins, fold-changes and p-values were calculated by Mann–Whitney U tests of the two groups. A volcano plot showing log2-fold-changes against minus log$_{10}$ p-values identified 46 proteins as being upregulated in the PPG and 54 proteins in the GPG (|log$_2$ fold-change| > 0.5; p-value < 0.05; Figure 2 and Table S3). These differentially expressed proteins included the six previously described candidate urinary biomarkers (APOE, CO3, COF1, NID1, OSTP-5, and PODXL) of glomerular or tubular injury [11].

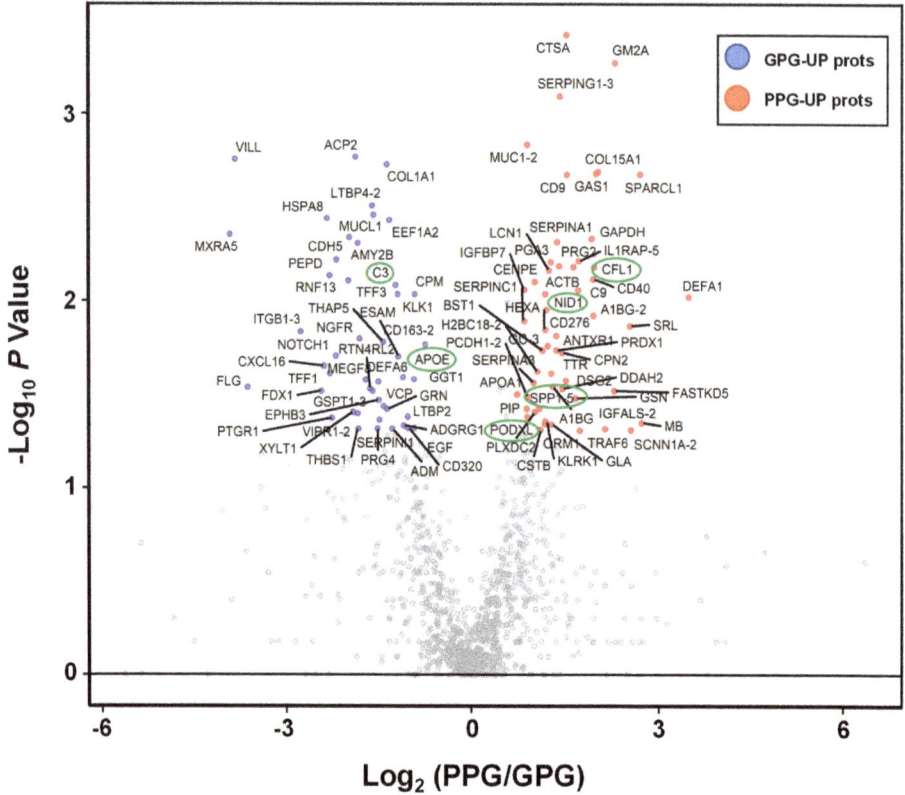

Figure 2. Volcano plot of urinary proteomic data. Volcano plots are depicted with the fold change of each protein abundance and the p value was calculated by performing a Mann–Whitney U-test. The averages of the urinary proteomic abundance data of good prognostic group (N = 35) were compared with the averages of the data for poor prognostic group (N = 19). Red circles show 54 urinary proteins that have significant increases in PPG. Blue circles show 46 urinary proteins which have significant decreases in PPG. Gray circles are urinary proteins without statistical meaning. Green circles are previously released as urinary protein markers for glomerular injury or tubular injury.

To determine whether urinary DAPs were associated with specific biological processes, up- and downregulated proteins in the PPG were subjected to gene ontology (GO) enrichment analysis. To integrate the three domains of GO and easily visualize the relationship between terms, ClueGO tools were applied with default settings (kappa score 0.4 and group merger of 50% of genes) to functionally organize the GO term networks [12].

Downregulated proteins in PPG were significantly enriched with an FDR < 0.01 (Figure 3A,B). Biological processes associated with these proteins included negative regulation of lipid localization, collagen catabolic process, positive regulation of neural precursor cell proliferation, and neuron projection regeneration. Resulting analysis of molecular function indicated that transforming growth factor beta binding and cargo receptor activity were annotated. The networks between proteins and functional GO terms showed that three proteins were negative regulators of lipid transport, as well as being associated with another GO term (Figure 3C). These included APOE, which is involved in neuron projection regeneration; THBS1, which is involved in transforming growth factor beta binding; and EGF, which is involved in positive regulation of neural precursor cell proliferation.

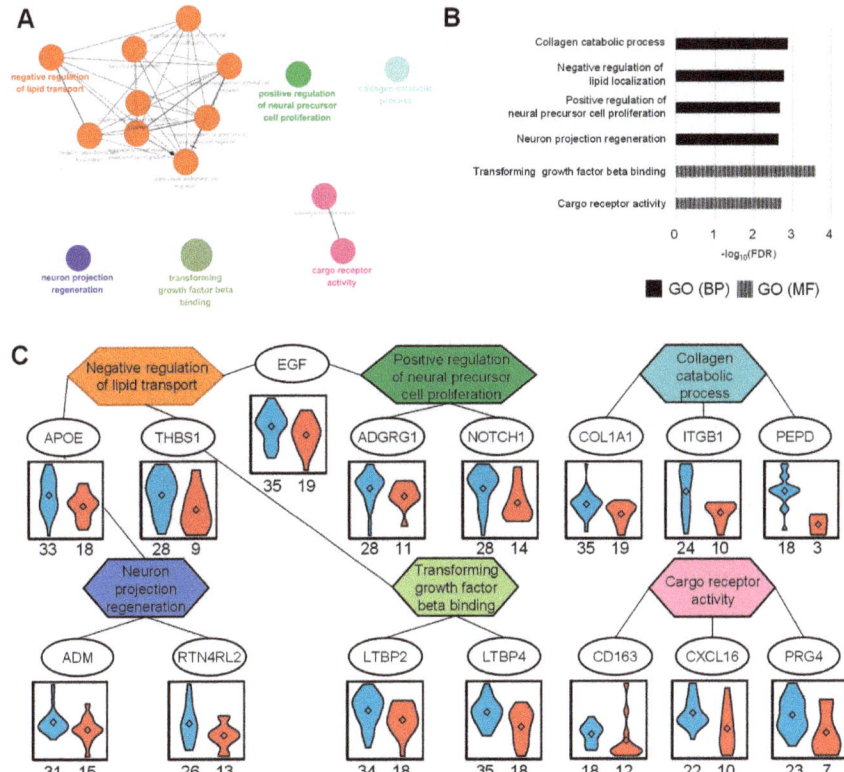

Figure 3. Up-regulated proteome in good prognosis group (GPG) and gene ontology (GO) analysis. (**A**) Functional GO network displaying grouping of GO terms enriched in GPG up-regulated proteins. (**B**) Enriched GO terms in biological process and molecular function. (**C**) The network between GO terms and corresponding proteins represents the relationship between GO terms via the proteins. The abundances of each protein represent the violin plots in two groups. The numbers listed below represent the measured numbers for each group.

Upregulated proteins in PPG were identified in enriched functional GO groups with an FDR < 0.01 (Figure 4A,B). Biological processes associated with these proteins included platelet degranulation, retina homeostasis, and heterotypic cell–cell adhesion. The molecular functional processes related with these proteins contained collagen binding. These urinary proteins were located in the lysosomal lumen and blood microparticles. The networks between proteins and functional GO terms indicated that the proteins in blood microparticles were functionally involved in platelet degranulation (Figure 4C). Platelets in patients with CKD are deficient in reactivity [13]. Leukocytes adhere to and destroy damaged kidney cell walls in patients with CKD [14], accompanied by bone marrow-derived kidney fibrosis, which is highly associated with cell–cell adhesion [15]. CKD is also associated with retinal abnormalities [16] and the possible destruction of retinal homeostasis, as confirmed in this study.

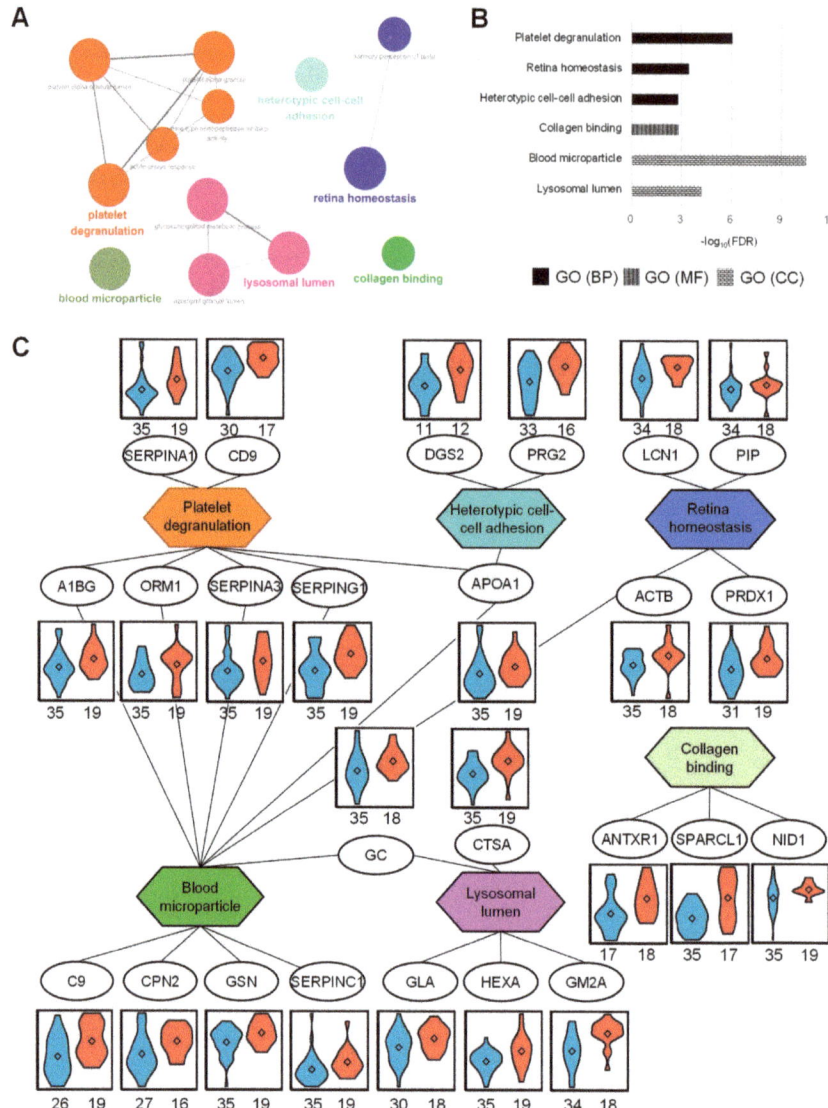

Figure 4. Up-regulated proteome in poor-prognostic group (PPG) and GO analysis. (**A**) Functional GO network displaying grouping of GO terms enriched in PPG up-regulated proteins. (**B**) Enriched GO terms in biological process, molecular function, and cellular component. (**C**) The network between GO terms and their contained proteins represents the relationship between GO terms via the proteins. The abundance of proteins represents the violin plots in two sample groups. The numbers listed below represent the measured numbers for each group.

2.4. Univariate ROC Analysis for Predicting Renal Outcome

To ensure statistical reliability, this study focused on 412 proteins quantified in more than 80% of urine samples [17], with missing values filled by local least squares imputation [18] (Table S4). To confirm that quantified urinary proteins could act as individual biomarkers, univariate receiver operating characteristic (ROC) analysis was performed in samples from the PPG and GPG, with the resulting histogram of AUC values shown in Figure 5. The AUC values of MUC1, CTSA, ACP2, SERPING1, AMY2B, GM2A, and COL1A1 were 0.791, 0.786, 0.773, 0.771, 0.768, 0.759, and 0.753, respectively. ACP2, AMY2B, and COL1A1 were significantly more abundant, whereas MUC1, CTSA, SERPING1, and GM2A were significantly less abundant, in the GPG than in the PPG (p-value < 0.05 each). The 66 urinary proteins showed significance with AUCs of 0.5 (p-value < 0.05; Table S5). Clinically, urinary albumin is a common marker of DKD [2,5]. The AUCs of 18 proteins were higher than that of albumin (0.722), but the differences were not statistically significant based on likelihood ratio tests.

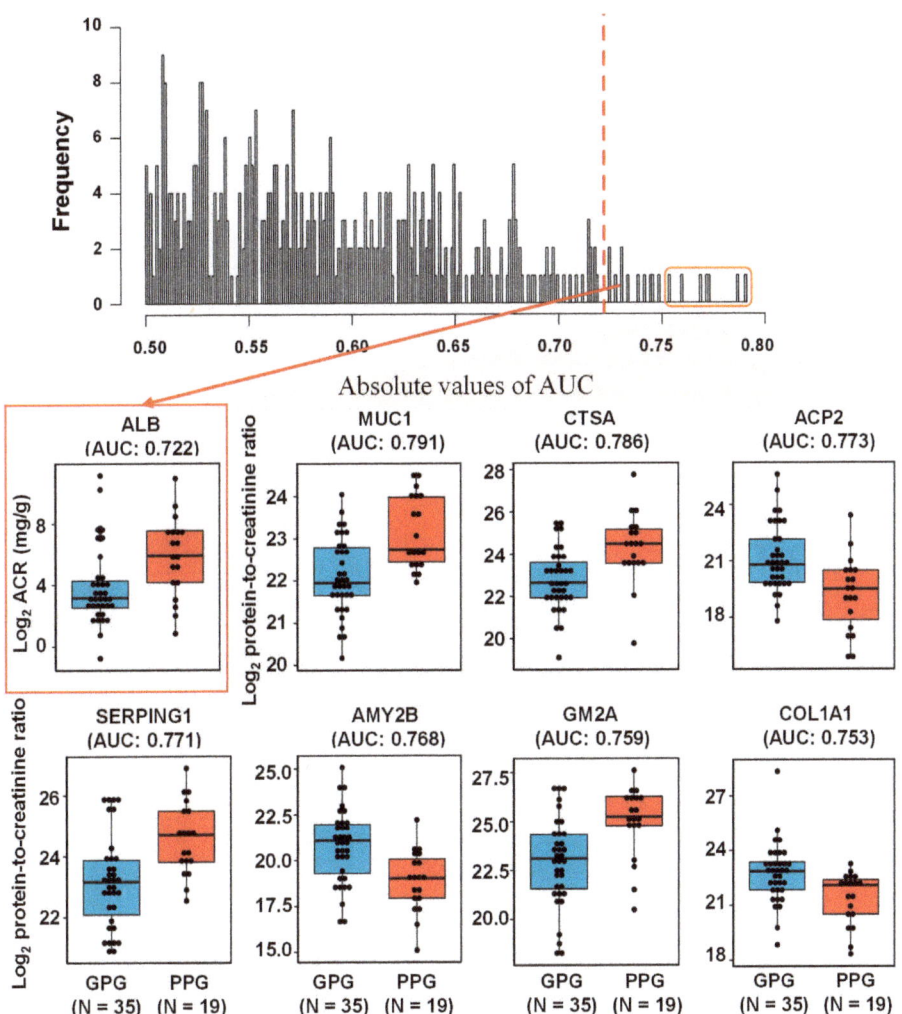

Figure 5. Histogram of area under the ROC curves (AUC) of 412 urinary proteins and ACR. Top seven proteins (MUC1, CTSA, ACP2, SERPING1, AMY2B, GM2A, and COL1A1) and ACR are represented with box plots.

2.5. Multivariate Analysis for Predicting Renal Outcome

To improve predictive performance and find a meaningful combination of proteins that could distinguish patients who were and were not at risk of disease progression, two classifiers of the 412 proteins were generated, one based on random forest (RF) [19] and the other on support vector machine (SVM) [20]. Both the RF and SVM methods selected five proteins (ACP2, CTSA, GM2A, MUC1, and SPARCL1) by an AUC-based RF backward-elimination process [21], according to a >0.3 importance of selection (Table 2). These variables were used to establish a RF model by generating 20,000 decision trees, and a linear SVM model by three repeated iterations of 10-fold cross-validation. Evaluation of the performance of these classifiers showed that the AUC values for RF and SVM were 1.000 and 0.935, respectively (Figure 6A). The nominal binary results of RF and SVM models were transformed in disease prediction scores, which ranged from 0 to 1 (Figure 6B and Table S6). The two classifiers differed significantly from albumin-to-creatinine ratio (likelihood ratio test: p-value < 0.05). These five proteins were located in extracellular exosomes, vesicles, or organelles, with three (ACP2, CTSA, and GM2A) located in the lysosomal lumen, MUC1 placed in plasma membrane, and SPARCL1 interacted with collagen in extracellular matrix.

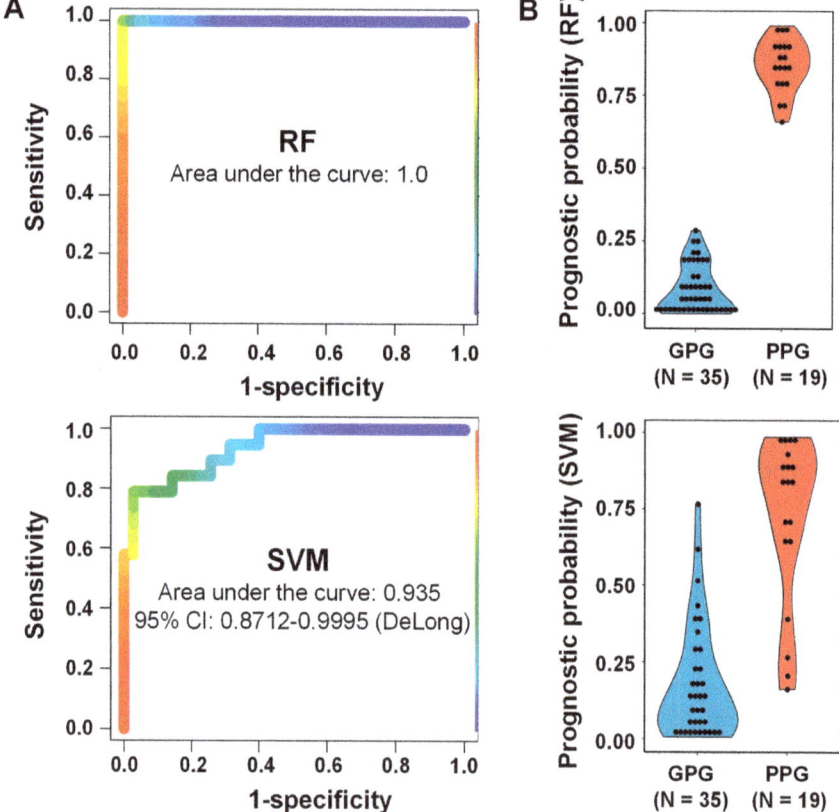

Figure 6. ROC curves of RF and SVM classifiers for five selected proteins (ACP2, CTSA, GM2A, MUC1 and SPARCL1). Performance of the two classifiers in the set of 54 samples, 35 from patients with good prognosis and 19 from patients with poor prognosis. (**A**) Areas under the curve (AUC) for the RF (1.0) and SVM (0.935) classifiers. (**B**) Clinical indices (0–1) of the two classifiers.

Table 2. AUC-based RF backward-elimination process-based selected feature proteins.

Uniprot Accession No.	Gene Name	Importance	Prob. Select	Selection	Univariate AUC
P10619	CTSA	0.422	0.700	Y	0.737
Q14515	SPARCL1	0.378	0.583	Y	0.659
P17900	GM2A	0.373	0.613	Y	0.726
P15941-2	MUC1	0.332	0.543	Y	0.791
P11117	ACP2	0.312	0.563	Y	0.718
P19961	AMY2B	0.299	0.510	N	0.779
P00734	F2	0.296	0.483	N	0.694
P06865	HEXA	0.274	0.466	N	0.651
P05155-3	SERPING1	0.275	0.377	N	0.771
P11142	HSPA8	0.238	0.330	N	0.734
P10451	SPP1	0.228	0.323	N	0.680

Probability of selection for each variable.

2.6. External Validation of Clinical Models in Public Studies

Since we were unable to find a benchmarking study in the discovery of urine protein biomarkers that could validate our statistical model, we validated the models with mRNA expression in the kidney, an organ that undoubtedly affects urine samples. The SVM and RF models consisting of five urine proteins were applied to four publicly available GEO datasets (GSE99339 [22], GSE47185 [23], GSE30122 [24], and GSE96804 [25,26]) without model adjustment. In the first GSE99339 dataset, mRNA expression in the renal glomerulus of 187 patients was studied, and the 11 disease groups are diabetic nephropathy (DN), rapidly progressive glomerulonephritis (RPGN), tumor nephrectomies (TN), hypertensive nephropathy (HT), IgA nephropathy, membranous glomerulonephritis (MGN), systemic lupus erythematosus (SLE), thin membrane disease (TMD), focal and segmental glomerulosclerosis (FSGS), focal and segmental glomerulosclerosis and minimal change disease (FSGS&MCD), and minimal change disease (MCD). The two classifiers' prognostic probabilities were highly correlated with each other in 187 samples ($\rho = 0.817$, Pearson correlation coefficient). In both models, the highest value in the DN group was higher than the other ten disease groups (Figure 7A). RF prediction values in the DN group were significantly higher than other eight groups except for RPGN and HT group (Mann-Whitney U Test: p-value < 0.05). SVM prediction values in the DN group were significantly higher than the other nine groups excluding the RPGN group (p-value < 0.05). In the second GSE99339 data set, there are a total of 223 kidney glomerulus ($N = 122$) and tubulointerstitia ($N = 101$) mRNA expression levels. The eight disease groups include DN, RPGN, TN, MGN, TMD, FSGS, FSGS&MCD, and MCD. The two classifiers' prognostic probabilities were also highly correlated in 223 samples ($r = 0.637$). The tendency of the predicted values was different depending on the cell type of the kidney (Figure 7B). In the glomeruli, the two model predictions are the highest in the DN group and are statistically significant with other seven groups. However, in the tubulointerstitium, the SVM model prediction values in DN were significant with four other groups except RPGN, TN, FSGS&MCD, and RF model prediction values in DN is only significant with MCD. It indicated that the five urine proteins are more closely related to the glomeruli than the kidney tubulointerstitium.

Meanwhile, we tried to verify whether the prognostic models could predict DKD. In the third GSE30122 data set, of the total of 69 samples, 26 of the 35 kidney glomerulus were normal obtained from living allograft donors, 9 of which were DKD, 34 of which were renal tubulus, of which 24 were normal and 10 were DKD. The results of the RF model in the glomeruli statistically were divided the normal and disease groups (p-value < 0.05), but the SVM model were not (p-value > 0.05; Figure 7C). The results of the both models in the tubulus statistically were not divided the normal and disease groups (p-value > 0.05). In the fourth GSE30122 dataset, 20 kidney glomerulus out of a total of 62 samples were glomerulus from the non-neoplastic part of tumor nephrectomies and 41 of them were from DN. The results of the both models statistically were not divided the normal and disease groups (*p*-value > 0.05; Figure 7D). It indicated that models for predicting kidney prognosis with urine protein markers in diabetics are difficult to distinguish DKD from normal groups by mRNA expression level in kidney.

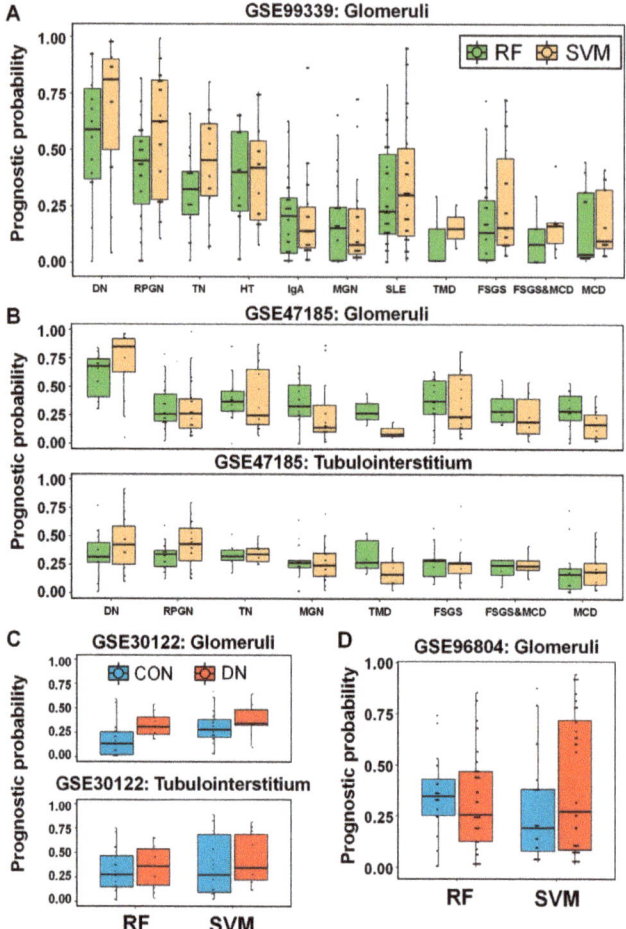

Figure 7. External validation of RF and SVM clinical models in public four GEO datasets (GSE99339, GSE47185, GSE30122 and GSE96804). (**A**) In the GSE99339 dataset, boxplot of the prognostic probabilities of the two classifiers in 11 disease groups including DN ($N = 14$), RPGN ($N = 23$), TN ($N = 14$), HT ($N = 15$), IgA nephropathy ($N = 26$), MGN ($N = 21$), SLE ($N = 30$), TMD ($N = 3$), FSGS ($N = 22$), FSGS&MCD ($N = 6$), and MCD ($N = 13$). (**B**) In the GSE30122 data set, the prognostic indexes of the two classifiers in the eight disease groups in the renal glomeruli with DN ($N = 14$), RPGN, ($N = 23$), TN ($N = 17$), MGN ($N = 21$), TMD ($N = 3$), FSGS ($N = 23$), FSGS&MCD ($N = 6$), and MCD ($N = 15$) and in the renal tubulointerstitia with DN ($N = 18$), RPGN ($N = 21$), TN ($N = 6$), MGN ($N = 18$), TMD ($N = 6$), FSGS ($N = 13$), FSGS&MCD ($N = 4$), and MCD ($N = 15$). (**C**) In the GSE30122 data set, the prediction values of the two classifiers in the control and disease groups in renal glomerulus ($N = 26$; control and $N = 9$; disease) and in renal tubulus ($N = 24$; control and $N = 10$; disease). (**D**) In the GSE30122 data set, the prediction probabilities of the two classifiers in the control ($N = 20$) and disease ($N = 41$) groups in renal glomeruli.

3. Discussion

Urine-based approaches for measuring internal biomolecules can be normalized. Ideally, urine should be collected for 24 h and urinary biomolecules measured. Because this method is practically difficult, urinary proteins in random spot samples were calibrated relative to creatinine concentrations [9]. Prolonged storage of urine samples for studying proteins is important because of the activity of urinary proteases depending on the temperature and pH [27]. In this retrospective study, urine samples were stored at −80 °C for 7–8 years before LC-MS/MS measurements. In general, it is known that it is stable without urine preservatives stored at −70 or −80 °C, and urine samples stored for more than 2.3 years have no significant change in not only most proteins including albumin but also metabolites including creatinine [28–31].

Proteins were extracted from urine samples using an equal volume-based approach similar to ELISA [32]. This procedure for protein standardization was suitable for downstream analysis. Urinary proteins normalized by this method showed lower sample-to-sample variation and higher correlation with immunoassay results.

Albuminuria is primarily used to detect DKD in clinical practice [2,5]. Because glomeruli filter blood, albumin is a good biomarker of chronic kidney disease (CKD) caused by glomerular abnormalities but is insufficient to determine subsequent prognosis [5]. Rather than this, it was determined that finding and measuring specific protein markers that affect pathological function is more clinically meaningful [33,34]. Although causality between albuminuria and prognostic values from the five-protein panel-based clinical models (RF and SVM) cannot be clarified in this retrospective study, it can be inferred by correlation analysis. Correlation analysis between two classifiers and ACR in the 54 enrolled patients reveals a little of bit correlation but no significance ($r = 0.086$; p-value > 0.05; SVM and $r = 0.094$; p-value > 0.05; RF). Therefore, it was confirmed that there was no causal relationship as well as a correlation. To consider closely at the relationship between them, we divided the three classes based on the ACR value (normal; <30 mg/g, microalbuminuria; 30–300 mg/g and macroalbuminuria; >300 mg/g) and plotted the predicted values of the SVM model according to the two prognostic groups (Figure S1). In T2D patients with normal range and microalbuminuria, SVM results were almost separated between two groups. Rather, it seems to have problems with predictive power in patients with macroalbuminuria. It means that SVM results did not depend on the development of albuminuria in T2D patients and showed the possibility to predict the earlier disease stage before the development of albuminuria. Moreover, the predicted value of RF results accurately separates two prognostic groups regardless of the ACR value.

As a rule, diabetics are persistently exposed to miscellaneous metabolic and hemodynamic risks [35], with DKD resulting from multiple pathophysiological processes. Multiple-biomarker approaches using proteomics and metabolomics may better reveal the complicated disease status thought to be associated with the onset of DKD [4,8]. CKD273, a panel consisting of 273 urinary peptides currently undergoing Phase 3 testing, was a high performance urine peptidomic classifier for CKD diagnosis [36]. Moreover, this classifier was recently validated as a predictor of the development of microalbuminuria in normoalbuminuric with diabetic patients [37]. These 273 intact peptides were derived from 30 independent proteins, 24 of which were quantified in this study. CKD273, which includes cleaved collagenase peptides and SERPINA1 peptides, is a good prognostic marker, showing that the concentrations of cleaved collagenase peptides decrease and those of SERPINA1 peptides increase in the urine of patients with CKD [38,39]. The present study showed a similar pattern of abundance in the urine of PPG patients despite artificial digestion. Our approach, based on protein concentrations in urine samples, could better explain the pathological pathway associated with DKD than the peptidome approach. Indicators of kidney dysfunction include increased blood particles in urine; lysosomal dysfunction in glomerular cells [40], which is related to the autophagy-lysosome pathway [41] abnormal heterotypic cell–cell adhesion among glomerular, tubular, and immune cell compartments, collagenase, and binding proteins (driven by rapid changes in glycolipids) [42] and platelet activation [43].

Our clinical models consist of five selected proteins, four proteins (CTSA, MUC1, GM2A, and SPARCL1) are high in PPG and other one protein (ACP2) is low in PPG. Cystatin A (CTSA), in the same protein family as cystatin C that can measure kidney function [44–46], has been found in our urinary biomarker discovery study. Muc1 is a multifaceted tumor protein, and its relationship with the kidney has recently been highlighted [47] and has been identified as a mutant that causes mendelian disorder medullary cystic kidney disease type 1 [48]. In a meta-analysis study of rat glomerular transcriptome profiling, it was confirmed that GM2A was highly expressed in various diabetic kidney disease rat [49]. Through the mouse kidney injury model experiment, SPARCL1 showed that mRNA expression was not changed in the acute phase, but the expression level was high in the fibrosis of the kidney [50], and it inhibited the movement and invasion of renal cell carcinoma [51]. Lastly, ACP 2, one of the lysosomal enzymes, is a protein used in peptiduria [52] or lysosomal enzymuria [53] that measures kidney disease in diabetic patients. Through the external kidney mRNA published studies, these urine biomarkers we found confirmed differential expression in kidney tissue with DKD.

This study had several limitations. First, the patient population in this study was homogeneous and of small sample size. These results require further validation in a multiethnic cohort including larger numbers of patients to assess applicability to a wider population with T2D, a study currently in progress. Second, DKD was clinically diagnosed in the absence of renal biopsies. Third, it is unclear which organ is derived from the urinary protein signatures. More research is needed to determine whether urinary protein signatures are biomarkers of tubular damage in pathological conditions with a glomerular protein load.

4. Materials and Methods

4.1. Patients and Urine Samples

Urine samples were collected from 54 outpatients with T2D and eGFR ≥ 60 mL/min/1.72 m^2 who were enrolled in the DKD study at Pusan National University Hospital, South Korea, from February 2010 to January 2011 and who met previously described inclusion and exclusion criteria [54]. After one year, patients were followed-up with until September 2017. Patients were managed according to standard guidelines, including treatment with RAS inhibitors, and eGFR was measured at least twice during a follow-up period ≥12 months. Renal function decline was defined as an eGFR < 60 mL/min/1.72 m^2, annual eGFR reduction > 3 mL/min/1.72 m^2, or CKD progression, defined as a reduction in GFR category, accompanied by a ≥ 25% deterioration in eGFR from baseline. The patients were divided into two groups—19 with renal outcomes (poor prognosis group (PPG)) and 35 without renal outcomes (good prognosis group (GPG)). The protocols and consent procedures were approved by the Institutional Review Board of Pusan National University Hospital (approval No. 2013033). Total proteinuria and albuminuria, as well as creatinine concentrations, were measured in random spot urine samples [55].

4.2. Measurements of Nephrology Parameters

eGFR was calculated using the equation eGFR = 141 × min (serum creatinine/kappa, 1) alpha × max (serum creatinine/kappa, 1) − 1.209 × 0.993 × age × sex × race. For females, sex = 1.018; alpha = −0.329; and kappa = 0.7; for males, sex = 1; alpha = −0.411; and kappa = 0.9. Renal outcomes were chronic kidney disease (CKD) progression based on guidelines of the International Society of Nephrology; accelerated eGFR decline, defined as an annual eGFR reduction > 3 mL/min/1.72 m^2; or the development of CKD stage ≥ 3. CKD stages 1, 2, 3a, 3b, 4, and 5 were defined as eGFRs of ≥ 90, 60–89, 45–59, 30–44, 15–29, and < 15 mL/min/1.73 m^2, respectively, and CKD progression was defined as a decline in eGFR category accompanied by a ≥ 25% deterioration in eGFR from baseline [56].

4.3. Urinary Protein Sample Preparation

Urine samples were centrifuged at 13,000 rpm for 30 min to remove debris, and 300 μL of each supernatant was mixed with 100 μL High Select™ HSA/Immunoglobulin Depletion Resin (Cat. No:

A36368, Thermo Fisher Scientific, Waltham, MA, USA) and incubated for 1 h at 4 °C to remove albumin and immunoglobulin. Following centrifugation at 13,000 rpm for 10 min, the supernatant was dried using a speed vac with a cold trap (CentriVap Cold Traps, Labconco, Kansas City, MO, USA).

4.4. Enzymatic Digestion in-Solution

Each dried urine sample was dissolved in 100 µL of 8 M urea, reduced with 20 mM dithiothreitol in 50 mM NH_4HCO_3 for 60 min at 25 °C, and alkylated with 40 mM iodoacetamide in 50 mM NH4HCO3 for 60 min in the dark. Urea concentration was diluted to less than 1.0 M. Each urine sample was incubated overnight at 37 °C with 12.5 µg sequencing grade modified trypsin/LysC (Promega, Madison, WI, USA) in 50 mM NH4HCO3 buffer (pH 7.8), followed by quenching with 10uL of 5% formic acid and lyophilization with a cold trap. The samples were re-suspended in 0.1% formic acid, desalted using C18 ZipTips (Millipore, Burlington, MA, USA), and dried for LC-MS analysis.

4.5. Nano-LC-ESI-MS/MS Analysis

Digested peptides were separated using a Dionex UltiMate 3000 RSLCnano system (Thermo Fisher Scientific, Waltham, MA, USA). Tryptic peptides from the bead column were reconstituted in 100 µL of 0.1% formic acid and separated on an Acclaim™ Pepmap 100 C18 column (500 mm × 75 µm i.d., 3 µm, 100 Å) equipped with a C18 Pepmap trap column (20 mm × 100 µm i.d., 5 µm, 100 Å; Thermo Fisher Scientific, Waltham, MA, USA) over 200 min (250 nL/min) using a 0–48% acetonitrile gradient in 0.1% formic acid and 5% DMSO for 150 min at 50 °C. The LC was coupled to a Q Exactive™ Plus Hybrid Quadrupole-Orbitrap™ mass spectrometer with a nano-ESI source. Mass spectra were acquired in a data-dependent mode with an automatic switch between a full scan and 10 data-dependent MS/MS scans. The target value for the full scan MS spectra, selected from a 350 to 1800 m/z, was 3,000,000 with a maximum injection time of 50 ms and a resolution of 70,000 at m/z 400. The selected ions were fragmented by higher-energy collisional dissociation in the following parameters: 2 Da precursor ion isolation window and 27% normalized collision energy. The ion target value for MS/MS was set to 1,000,000 with a maximum injection time of 100 ms and a resolution of 17,500 at m/z 400. Repeated peptides were dynamically excluded for 20 s. All MS data were measured once per sample and have been deposited in the PRIDE archive (www.ebi.ac.uk/pride/archive/projects/PXD016571) [57] under Project 1-20191129-77373 12.

4.6. Database Searching and Label-Free Quantitation

The SwissProt human database (May 2017) was searched for acquired MS/MS spectra using SequestHT on Proteome discoverer (version 2.2, Thermo Fisher Scientific, USA) [58]. The search parameters were set as default including cysteine carbamidomethylation as a fixed modification, and N-terminal acetylation and methionine oxidation as variable modifications with two miscleavages. Peptides were identified based on a search with an initial mass deviation of the precursor ion of up to 10 ppm, with the allowed fragment mass deviation set to 20 ppm. When assigning proteins to peptides, both unique and razor peptides were used. Label-free quantitation (LFQ) was performed using peak intensity for unique peptides of each protein.

4.7. Normalization of Protein Abundance

To correct for sampling variations resulting from random spot urine collection, the raw LFQ values for each protein were divided by the amounts of total protein and creatinine in each sample, followed by normalization of the corrected LFQ values by endogenous proteins without spike-in standards [59]. To identify endogenous urinary proteins for normalization, the 112 initial completely quantified proteins were considered, with six selected based on the following criteria: (1) quantified in all 54 samples; (2) corrected LFQ values did not differ significantly in the poor and good prognosis groups by the Mann–Whitney U Test (p-value > 0.05); and (3) had nearly persistent urine concentrations throughout the sample as top-ranked by NormFinder stability value [60].

The corrected LFQ values of the six selected normalization proteins in each sample were divided by their median value in all samples. The median of these six ratios was defined as the normalization scaling factor (NSF) for that sample. For example, NSF for sample s can be determined using the equation:

$$NSF_s = median\left(\frac{N_{1,s}}{\hat{N}_1}, \frac{N_{2,s}}{\hat{N}_2}, \cdots, \frac{N_{6,s}}{\hat{N}_6}\right) \quad (1)$$

where $N_{i,s}$ is the corrected LFQ value of normalization protein i in sample s and $\hat{N}_i$ is the median corrected LFQ value of normalization protein i in all samples. Except for the six normalization proteins in a sample, the normalized LFQ value of each protein was calculated by dividing its corrected LFQ value by NSF.

$$L\check{F}Q_{j,s} = \frac{LFQ_{j,s}}{NSF_s} \quad (2)$$

where $L\check{F}Q_{j,s}$ is the normalized LFQ of urinary protein j in sample s and $LFQ_{j,s}$ is the corrected LFQ of the corresponding protein [61].

4.8. Differential Data Analysis by Filling Missing Data

For clinical utility, the LFQ data were filtered to <20% of quantified proteins in each sample group to analyze the differential urinary proteins in these groups, with the missing data filled by the local least squared imputation method at the normalized abundance [18].

4.9. GO Analysis

Differential abundant proteins (DAPs) in the poor and good prognosis groups were analyzed using the ClueGO (version 2.5.1) [12] plugin for Cytoscape (version 3.6.1) [62]. To group GO terms, the kappa score was set at 0.4 and the number of overlapping genes to combine groups was set at 50%.

4.10. Statistical Clinical Model Generation Based on Feature Selection

The process of feature selection was to find the best subset for classifying two disease progression groups out of 412 proteins. There are two steps. In the first step, 50,000 decision trees containing eight variables were randomly generated 50,000 trees and had AUC values. Based on the AUCs values, the optimal number of proteins were determined by out-of-bag error estimation and the value is 11. Second, through the 100 iterations with three-fold cross-validation for from the selected 11 optimal variables, the probability and importance that each variable was included in the model was calculated. We selected five proteins (>0.3 importance). Prior to model building, centering and scaling were performed as preprocessing on the data. In the clinical models, SVM model with linear kernel was generated by a 10 repeated three-fold cross validation method (parameter C = 0.1052) and The RF model was made by a three-fold cross validation method repeated 100 times with 1000 trees, mtry = 5 and nodesize = 5.

4.11. Mining Public Microarray Data

We downloaded the mRNA expression data (series accession number: GSE99339, GSE47185, GSE30122, and GSE96804) in the Gene Expression Omnibus database [63]. Then, using GEO2R interactive web tool, five identifiers matching the five selected genes according to the platform record and their expression values were extracted.

4.12. Statistical Analysis

Data were analyzed using RStudio (version 1.1.456) including R (version 3.6.0). Statistical R software packages included ggplot2 for drawing box, scattering, volcano and violin plots, permcor for calculating permutation-based *p*-values for Pearson correlation [64], pcaMethods for missing value estimation [65], pROC for univariate ROC analysis [66], ROCR for multivariate ROC analysis,

AUCRF for feature selection [21], caret for building statistical classifiers [67], randomForest for building a RF classifier, and e1071 for building a SVM classifier.

5. Conclusions

These results suggest that measurement of urinary proteome was more promising than albuminuria alone for predicting renal outcomes in patients with type 2 diabetes. A panel of five proteins had the potential for use as a biomarker in clinical practice.

Supplementary Materials: Supplementary materials can be found at http://www.mdpi.com/1422-0067/21/12/4236/s1. Figure S1. Prognostic probability of 54 patients by RF and SVM classifier divided into three groups by albumin-to-creatinine ratio.; Table S1. Demographic and clinical characteristics of the 54 patients with type 2 diabetes.; Table S2. Search result of MS/MS spectra of protein sequences obtained from the 54 urine samples in the Human Swissprot proteome database using the SequestHT search engine.; Table S3. Results of volcano plot analysis.; Table S4. Normalized abundance of 412 urinary proteins in the 54 patients with type 2 diabetes.; Table S5. Univariate receiver operating curve analysis of the areas under the curves of 412 urinary proteins.; Table S6. Prognostic probability by RF and SVM classifier of 54 patients.

Author Contributions: Conceptualization, J.H.K., S.H.S., S.S.K., I.J.K., and K.K.; methodology, H.J.; formal analysis, H.-S.A.; investigation, J.Y. (Jiyoung Yu); data curation, H.-S.A., S.S.K., and I.J.K.; writing—original draft preparation, H.-S.A. and K.K.; writing—review and editing, J.H.K., J.Y. (Jiyoung Yu), J.Y. (Jeonghun Yeom), S.H.S., S.S.K., and I.J.K; visualization, H.-S.A.; supervision, I.J.K and K.K.; funding acquisition, J.H.K. All authors have read and agreed to the published version of the manuscript.

Funding: This research was funded by a Biomedical Research Institute Grant (2017-20) from Pusan National University Hospital.

Acknowledgments: The authors thank the Department of Biostatistics, Clinical Trial Center, Biomedical Research Institute, Pusan National University Hospital.

Conflicts of Interest: The authors declare no conflict of interest.

Abbreviations

T2D	Type 2 diabetes
eGFR	Estimated glomerular filtration rate
DKD	Diabetic kidney disease
BMI	Body mass index
SBP	Systolic blood pressure
HbA1c	Glycated hemoglobin concentration
LDL	Low-density lipoprotein
HDL	High-density lipoprotein
ACR	Albumin-to-creatinine ratio
NAPCR	Nonalbumin protein-to-creatinine ratio
PCR	Urine protein-to-creatinine ratio
GPG	Good-prognostic group
PPG	Poor-prognostic group
LC-MS	Liquid chromatography–mass spectrometry
DAP	Differential abundant protein
GO	Gene ontology
FDR	False discovery rate
ROC	Receiver operating characteristic
AUC	Area under the receiver operating characteristic curve
RF	Random forest
SVM	Support vector machine
ELISA	Enzyme-linked immunosorbent assay
CKD	Chronic kidney disease
MS/MS	Tandem mass spectrometry
LFQ	Label-free quantitation
NSF	Normalization scaling factor

DN	Diabetic nephropathy
FSGS	Focal and segmental glomerulosclerosis
FSGS&MCD	Focal and segmental glomerulosclerosis and minimal change disease
HT	Hypertensive nephropathy
MCD	Minimal change disease
MGN	Membranous glomerulonephritis
RPGN	Rapidly progressive glomerulonephritis
SLE	Systemic lupus erythematosus
TMD	Thin membrane disease
TN	Tumor nephrectomies

References

1. Ahn, J.H.; Yu, J.H.; Ko, S.H.; Kwon, H.S.; Kim, D.J.; Kim, J.H.; Kim, C.S.; Song, K.H.; Won, J.C.; Lim, S.; et al. Prevalence and determinants of diabetic nephropathy in Korea: Korea national health and nutrition examination survey. *Diabetes Metab. J.* **2014**, *38*, 109–119. [CrossRef]
2. Tuttle, K.R.; Bakris, G.L.; Bilous, R.W.; Chiang, J.L.; de Boer, I.H.; Goldstein-Fuchs, J.; Hirsch, I.B.; Kalantar-Zadeh, K.; Narva, A.S.; Navaneethan, S.D.; et al. Diabetic kidney disease: A report from an ADA Consensus Conference. *Diabetes Care* **2014**, *37*, 2864–2883. [CrossRef] [PubMed]
3. Collins, A.J.; Foley, R.N.; Chavers, B.; Gilbertson, D.; Herzog, C.; Johansen, K.; Kasiske, B.; Kutner, N.; Liu, J.; St Peter, W.; et al. United States Renal Data System 2011 Annual Data Report: Atlas of chronic kidney disease & end-stage renal disease in the United States. *Am. J. Kidney Dis.* **2012**, *59*, A7. [CrossRef] [PubMed]
4. Currie, G.; Delles, C. Urinary Proteomics for Diagnosis and Monitoring of Diabetic Nephropathy. *Curr. Diabetes Rep.* **2016**, *16*, 104. [CrossRef] [PubMed]
5. KDIGO Working Group. KDIGO clinical practice guideline for the evaluation and management of chronic kidney disease. Chapter 2: Definition, identification, and prediction of CKD progression. *Kidney Int. Suppl.* **2013**, *3*, 63–72. [CrossRef]
6. Barratt, J.; Topham, P. Urine proteomics: The present and future of measuring urinary protein components in disease. *CMAJ* **2007**, *177*, 361–368. [CrossRef] [PubMed]
7. Retnakaran, R.; Cull, C.A.; Thorne, K.I.; Adler, A.I.; Holman, R.R.; Group, U.S. Risk factors for renal dysfunction in type 2 diabetes: U.K. Prospective Diabetes Study 74. *Diabetes* **2006**, *55*, 1832–1839. [CrossRef] [PubMed]
8. Kamijo-Ikemori, A.; Sugaya, T.; Kimura, K. Novel urinary biomarkers in early diabetic kidney disease. *Curr. Diabetes Rep.* **2014**, *14*, 513. [CrossRef]
9. Abitbol, C.; Zilleruelo, G.; Freundlich, M.; Strauss, J. Quantitation of proteinuria with urinary protein/creatinine ratios and random testing with dipsticks in nephrotic children. *J. Pediatr.* **1990**, *116*, 243–247. [CrossRef]
10. Lemann, J., Jr.; Doumas, B.T. Proteinuria in health and disease assessed by measuring the urinary protein/creatinine ratio. *Clin. Chem.* **1987**, *33*, 297–299. [CrossRef]
11. Zhao, M.; Li, M.; Yang, Y.; Guo, Z.; Sun, Y.; Shao, C.; Li, M.; Sun, W.; Gao, Y. A comprehensive analysis and annotation of human normal urinary proteome. *Sci. Rep.* **2017**, *7*, 3024. [CrossRef] [PubMed]
12. Bindea, G.; Mlecnik, B.; Hackl, H.; Charoentong, P.; Tosolini, M.; Kirilovsky, A.; Fridman, W.H.; Pages, F.; Trajanoski, Z.; Galon, J. ClueGO: A Cytoscape plug-in to decipher functionally grouped gene ontology and pathway annotation networks. *Bioinformatics* **2009**, *25*, 1091–1093. [CrossRef] [PubMed]
13. Van Bladel, E.R.; de Jager, R.L.; Walter, D.; Cornelissen, L.; Gaillard, C.A.; Boven, L.A.; Roest, M.; Fijnheer, R. Platelets of patients with chronic kidney disease demonstrate deficient platelet reactivity in vitro. *BMC Nephrol.* **2012**, *13*, 127. [CrossRef] [PubMed]
14. Prozialeck, W.C.; Edwards, J.R. Cell adhesion molecules in chemically-induced renal injury. *Pharmacol. Ther.* **2007**, *114*, 74–93. [CrossRef]
15. Yan, J.; Zhang, Z.; Jia, L.; Wang, Y. Role of Bone Marrow-Derived Fibroblasts in Renal Fibrosis. *Front. Physiol.* **2016**, *7*, 61. [CrossRef]

16. Deva, R.; Alias, M.A.; Colville, D.; Tow, F.K.; Ooi, Q.L.; Chew, S.; Mohamad, N.; Hutchinson, A.; Koukouras, I.; Power, D.A.; et al. Vision-threatening retinal abnormalities in chronic kidney disease stages 3 to 5. *Clin. J. Am. Soc. Nephrol.* **2011**, *6*, 1866–1871. [CrossRef]
17. Dziura, J.D.; Post, L.A.; Zhao, Q.; Fu, Z.; Peduzzi, P. Strategies for dealing with missing data in clinical trials: From design to analysis. *Yale J. Biol. Med.* **2013**, *86*, 343–358.
18. Karpievitch, Y.V.; Dabney, A.R.; Smith, R.D. Normalization and missing value imputation for label-free LC-MS analysis. *BMC Bioinform.* **2012**, *13* (Suppl. 16), S5. [CrossRef]
19. Breiman, L. Random forests. *Mach Learn* **2001**, *45*, 5–32. [CrossRef]
20. Cortes, C.; Vapnik, V. Support-Vector Networks. *Mach. Learn.* **1995**, *20*, 273–297. [CrossRef]
21. Calle, M.L.; Urrea, V.; Boulesteix, A.L.; Malats, N. AUC-RF: A new strategy for genomic profiling with random forest. *Hum. Hered.* **2011**, *72*, 121–132. [CrossRef] [PubMed]
22. Shved, N.; Warsow, G.; Eichinger, F.; Hoogewijs, D.; Brandt, S.; Wild, P.; Kretzler, M.; Cohen, C.D.; Lindenmeyer, M.T. Transcriptome-based network analysis reveals renal cell type-specific dysregulation of hypoxia-associated transcripts. *Sci. Rep.* **2017**, *7*, 8576. [CrossRef] [PubMed]
23. Ju, W.; Greene, C.S.; Eichinger, F.; Nair, V.; Hodgin, J.B.; Bitzer, M.; Lee, Y.S.; Zhu, Q.; Kehata, M.; Li, M.; et al. Defining cell-type specificity at the transcriptional level in human disease. *Genome Res.* **2013**, *23*, 1862–1873. [CrossRef] [PubMed]
24. Woroniecka, K.I.; Park, A.S.; Mohtat, D.; Thomas, D.B.; Pullman, J.M.; Susztak, K. Transcriptome analysis of human diabetic kidney disease. *Diabetes* **2011**, *60*, 2354–2369. [CrossRef] [PubMed]
25. Shi, J.S.; Qiu, D.D.; Le, W.B.; Wang, H.; Li, S.; Lu, Y.H.; Jiang, S. Identification of Transcription Regulatory Relationships in Diabetic Nephropathy. *Chin. Med. J.* **2018**, *131*, 2886–2890. [CrossRef] [PubMed]
26. Pan, Y.; Jiang, S.; Hou, Q.; Qiu, D.; Shi, J.; Wang, L.; Chen, Z.; Zhang, M.; Duan, A.; Qin, W.; et al. Dissection of Glomerular Transcriptional Profile in Patients With Diabetic Nephropathy: SRGAP2a Protects Podocyte Structure and Function. *Diabetes* **2018**, *67*, 717–730. [CrossRef]
27. Kania, K.; Byrnes, E.A.; Beilby, J.P.; Webb, S.A.; Strong, K.J. Urinary proteases degrade albumin: Implications for measurement of albuminuria in stored samples. *Ann. Clin. Biochem.* **2010**, *47*, 151–157. [CrossRef]
28. Parekh, R.S.; Kao, W.H.; Meoni, L.A.; Ipp, E.; Kimmel, P.L.; La Page, J.; Fondran, C.; Knowler, W.C.; Klag, M.J.; Family Investigation of Nephropathy and Diabetes; et al. Reliability of urinary albumin, total protein, and creatinine assays after prolonged storage: The Family Investigation of Nephropathy and Diabetes. *Clin. J. Am. Soc. Nephrol.* **2007**, *2*, 1156–1162. [CrossRef]
29. Chapman, D.P.; Gooding, K.M.; McDonald, T.J.; Shore, A.C. Stability of urinary albumin and creatinine after 12 months storage at −20 degrees C and −80 degrees C. *Pract. Lab. Med.* **2019**, *15*, e00120. [CrossRef]
30. Herrington, W.; Illingworth, N.; Staplin, N.; Kumar, A.; Storey, B.; Hrusecka, R.; Judge, P.; Mahmood, M.; Parish, S.; Landray, M.; et al. Effect of Processing Delay and Storage Conditions on Urine Albumin-to-Creatinine Ratio. *Clin. J. Am. Soc. Nephrol.* **2016**, *11*, 1794–1801. [CrossRef]
31. Klasen, I.S.; Reichert, L.J.; de Kat Angelino, C.M.; Wetzels, J.F. Quantitative determination of low and high molecular weight proteins in human urine: Influence of temperature and storage time. *Clin. Chem.* **1999**, *45*, 430–432. [CrossRef] [PubMed]
32. Voller, A.; Bartlett, A.; Bidwell, D.E. Enzyme immunoassays with special reference to ELISA techniques. *J. Clin. Pathol.* **1978**, *31*, 507–520. [CrossRef] [PubMed]
33. Frantzi, M.; Bhat, A.; Latosinska, A. Clinical proteomic biomarkers: Relevant issues on study design & technical considerations in biomarker development. *Clin. Transl. Med.* **2014**, *3*, 7. [CrossRef] [PubMed]
34. Borrebaeck, C.A. Precision diagnostics: Moving towards protein biomarker signatures of clinical utility in cancer. *Nat. Rev. Cancer* **2017**, *17*, 199–204. [CrossRef]
35. Thomas, M.C.; Burns, W.C.; Cooper, M.E. Tubular changes in early diabetic nephropathy. *Adv. Chronic Kidney Dis.* **2005**, *12*, 177–186. [CrossRef]
36. Good, D.M.; Zurbig, P.; Argiles, A.; Bauer, H.W.; Behrens, G.; Coon, J.J.; Dakna, M.; Decramer, S.; Delles, C.; Dominiczak, A.F.; et al. Naturally occurring human urinary peptides for use in diagnosis of chronic kidney disease. *Mol. Cell. Proteomics* **2010**, *9*, 2424–2437. [CrossRef]
37. Lindhardt, M.; Persson, F.; Zurbig, P.; Stalmach, A.; Mischak, H.; de Zeeuw, D.; Lambers Heerspink, H.; Klein, R.; Orchard, T.; Porta, M.; et al. Urinary proteomics predict onset of microalbuminuria in normoalbuminuric type 2 diabetic patients, a sub-study of the DIRECT-Protect 2 study. *Nephrol. Dial. Transplant.* **2017**, *32*, 1866–1873. [CrossRef]

38. Rodriguez-Ortiz, M.E.; Pontillo, C.; Rodriguez, M.; Zurbig, P.; Mischak, H.; Ortiz, A. Novel Urinary Biomarkers For Improved Prediction Of Progressive Egfr Loss In Early Chronic Kidney Disease Stages And In High Risk Individuals Without Chronic Kidney Disease. *Sci. Rep.* **2018**, *8*, 15940. [CrossRef]
39. Pontillo, C.; Mischak, H. Urinary peptide-based classifier CKD273: Towards clinical application in chronic kidney disease. *Clin. Kidney J.* **2017**, *10*, 192–201. [CrossRef] [PubMed]
40. Surendran, K.; Vitiello, S.P.; Pearce, D.A. Lysosome dysfunction in the pathogenesis of kidney diseases. *Pediatr. Nephrol.* **2014**, *29*, 2253–2261. [CrossRef] [PubMed]
41. Liu, W.J.; Shen, T.T.; Chen, R.H.; Wu, H.L.; Wang, Y.J.; Deng, J.K.; Chen, Q.H.; Pan, Q.; Huang Fu, C.M.; Tao, J.L.; et al. Autophagy-Lysosome Pathway in Renal Tubular Epithelial Cells Is Disrupted by Advanced Glycation End Products in Diabetic Nephropathy. *J. Biol. Chem.* **2015**, *290*, 20499–20510. [CrossRef]
42. Rops, A.L.; van der Vlag, J.; Lensen, J.F.; Wijnhoven, T.J.; van den Heuvel, L.P.; van Kuppevelt, T.H.; Berden, J.H. Heparan sulfate proteoglycans in glomerular inflammation. *Kidney Int.* **2004**, *65*, 768–785. [CrossRef] [PubMed]
43. Landray, M.J.; Wheeler, D.C.; Lip, G.Y.; Newman, D.J.; Blann, A.D.; McGlynn, F.J.; Ball, S.; Townend, J.N.; Baigent, C. Inflammation, endothelial dysfunction, and platelet activation in patients with chronic kidney disease: The chronic renal impairment in Birmingham (CRIB) study. *Am. J. Kidney Dis.* **2004**, *43*, 244–253. [CrossRef] [PubMed]
44. Shlipak, M.G.; Matsushita, K.; Arnlov, J.; Inker, L.A.; Katz, R.; Polkinghorne, K.R.; Rothenbacher, D.; Sarnak, M.J.; Astor, B.C.; Coresh, J.; et al. Cystatin C versus creatinine in determining risk based on kidney function. *N. Engl. J. Med.* **2013**, *369*, 932–943. [CrossRef]
45. Inker, L.A.; Schmid, C.H.; Tighiouart, H.; Eckfeldt, J.H.; Feldman, H.I.; Greene, T.; Kusek, J.W.; Manzi, J.; Van Lente, F.; Zhang, Y.L.; et al. Estimating glomerular filtration rate from serum creatinine and cystatin C. *N. Engl. J. Med.* **2012**, *367*, 20–29. [CrossRef] [PubMed]
46. Ingelfinger, J.R.; Marsden, P.A. Estimated GFR and risk of death–is cystatin C useful? *N. Engl. J. Med.* **2013**, *369*, 974–975. [CrossRef] [PubMed]
47. Al-Bataineh, M.M.; Sutton, T.A.; Hughey, R.P. Novel roles for mucin 1 in the kidney. *Curr. Opin. Nephrol. Hypertens.* **2017**, *26*, 384–391. [CrossRef]
48. Kirby, A.; Gnirke, A.; Jaffe, D.B.; Baresova, V.; Pochet, N.; Blumenstiel, B.; Ye, C.; Aird, D.; Stevens, C.; Robinson, J.T.; et al. Mutations causing medullary cystic kidney disease type 1 lie in a large VNTR in MUC1 missed by massively parallel sequencing. *Nat. Genet.* **2013**, *45*, 299–303. [CrossRef]
49. Tryggvason, S.H.; Guo, J.; Nukui, M.; Norlin, J.; Haraldsson, B.; Jornvall, H.; Tryggvason, K.; He, L. A meta-analysis of expression signatures in glomerular disease. *Kidney Int.* **2013**, *84*, 591–599. [CrossRef]
50. Feng, D.; Ngov, C.; Henley, N.; Boufaied, N.; Gerarduzzi, C. Characterization of Matricellular Protein Expression Signatures in Mechanistically Diverse Mouse Models of Kidney Injury. *Sci. Rep.* **2019**, *9*, 16736. [CrossRef]
51. Ye, H.; Wang, W.G.; Cao, J.; Hu, X.C. SPARCL1 suppresses cell migration and invasion in renal cell carcinoma. *Mol. Med. Rep.* **2017**, *16*, 7784–7790. [CrossRef] [PubMed]
52. Gudehithlu, K.P.; Hart, P.D.; Vernik, J.; Sethupathi, P.; Dunea, G.; Arruda, J.A.L.; Singh, A.K. Peptiduria: A potential early predictor of diabetic kidney disease. *Clin. Exp. Nephrol.* **2019**, *23*, 56–64. [CrossRef]
53. Gatsing, D.; Garba, I.H.; Adoga, G.I. The use of lysosomal enzymuria in the early detection and monitoring of the progression of diabetic nephropathy. *Indian J. Clin. Biochem.* **2006**, *21*, 42–48. [CrossRef]
54. Kim, S.S.; Song, S.H.; Kim, I.J.; Yang, J.Y.; Lee, J.G.; Kwak, I.S.; Kim, Y.K. Clinical implication of urinary tubular markers in the early stage of nephropathy with type 2 diabetic patients. *Diabetes Res. Clin. Pract.* **2012**, *97*, 251–257. [CrossRef] [PubMed]
55. Lane, C.; Brown, M.; Dunsmuir, W.; Kelly, J.; Mangos, G. Can spot urine protein/creatinine ratio replace 24 h urine protein in usual clinical nephrology? *Nephrology* **2006**, *11*, 245–249. [CrossRef] [PubMed]
56. Summary of Recommendation Statements. *Kidney Int* **2013**, *3*, 5–14. [CrossRef] [PubMed]
57. Deutsch, E.W.; Bandeira, N.; Sharma, V.; Perez-Riverol, Y.; Carver, J.J.; Kundu, D.J.; Garcia-Seisdedos, D.; Jarnuczak, A.F.; Hewapathirana, S.; Pullman, B.S.; et al. The ProteomeXchange consortium in 2020: Enabling 'big data' approaches in proteomics. *Nucleic Acids Res.* **2019**. [CrossRef] [PubMed]
58. The UniProt Consortium. UniProt: The universal protein knowledgebase. *Nucleic Acids Res.* **2017**, *45*, D158–D169. [CrossRef]

59. Wisniewski, J.R.; Hein, M.Y.; Cox, J.; Mann, M. A "proteomic ruler" for protein copy number and concentration estimation without spike-in standards. *Mol. Cell. Proteomics* **2014**, *13*, 3497–3506. [CrossRef]
60. Andersen, C.L.; Jensen, J.L.; Orntoft, T.F. Normalization of real-time quantitative reverse transcription-PCR data: A model-based variance estimation approach to identify genes suited for normalization, applied to bladder and colon cancer data sets. *Cancer Res.* **2004**, *64*, 5245–5250. [CrossRef] [PubMed]
61. Ahn, H.S.; Sohn, T.S.; Kim, M.J.; Cho, B.K.; Kim, S.M.; Kim, S.T.; Yi, E.C.; Lee, C. SEPROGADIC—Serum protein-based gastric cancer prediction model for prognosis and selection of proper adjuvant therapy. *Sci. Rep.* **2018**, *8*, 16892. [CrossRef] [PubMed]
62. Saito, R.; Smoot, M.E.; Ono, K.; Ruscheinski, J.; Wang, P.L.; Lotia, S.; Pico, A.R.; Bader, G.D.; Ideker, T. A travel guide to Cytoscape plugins. *Nat. Methods* **2012**, *9*, 1069–1076. [CrossRef] [PubMed]
63. Barrett, T.; Edgar, R. Gene expression omnibus: Microarray data storage, submission, retrieval, and analysis. *Methods Enzymol.* **2006**, *411*, 352–369. [CrossRef] [PubMed]
64. Legendre, P. Comparison of permutation methods for the partial correlation and partial Mantel tests. *J Stat Comput. Sim.* **2000**, *67*, 37–73. [CrossRef]
65. Stacklies, W.; Redestig, H.; Scholz, M.; Walther, D.; Selbig, J. pcaMethods–a bioconductor package providing PCA methods for incomplete data. *Bioinformatics* **2007**, *23*, 1164–1167. [CrossRef]
66. Robin, X.; Turck, N.; Hainard, A.; Tiberti, N.; Lisacek, F.; Sanchez, J.C.; Muller, M. pROC: An open-source package for R and S+ to analyze and compare ROC curves. *BMC Bioinformatics* **2011**, *12*, 77. [CrossRef]
67. Kuhn, M. Building Predictive Models in R Using the caret Package. *J. Stat. Softw* **2008**, *28*, 1–26. [CrossRef]

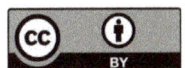

© 2020 by the authors. Licensee MDPI, Basel, Switzerland. This article is an open access article distributed under the terms and conditions of the Creative Commons Attribution (CC BY) license (http://creativecommons.org/licenses/by/4.0/).

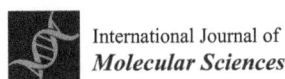

Article

Trichostatin A Alleviates Renal Interstitial Fibrosis Through Modulation of the M2 Macrophage Subpopulation

Wei-Cheng Tseng [1,2,3,4], **Ming-Tsun Tsai** [1,2,3], **Nien-Jung Chen** [5] **and Der-Cherng Tarng** [1,2,3,4,6,7,*]

1. Division of Nephrology, Department of Medicine, Taipei Veterans General Hospital, Taipei 11217, Taiwan; wctseng@gmail.com (W.-C.T.); mingtsun74@gmail.com (M.-T.T.)
2. Faculty of Medicine, School of Medicine, National Yang-Ming University, Taipei 11221, Taiwan
3. Institute of Clinical Medicine, School of Medicine, National Yang-Ming University, Taipei 11221, Taiwan
4. Center for Intelligent Drug Systems and Smart Bio-devices (IDS2B), National Chiao-Tung University, Hsinchu 30010, Taiwan
5. Institute of Microbiology and Immunology, School of Life Sciences, National Yang-Ming University, Taipei 11221, Taiwan; njchen@ym.edu.tw
6. Department and Institute of Physiology, School of Medicine, National Yang-Ming University, Taipei 11221, Taiwan
7. Department of Biological Science and Technology, College of Biological Science and Technology, National Chiao-Tung University, Hsinchu 30010, Taiwan
* Correspondence: dctarng@vghtpe.gov.tw; Tel.: +886-2-28757517; Fax: +886-2-28757841

Received: 13 August 2020; Accepted: 16 August 2020; Published: 19 August 2020

Abstract: Mounting evidence indicates that an increase in histone deacetylation contributes to renal fibrosis. Although inhibition of histone deacetylase (HDAC) can reduce the extent of fibrosis, whether HDAC inhibitors exert the antifibrotic effect through modulating the phenotypes of macrophages, the key regulator of renal fibrosis, remains unknown. Moreover, the functional roles of the M2 macrophage subpopulation in fibrotic kidney diseases remain incompletely understood. Herein, we investigated the role of HDAC inhibitors on renal fibrogenesis and macrophage plasticity. We found that HDAC inhibition by trichostatin A (TSA) reduced the accumulation of interstitial macrophages, suppressed the activation of myofibroblasts and attenuated the extent of fibrosis in obstructive nephropathy. Moreover, TSA inhibited M1 macrophages and augmented M2 macrophage infiltration in fibrotic kidney tissue. Interestingly, TSA preferentially upregulated M2c macrophages and suppressed M2a macrophages in the obstructed kidneys, which was correlated with a reduction of interstitial fibrosis. TSA also repressed the expression of proinflammatory and profibrotic molecules in cultured M2a macrophages and inhibited the activation of renal myofibroblasts. In conclusion, our study was the first to show that HDAC inhibition by TSA alleviates renal fibrosis in obstructed kidneys through facilitating an M1 to M2c macrophage transition.

Keywords: macrophage subpopulation; renal fibrosis; trichostatin A

1. Introduction

Chronic kidney disease (CKD) is an emerging global public health issue with a prevalence rate of 10% to 12% worldwide [1]. Regardless of the etiologies of renal diseases, unresolved renal insult engages an excessive deposition of extracellular matrix in the tubulointerstitium, thereby bringing about end-stage renal disease [2]. Tubulointerstitial fibrosis is the final common pathway of all kidney diseases and, also, represents the major determinant of renal function decline [2]. A wealth of studies has indicated that renal function decline correlates well with the increasing risks for all-cause mortality, cardiovascular events and hospitalization [1,3,4]. Despite that current available therapies have targeted traditional risk factors for renal function decline—namely, hypertension, hyperglycemia and hyperlipidemia, nearly half of CKD patients still experience progressive renal function decline and eventual end-stage renal disease [5]. Hence, a novel treatment modality to tackle renal fibrosis and halt the progression of CKD is urgently needed.

Infiltrated renal macrophages play pivotal roles in the homeostasis of renal fibrogenesis following initial renal insult, either ischemic, immunologic, mechanical or toxic damage [6]. Macrophages are highly plastic and differentiate into different phenotypes in response to the local environments. Macrophage phenotypes can be broadly categorized into the proinflammatory "M1" macrophages (characterized by inducible nitric oxide synthase (iNOS)) and the anti-inflammatory, reparative "M2" macrophages (characterized by arginase-1 (Arg1)) [6]. M2 macrophages can be further classified into M2a and M2c subpopulations by the presence of C-type lectin domain family 7 member A (CLEC7A) and signaling lymphocytic activation molecule (SLAM), respectively [7]. These macrophage subsets play distinct roles in the wound-healing process following tissue injury [8]. During the normal wound-healing process, the initial proinflammatory milieu recruits M1 macrophages to induce apoptosis and eliminate the pathogen and necrotic tissue. Thereafter, anti-inflammatory M2 macrophages predominate in the later tissue repair stage to activate re-epithelialization and neoangiogenesis in the injured area. Finally, a resolution stage ends the whole healing process by promoting the apoptosis of recruited immune cells, suppression of inflammation and tissue remodeling [8]. Nonetheless, dysregulation of the M1-to-M2 transition in a normal wound-healing process would lead to pathologic fibrosis and tissue scarring [8]. Recent studies further suggest that the excessive activation of M1 macrophages and certain profibrotic M2 macrophages both contribute to the development of fibrosis formation [9].

M2 macrophages may function as a double-edged sword in regulating renal fibrosis. M2 macrophages help control inflammation through releasing interleukin (IL)-10, Arg1, transforming growth factor-β (TGF-β) and heme oxygenase-1 [9]. On the other hand, the chronic activation of M2 macrophages can activate resident fibroblasts through the release of TGF-β, platelet-derived growth factor, vascular endothelium growth factor, insulin-like growth factor-1 and galactin-3 [9]. In this regard, M2 macrophages are proposed to be profibrotic in the renal fibrosis model of unilateral ureteral obstruction (UUO), and depletion of these M2 macrophages in UUO should be beneficial [9,10]. However, not all macrophage depletion strategies result in a reduction in fibrosis in UUO [10]. Inhibition of the c-fms kinase almost suppresses all infiltrating macrophage numbers in day 14 obstructed kidneys but does not change the course of fibrosis, suggesting some antifibrotic M2 macrophages are also depleted [11]. Until now, the functional roles of the M2 macrophage subpopulation in renal fibrogenesis remained unclear and conflicting. M2a and M2c macrophages are initially found to be anti-inflammatory and reparative in murine Adriamycin nephrosis [12]. Nonetheless, two recent studies indicate that M2a macrophages are upregulated in endometrial fibrosis and skeletal muscle fibrosis [13,14], suggesting M2a macrophages may exhibit a profibrotic feature in chronic fibrotic diseases. Therefore, further elucidating the roles of the M2a and M2c subsets may help delineate the complex fibrogenic process in UUO.

Emerging evidence indicates that epigenetic modulation of the chromatin state is crucial in determining the progression of CKD and macrophage polarization [15,16]. The histone acetylation status has recently been found to associate with certain kidney diseases and renal fibrogenesis [17]. Histone deacetylases (HDACs) are a group of enzymes that exert epigenetic effects by altering the acetylation status of histone and nonhistone proteins [18]. Although potential favorable effects of HDAC inhibitors have been found in animal models of acute kidney injury [19], diabetic nephropathy [20] and Adriamycin nephropathy [21], the roles of HDAC inhibitors in UUO and macrophage plasticity remain incompletely understood. Marumo et al. found that the expression of HDAC1 and HDAC2 are upregulated in obstructed kidneys and contribute to proinflammatory and fibrotic responses [22]. Nonetheless, whether HDAC inhibition regulates the phenotypic change of renal interstitial macrophages in UUO is still unclear. Previously, HDAC3-deficient bone marrow-derived macrophages displayed an M2-polarized IL-4-induced alternatively activated phenotype [11], implying HDAC inhibition may contribute to M2 macrophage polarization. Currently, there is no study exploring the interaction between histone acetylation and macrophage subsets in kidney diseases. Hence, we aimed to investigate whether HDAC inhibition attenuates renal fibrosis through modulating the phenotype of renal interstitial macrophages.

In this study, we found the distinct expression of M2a and M2c subset macrophages in obstructed kidneys. An increased M2a macrophage infiltrate correlated with a higher extent of renal interstitial fibrosis. Interestingly, the administration of trichostatin A (TSA), an HDAC inhibitor, suppressed M2a macrophage infiltration, enhanced M2c macrophage expression and attenuated renal fibrosis in UUO. TSA also repressed the expression of proinflammatory and profibrotic molecules in cultured M2a macrophages and inhibited the activation of renal myofibroblasts. Our study is the first to demonstrate that TSA modulates the renal macrophage M2 subpopulation to inhibit renal fibrosis.

2. Results

2.1. Infiltration of Interstitial Macrophages Correlates with Fibrosis in Obstructed Kidneys

To investigate the role of macrophage infiltration in renal fibrosis, we compared five mice kidneys harvested seven days after UUO to five mice kidneys harvested 14 days after UUO. Masson trichrome staining indicated that the area of renal tubulointerstitial fibrosis increased with the time of UUO. Moreover, immunohistochemistry showed α-smooth muscle actin (α-SMA)-positive myofibroblasts progressively increased in the day 14 obstructed kidneys as compared to the day 7 ones. Notably, the area of F4/80 (pan-macrophage marker)-positive macrophage infiltrate also correspondingly increased in the day 14 obstructed kidneys (Figure 1), indicating that interstitial macrophages did play an essential role in the development of renal fibrosis.

2.2. Preferential Accumulation of M1 and M2a Macrophages in Obstructed Kidneys

As macrophage plasticity is critical for regulating renal fibrosis [8], next, we analyzed the phenotypes of macrophages at different time points of UUO. Immunohistochemistry showed that both iNOS-positive M1 macrophages and Arg1-positive M2 macrophages progressively accumulated in the day 14 obstructed kidneys. Thereafter, we explored the M2 macrophage subpopulation in UUO. Interestingly, CLEC7A-positive M2a macrophages predominantly expressed in the day 14 obstructed kidneys. By contrast, the number of SLAM-positive M2c macrophages was only slightly increased over time (Figure 2A,B). Western blot analyses also showed the consistent results that the expression of M1 and M2a markers progressively increased with the time of UUO (Figure 2C,D). These data suggest that M1 and M2a macrophages are involved in the development of renal fibrosis.

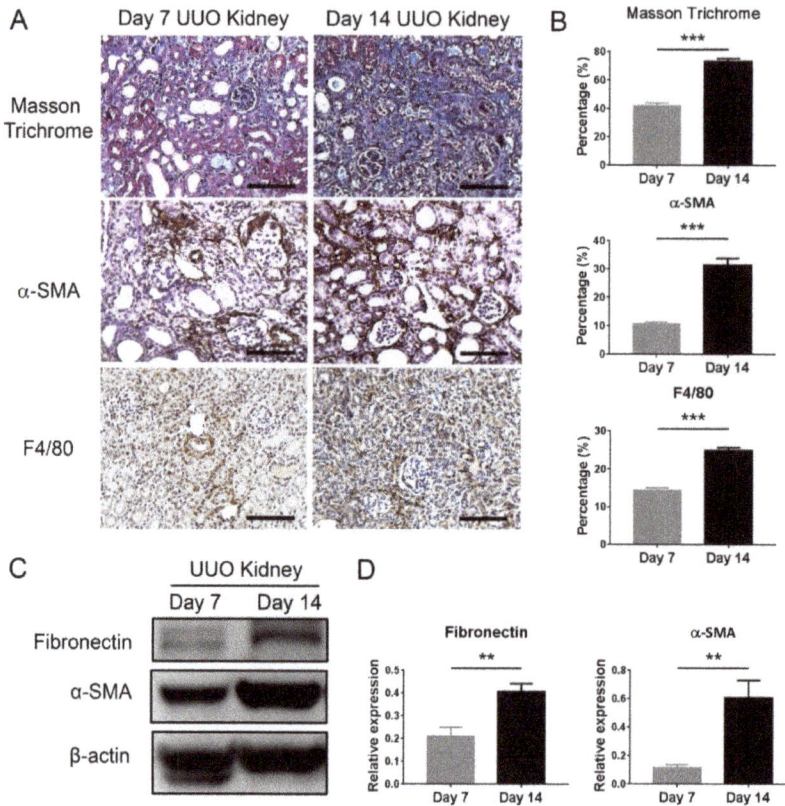

Figure 1. Macrophage infiltration correlates with renal interstitial fibrosis following a unilateral ureteral obstruction (UUO) injury. (**A**) Representative images of the Masson trichrome staining showed that the extent of fibrosis (blue staining) progressively increased in day 14 UUO kidneys as compared to day 7 ones. Immunohistochemistry demonstrated that more α-smooth muscle actin (α-SMA)-positive myofibroblasts and F4/80-positive macrophages accumulated in day 14 UUO kidneys. Scale bar = 100 μm. (**B**) Quantification of the fibrosis extent, α-SMA-positive and F4/80-positive areas. ** $p < 0.01$ and *** $p < 0.001$ by the unpaired Student's t-test; $n = 5$ for each group. (**C**) Western blot analysis of fibronectin and α-SMA expression in day 7 and day 14 obstructed kidneys. β-actin served as the loading control. (**D**) Quantification of the Western blot analyses. ** $p < 0.01$ and *** $p < 0.001$ by the unpaired Student's t-test; $n = 5$ for each group.

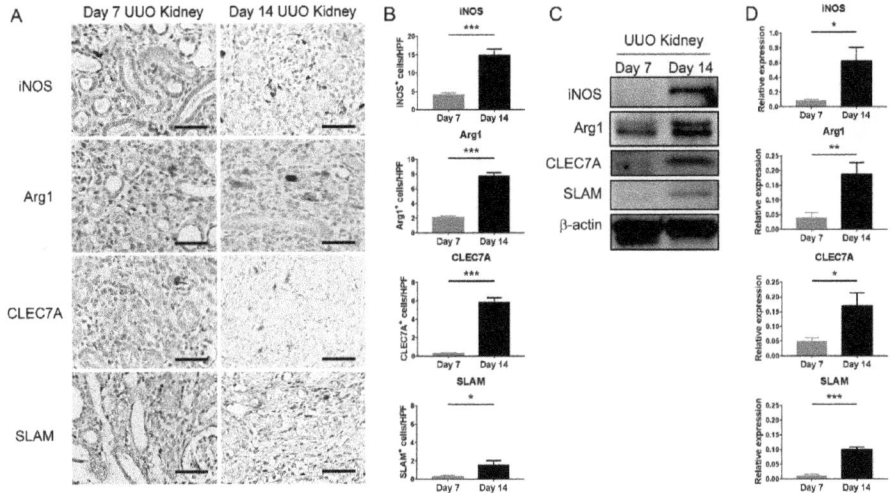

Figure 2. M1 and M2a macrophage infiltrates predominate in the late stage of unilateral ureteral obstruction (UUO). (**A**) Representative immunohistochemical photomicrographs of inducible nitric oxide synthase (iNOS), arginase-1 (Arg1), C-type lectin domain family 7 member A (CLEC7A) and signaling lymphocytic activation molecule (SLAM) in day 7 and day 14 obstructed kidneys. Scale bar = 25 μm. (**B**) Quantification of the iNOS-, Arg1-, CLEC7A- and SLAM-positive interstitial cells in day 7 and day 14 obstructed kidneys. * $p < 0.05$ and *** $p < 0.001$ by the unpaired Student's t-test; $n = 5$ for each group. (**C**) Western blot analyses of iNOS, Arg1, CLEC7A and SLAM expressions in day 7 and day 14 obstructed kidneys. β-actin served as the loading control. (**D**) Quantification of the Western blot analyses. * $p < 0.05$, ** $p < 0.01$ and *** $p < 0.001$ by the unpaired Student's t-test; $n = 5$ for each group.

2.3. HDAC Inhibition Represses Renal Fibrosis and Macrophage Infiltration in UUO

Given that increased histone deacetylation may be associated with renal fibrogenesis [17], we then investigated the therapeutic effect of TSA in UUO. The administration of TSA significantly reduced the extent of α-SMA-positive myofibroblasts and the area of renal interstitial fibrosis in UUO. Moreover, TSA also decreased the extent of interstitial macrophage infiltrate (Figure 3A,B). Western blot analysis also found that TSA reduced the expression of the extracellular matrix (fibronectin) and α-SMA in obstructed kidneys (Figure 3C,D).

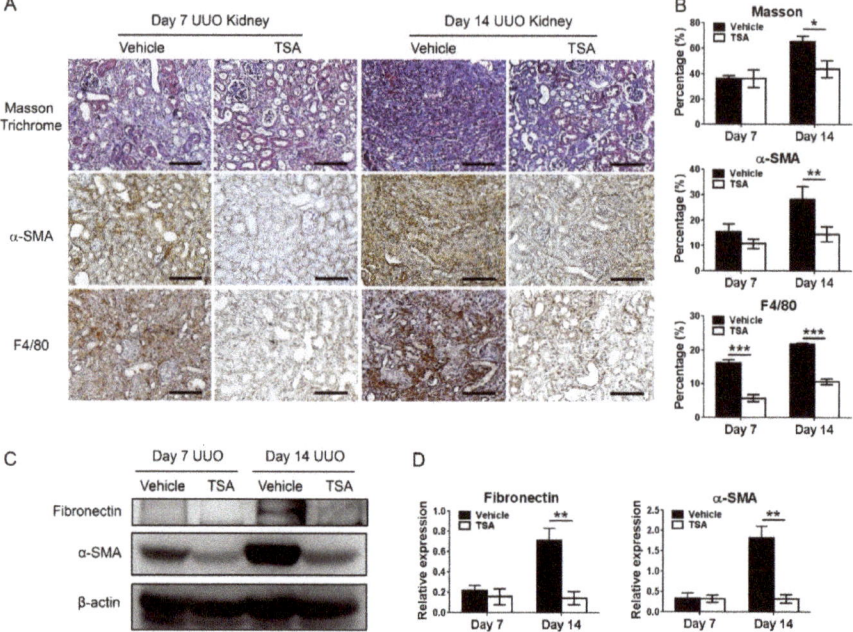

Figure 3. Trichostatin A (TSA) ameliorates renal inflammation and fibrosis in unilateral ureteral obstruction (UUO). (**A**) Representative images of Masson trichrome staining of obstructed kidneys at 7 days and 14 days following UUO in the vehicle and TSA groups. The TSA treatment markedly reduced the extent of interstitial fibrosis (blue area). Immunohistochemical staining for α-smooth muscle actin (α-SMA, myofibroblast marker) and F4/80 (pan-macrophage marker) in day 7 and day 14 obstructed kidneys. Scale bar = 100 μm. (**B**) Quantification of the fibrosis extent, α-SMA-positive and F4/80-positive areas. * $p < 0.05$, ** $p < 0.01$ and *** $p < 0.001$ by the unpaired Student's t-test; $n = 5$ for each group. (**C**) Western blots of fibronectin and α-SMA in day 7 and day 14 UUO kidneys treated with the vehicle or TSA. β-actin served as the loading control. (**D**) Quantification of fibronectin and α-SMA expression levels. ** $p < 0.01$ by the unpaired Student's t-test; $n = 5$ for each group.

2.4. HDAC Inhibition Promotes an M1-to-M2 Phenotypic Transition and Skews the M2 Macrophage Phenotype Towards an M2c Feature

To explore the role of HDAC inhibition on macrophage plasticity, we analyzed the phenotypes of interstitial macrophages in UUO after the administration of TSA. Upon treatment with TSA, immunohistochemistry showed that the infiltration of iNOS-positive M1 macrophages significantly decreased as compared to the vehicle group. Conversely, Arg1-positive macrophages were significantly upregulated in the TSA-treated kidneys following 14 days of obstruction (Figure 4A,B). Remarkably, TSA increased the number of SLAM-positive M2c macrophages but decreased the number of M2a macrophages. Immunofluorescent staining showed that both CLEC7A and SLAM colocalized with F4/80+CD206+ cells in obstructed kidneys, supporting that CLEC7A-positive and SLAM-positive cells represented M2a and M2c macrophages, respectively. Immunoblot confirmed that TSA downregulated the expression of iNOS and CLEC7A, as well as upregulated the expression of Arg1 and CLEC7A (Figure 4C–F). These data indicated that TSA suppressed the accumulation of proinflammatory M1 macrophages and profibrotic M2a macrophages in UUO. Instead, TSA increased the anti-inflammatory M2c macrophage infiltration, which limited the extent of inflammation and inhibited the activation of myofibroblasts and deposition of the extracellular matrix.

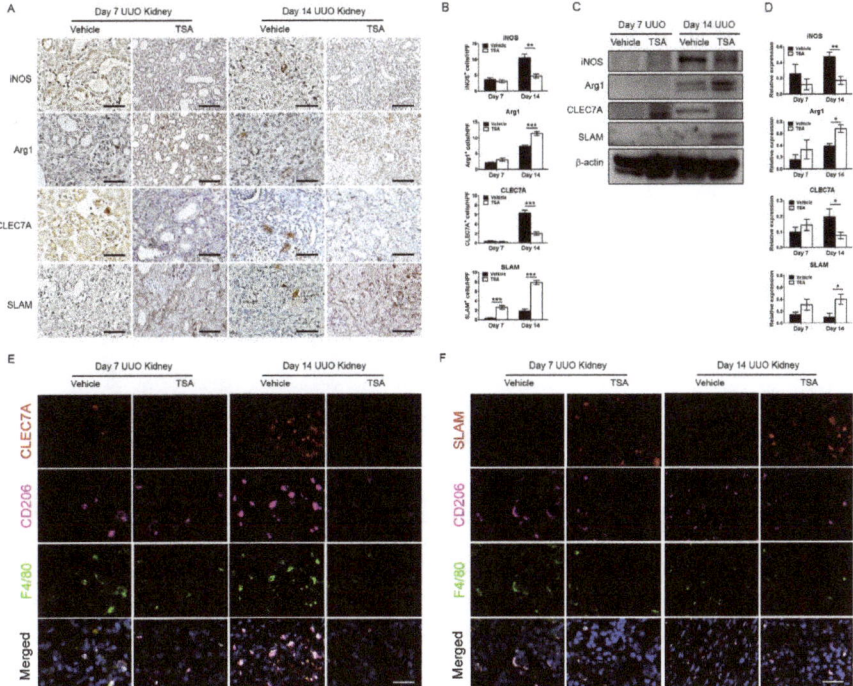

Figure 4. Trichostatin A (TSA) suppresses M1 and M2a macrophage infiltration but promotes M2c macrophage infiltration in unilateral ureteral obstruction (UUO). (**A**) Representative immunohistochemical images of inducible nitric oxide synthase (iNOS, M1 macrophage marker), arginase-1 (Arg1, pan-M2 macrophage marker), C-type lectin domain family 7 member A (CLEC7A, M2a macrophage marker) and signaling lymphocytic activation molecule (SLAM, M2c macrophage marker) in day 7 and day 14 obstructed kidneys either treated with the vehicle or TSA. Scale bar = 25 µm. (**B**) Quantification of the iNOS-, Arg1-, CLEC7A- and SLAM-positive interstitial cells in day 7 and day 14 obstructed kidneys treated with the vehicle or TSA. ** $p < 0.01$ and *** $p < 0.001$ by the unpaired Student's t-test; $n = 5$ for each group. (**C**) Western blots of iNOS, Arg1, CLEC7A and SLAM in day 7 and day 14 obstructed kidneys either treated with the vehicle or TSA. β-actin served as the loading control. (**D**) Quantification of iNOS, Arg1, CLEC7A and SLAM expression levels in obstructed kidneys. * $p < 0.05$ and ** $p < 0.01$ by the unpaired Student's t-test; $n = 5$ for each group. (**E**) Immunofluorescent staining of CLEC7A, CD206 and F4/80 in obstructed kidneys. Scale bar = 25 µm. (**F**) Immunofluorescent staining of SLAM, CD206 and F4/80 in obstructed kidneys. Scale bar = 25 µm. White color indicates colocalization in the merged panels.

2.5. HDAC Inhibition Suppresses Proinflammatory and Profibrotic Phenotypes in Cultured M2 Macrophages

To further clarify the effect of HDAC inhibition on the proinflammatory and profibrotic phenotypes of macrophages, J774A.1 macrophages were stimulated with IL-4/IL-13 or IL-10/TGF-b1 in the presence or absence of TSA for 24 h. IL-4/IL-13 induced the expression of Arg1 and CLEC7A in J774A.1 macrophages and polarized the cells towards an M2a phenotype. M2a J774A.1 macrophages increased the expression of profibrotic α-SMA and fibronectin, which were suppressed by TSA treatment. Furthermore, the amounts of proinflammatory tumor necrosis factor-α and iNOS in the M2a macrophages were also downregulated by TSA (Figure 5A,B). In contrast, IL-10/TGF-β1 induced the SLAM expression in J774A.1 macrophages and skewed the cells towards an M2c phenotype. The TSA treatment enhanced the SLAM expression in M2c J774A.1 macrophages and also further suppressed the amounts of TNF-α, iNOS, α-SMA and fibronectin in a dose-dependent manner (Figure 5C,D).

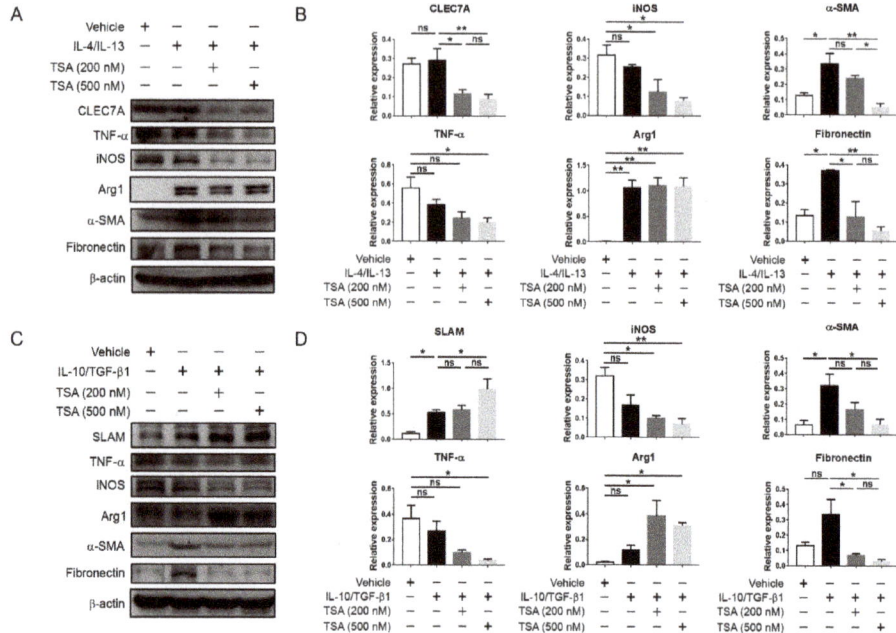

Figure 5. The effect of trichostatin A (TSA) on proinflammatory and profibrotic phenotypes of M2a and M2c macrophages. (A) Western blots of C-type lectin domain family 7 member A (CLEC7A), proinflammatory (tumor necrosis factor-α (TNF-α) and inducible nitric oxide synthase (iNOS)) and profibrotic (α-smooth muscle actin (α-SMA) and fibronectin) expressions in J774A.1 macrophages treated with the indicated conditions for 24 h. Concentrations of interleukin (IL)-4 and IL-13 were both 20 ng/mL. β-actin served as the loading control. (B) Quantification for the levels of indicated proteins. * $p < 0.05$ and ** $p < 0.01$ by ANOVA, followed by Tukey's post hoc multiple comparison test; $n = 3$ for each group. (C) Western blots of SLAM, proinflammatory (TNF-α and iNOS) and profibrotic (α-SMA and fibronectin) expressions in J774A.1 macrophages treated with the indicated conditions for 24 h. Concentrations of IL-10 and transforming growth factor (TGF)-β1 were both 20 ng/mL. β-actin served as the loading control. (D) Quantification for the levels of indicated proteins. * $p < 0.05$ and ** $p < 0.01$ by ANOVA, followed by Tukey's post hoc multiple comparison test; $n = 3$ for each group.

2.6. HDAC Inhibition Attenuates TGF-β1-Activated Renal Tubular Epithelial Cells and Fibroblasts

TGF-β1 is a well-known predominant mediator of the activation of renal myofibroblasts and resultant fibrogenesis in UUO [23]. To substantiate the role of HDAC inhibition on TGF-β1-induced renal fibrosis, renal tubular epithelial NRK-52E cells and renal NRK-49F fibroblasts were stimulated with TGF-β1 in the presence or absence of TSA. Western blotting revealed that TGF-β1 upregulated the expression of α-SMA and fibronectin in NRK-52E cells in a time-dependent manner. The treatment with TSA abrogated TGF-β1-induced fibrogenesis in NRK-52E cells (Figure 6A,B). These effects were further confirmed by immunofluorescent staining (Figure 6C,D). In NRK-49F fibroblasts, the TSA treatment also repressed TGF-β1-induced α-SMA expression (Supplementary Figure S1). These data indicate that TSA reduced renal fibrosis through attenuating the activation of myofibroblasts by TGF-β1.

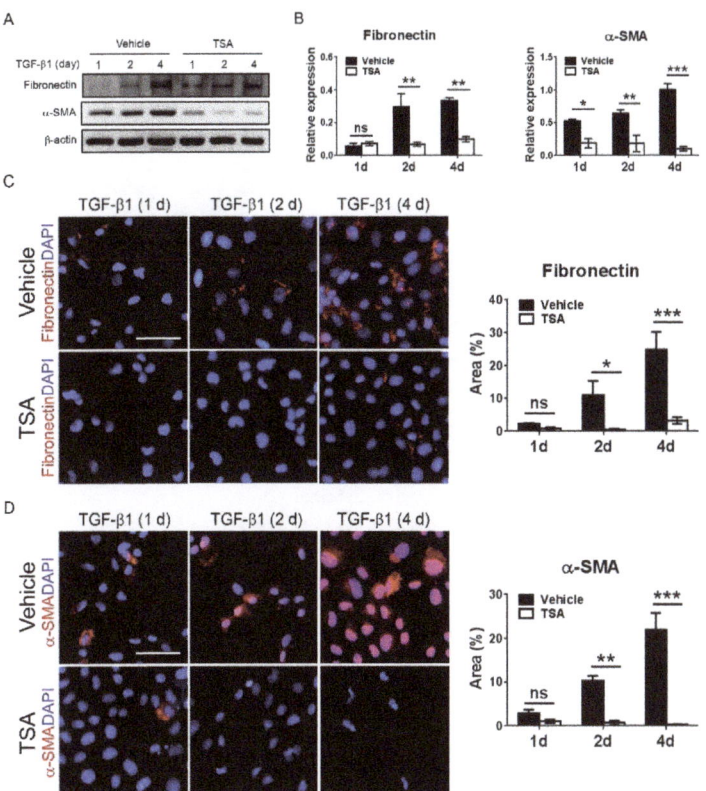

Figure 6. The effect of trichostatin A (TSA) on the activation of renal myofibroblasts. (**A**) Western blots of fibronectin and α-smooth muscle actin (a-SMA) expressions in transforming growth factor-β1 (TGF- β1, 20 ng/mL)-stimulated renal tubular epithelial NRK-52E cells at the indicated time. β-actin served as the loading control. (**B**) Quantification for the levels of indicated proteins. * $p < 0.05$, ** $p < 0.01$ and *** $p < 0.001$ by ANOVA, followed by Tukey's post hoc multiple comparison test. ns, nonsignificance. $n = 3$ for each group. (**C,D**) Immunofluorescent staining of fibronectin and α-SMA in the TGF-β1-treated NRK-52E cells at the indicated time. Scale bar = 50 μm. * $p < 0.05$, ** $p < 0.01$ and *** $p < 0.001$ by ANOVA, followed by Tukey's post hoc multiple comparison test. ns, nonsignificance. $n = 3$ for each group.

Our findings are summarized schematically in Figure 7. In renal fibrogenesis, the accumulation of M1 and M2a macrophages enhances inflammation and activates myofibroblasts. Trichostatin A suppresses the infiltration of proinflammatory M1 and M2a macrophages and increases the infiltration of anti-inflammatory M2c macrophages, thereby inhibiting the activation of renal myofibroblasts and resultant renal fibrosis.

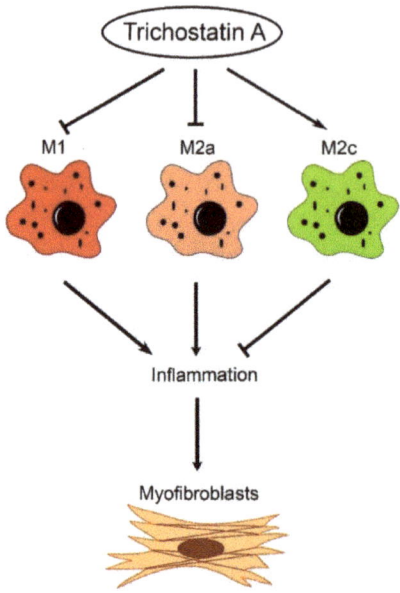

Figure 7. Proposed immunomodulatory and antifibrotic mechanism by trichostatin A in renal fibrosis. In a mice model of unilateral ureteral obstruction, the administration of trichostatin A suppresses the infiltration of proinflammatory M1a and M2a macrophages, as well as promotes the accumulation of anti-inflammatory M2c macrophages, thereby limiting excessive inflammation. Accordingly, the activation of myofibroblasts is limited, and renal fibrosis is attenuated.

3. Discussion

This present study showed that HDAC inhibition by TSA reduced renal fibrosis through modulating the M2 macrophage subpopulation. We found that a TSA treatment significantly decreased the extent of interstitial fibrosis, myofibroblast accumulation and macrophage infiltration in the obstructed kidneys. Interestingly, TSA downregulated iNOS expression and upregulated Arg1 expression in the whole kidney protein expression levels. Consistently, immunochemistry also found that TSA suppressed the infiltration of iNOS-positive M1 macrophages and promoted the accumulation of Arg1-positive M2 macrophages in the obstructed renal interstitial areas. Specifically, TSA suppressed the accumulation of CLEC7A-positive M2a macrophages but increased the number of SLAM-positive M2c macrophages. These data indicated that the increment of M2 macrophages by TSA in UUO was preferentially attributed to the increased accumulation of M2c macrophages. Consistently, we also found that TSA suppressed CLEC7A expression in M2a macrophages and enhanced SLAM expression in M2c macrophages in vitro. Notably, TSA further downregulated the expression of proinflammatory and profibrotic factors in M2a macrophages. Moreover, TSA attenuated the TGF-β1-induced expression of α-SMA and fibronectin in cultured renal tubular epithelial cells and fibroblasts, indicating that TSA also attenuated the activation of renal myofibroblasts through inhibiting the epithelial-mesenchymal transition. Collectively, our findings indicated that TSA suppressed renal fibrogenesis through increasing the anti-inflammatory and antifibrotic M2 subpopulation.

Conflicting results exist regarding the role of M2 macrophages on renal fibrosis in UUO [9], probably related to the heterogeneity of the M2 subpopulation. Previously, M2 macrophages were proposed to be profibrotic, because the macrophage infiltrate in the UUO-kidney has a predominant M2 phenotype and the percentage of M2 macrophages increases along with the duration of obstruction [10]. If this is the case, the depletion of all macrophages in the later stage of UUO should mitigate renal fibrosis. However, not all macrophage ablation strategies result in the improvement of renal fibrosis in UUO [10]. The depletion of infiltrating macrophages through targeting the c-fms kinase fails to attenuate the extent of renal fibrosis in day 14 obstructed kidneys [11], suggesting certain antifibrotic M2 macrophages are also depleted and also highlighting the complex functional heterogeneity of the M2 macrophage population [24]. Our study found that the TSA treatment resulted in fibrosis reduction, the downregulation of iNOS-positive M1 macrophages and CLEC7A-positive M2a macrophages and the upregulation of SLAM-positive M2c macrophages. In line with our observations, Wang et al. found that M2a macrophages are associated with the accumulation of collagen and muscle fibrosis [14]. Moreover, Duan et al. showed that the adoptive transfer of M2a macrophages significantly increased the extent of fibrosis in endometriosis [13], suggesting that M2a macrophages are profibrotic and critically involved in fibrogenesis. The controversy regarding the profibrotic or antifibrotic roles of M2 macrophages may be reconciled by the balance of distinct M2a and M2c macrophages in chronic fibrotic disorders.

Recent attention has focused on the significance of post-translational histone modifications in determining the progression of CKD and macrophage polarization [15,16]. Nonetheless, the role of epigenetic regulation on macrophage phenotypes in UUO remains elusive. The present study found that HDAC inhibition by TSA significantly alleviated renal inflammation and fibrosis. We also found that TSA inhibited the infiltration of M1 and M2a macrophages, enhanced the infiltration of M2c macrophages and directed an M1-to-M2c switch. The TSA-induced upregulation of M2c macrophages correlated with a reduction of renal interstitial fibrosis, and TSA also enhanced the SLAM expression and suppressed profibrotic and proinflammatory phenotypes in cultured M2c macrophages. These data supported that TSA repressed renal fibrosis through augmenting the expression of antifibrotic M2 macrophages. Although we found that TSA reduced UUO-induced renal fibrosis through modulation of the M2 macrophage subpopulation, our findings may not be extrapolated to renal fibrosis attributed to other insults, such as toxin, diabetes or autoimmune diseases. Clearly, more studies will be required to confirm the immunomodulatory and antifibrotic effects of TSA in other models of kidney diseases. In consistency with our findings, Pang et al. found that TSA can mitigate the extent of renal fibrosis in obstructive nephropathy, but the role of TSA on renal inflammation is undefined in their study [25]. A later study by Marumo et al. also found that TSA suppressed tubulointerstitial fibrosis in obstructed kidneys and further showed that TSA reduced renal inflammation in terms of the downregulation of EMR1 and MCP1 expressions, as well as decreased the number of infiltrated macrophages [22]. However, the effect of HDAC inhibition on the phenotypic transition of macrophages was not examined [22]. Taken together, our study provided novel evidence that TSA attenuated renal fibrosis through suppressing the profibrotic M2a macrophage and promoting anti-inflammatory, antifibrotic M2c macrophages. In conclusion, our study showed that HDAC inhibition by TSA significantly attenuated renal fibrosis through promoting an M1-to-M2c macrophage transition in obstructed kidneys. Our study not only added to the knowledge of antifibrotic M2 macrophages but, also, provided the bench evidence that pharmacological HDAC inhibitors can be applied to clinical treatments of renal fibrosis in the future.

4. Materials and Methods

4.1. Animals

Male 6-to-8-week-old C57BL/6J mice weighing 20-25 g were purchased from the National Laboratory Animal Center (Taipei, Taiwan) and housed at the Laboratory Animal Center of the National Yang-Ming University (Taipei, Taiwan). The mice were raised in a sound-attenuated, temperature-controlled (22 ± 1 °C) room with a 12-h light/dark cycle. Standard rodent chow and drinking water were supplied ad libitum. All experimental procedures conformed to the Guide for the Care and Use of Laboratory Animals published by the National Institutes of Health. The study was approved by the Institutional Animal Care and Use Committee of the National Yang-Ming University under the license number 1041244.

4.2. Cell Culture and Treatment

Mouse J774A.1 macrophages (Bioresource Collection and Research Center, Hsin-Chu, Taiwan) were cultured in Dulbecco's modified Eagle's medium (10-013-CM, Corning Inc., Corning, NY, USA) supplemented with 10% fetal bovine serum (Gibco, Grand Island, NY, USA) in a 5% CO_2, 37 °C humidified incubator. To examine the effect of TSA on the macrophage subpopulation, J774A.1 macrophages were first seeded in 6-well dishes (5×10^6 cells/well). Afterwards, J774A.1 macrophages were polarized into the M2a phenotype by stimulation with IL-4 (20 ng/mL, PeproTech, Rocky Hill, NJ, USA) and IL-13 (20 ng/mL, PeproTech) or into the M2c phenotype by stimulation with IL-10 (20 ng/mL, PeproTech) and TGF-b1 (20 ng/mL, PeproTech) for 24 h in the presence or absence of TSA (200 nM and 500 nM, T8552, Sigma-Aldrich, St. Louis, MO, USA) at different concentrations.

Normal rat renal tubular NRK-52E cells (Bioresource Collection and Research Center) were cultured in the low-glucose Dulbecco's modified Eagle's medium (10-014-CV, Corning Inc.) supplemented with 5% fetal bovine serum (Gibco). To determine the effect of TSA on renal myofibroblasts, NRK-52E were stimulated with TGF-β1 (20 ng/mL, PeproTech) for 1, 2 and 4 days in the presence or absence of TSA (500 nM, Sigma-Aldrich).

4.3. Experimental UUO Model

After anesthesia, the UUO model was performed in mice by ligation of the left ureter with 5-O silk through a flank incision, as previously described [26]. After the surgery, the mice were recovered under a warming lamp. For HDAC inhibition experiments, TSA (1 mg/kg, Sigma-Aldrich) or the vehicle were injected intraperitoneally daily. The animals were euthanized, and the obstructed kidneys were harvested 7 and 14 days after UUO for further analyses.

4.4. Histological Analysis of the Kidneys

The kidney tissue was fixed with 4% phosphate-buffered formalin solution (Macron Chemicals, Center Valley, PA, USA), embedded in paraffin block and cut into 4-μm sections. For histological analysis, after deparaffinization and rehydration by xylene and graded alcohols, the sections were subjected to Masson trichrome staining according to the manufacturer's instructions (Accustain, Sigma-Aldrich). Twenty randomly selected nonoverlapping high-power fields (40× objective) were evaluated for each mouse, and the average for each group was then analyzed. The fibrotic area was quantified by ImageJ software (1.52a, US National Institutes of Health, Bethesda, MD, USA).

4.5. Immunohistochemical Staining

Immunohistochemical staining was performed on formalin-fixed paraffin-embedded sections of obstructed kidneys, as previously described [27]. Briefly, after deparaffinization by xylene and rehydration by graded alcohols, consecutive 4-μm sections of kidneys were subjected to heat antigen retrieval in a microwave oven (650W, 12 min) in a 10-mM sodium citrate buffer (pH 6.0). Afterwards, endogenous peroxidase activity was quenched by 3% hydrogen peroxide (Sigma-Aldrich) for 10 min. Thereafter, tissue sections were incubated with the primary antibodies at 4 °C overnight and then with the secondary antibody (Envision$^+$Dual Link System-HRP, Dako, Glostrup, Denmark) for 30 min at room temperature. Signals were developed with diaminobenzidine substrate-chromogen (DAB, Dako), which resulted in a brown-colored precipitate at the antigen site. Finally, sections were counterstained with a Gill's hematoxylin (Merck, Darmstadt, Germany). Primary antibodies included F4/80 (1:100, Cat#sc-25830, Santa Cruz Biotechnology, Santa Cruz, CA, USA), iNOS (1:200, Cat#sc-651, Santa Cruz Biotechnology), Arg1 (1:200, Cat#sc-20150, Santa Cruz Biotechnology), α-SMA (1:200, Cat#ab5694, Abcam, Cambridge, UK), CLEC7A (1:50, Cat#TA322197, OriGene Technologies, Rockville, MD, USA) and SLAM (1:100, Cat#ab156288, Abcam). Twenty randomly selected nonoverlapping high-power fields (40× objective) at the renal cortex were evaluated for each mouse. Analysis of the

DAB-positive area was carried out using Image J with the "Threshold Colour" plug-in (version 1.16, https://imagejdocu.tudor.lu/plugin/color/threshold_colour/start#threshold_colour).

4.6. Western Blotting

Western blotting analysis was performed as previously described [28]. Briefly, protein from the obstructed kidney tissue or cells was extracted in a radioimmunoprecipitation assay buffer containing a protease inhibitor cocktail (cOmplete-Mini, Roche, Indianapolis, IN, USA). The protein concentration was determined by a Bradford assay (Bio-Rad Laboratories, Montreal, Quebec, Canada), separated by sodium dodecyl sulfate-polyacrylamide gel electrophoresis and, subsequently, transferred to polyvinylidene fluoride membranes. The membranes were then probed with primary antibodies against fibronectin (1:1000, Cat#15613-1-AP, Proteintech Group, Chicago, IL, USA), α-SMA (1:5000, Cat#14395-1-AP, Proteintech Group), iNOS (1:1000, Cat#ab3523, Abcam), Arg1 (1:1000, Cat#93668S, Cell Signaling Technology, Boston, MA, USA), CLEC7A (1:500, Cat#TA322197, OriGene Technologies), SLAM (1:1000, Cat#ab156288, Abcam), TNF-α (1:1000, Cat#ab66579, Abcam) and β-actin (1:5000, Cat#60008, Proteintech Group) at 4 °C overnight. Afterwards, the membranes were incubated with horseradish peroxidase-conjugated secondary antibodies (Jackson ImmunoResearch, West Grove, PA, USA) at room temperature for 1.5 h, and the signals were developed using a West Femto Chemiluminescent Substrate kit (Thermo Fisher Scientific, Hudson, NH, USA). Bands were visualized and quantified using a ChemiDoc-It Imaging system (UVP, Cambridge, UK). Data were normalized to the β-actin expression.

4.7. Immunofluorescence

For in vivo experiments, paraffin-embedded 4-μm sections of obstructed kidneys were deparaffinized with xylene, rehydrated with graded alcohols and boiled in a 10-mM citrate buffer. Thereafter, the sections were blocked with hydrogen peroxide and then reacted with primary antibodies against F4/80 (1:100, Cat#MCA497R, Abd Serotec, Oxford, UK), CD206 (1:100, Cat#60143-1-Ig, Proteintech Group), CLEC7A (1:50, Cat#MBS9414183, MyBiosource, San Diego, CA, USA) or SLAM (1:100, Cat#ab156288, Abcam) at 4 °C overnight. Fluorescein isothiocyanate-conjugated goat anti-rat immunoglobulin G (IgG, 1:250, Cat#112-095-003, Jackson ImmunoResearch) and Alexa Fluor 647-conjugated donkey anti-mouse IgG (1:250, Cat# 715-605-151, Jackson ImmunoResearch) were used to visualize the location of F4/80 and CD206, respectively. Alexa Fluor 568-conjugated goat anti-rabbit IgG (1:250, Cat#A11011, Thermo Fisher Scientific) was used to visualize the location of CLEC7A and SLAM. Slides were then mounted with Fluoroshield Mounting Medium with DAPI (ab104139, Abcam).

For in vitro experiments, TGF-β1-stimulated NRK-52E cells were plated in chamber slides (μ-Slide 8-Well, Ibidi, Munich, Germany) for 1, 2 and 4 days in the presence or absence of trichostatin. Afterwards, the chamber slides were fixed with 4% paraformaldehyde for 10 min and blocked with 1% bovine serum albumin for 30 min. Thereafter, slides were incubated with primary antibodies against α-SMA (1:200, ab5694, Abcam) or fibronectin (1:200, 15613-1-AP, Proteintech) at 4 °C overnight, reacted with Alexa Fluor 568-conjugated goat anti-rabbit secondary antibody (1:200, Cat#A11011, Thermo Fisher Scientific) and then counterstained with DAPI (ab104139, Abcam).

4.8. Statistical Analysis

All values are expressed as mean ± SEM. Between-group comparisons were determined by the unpaired Student's t-tests or ANOVA, followed by Tukey's post hoc multiple comparison test. Statistical analysis was performed using the Statistical Analysis System (SAS, Version 9.4, SAS Institute, Cary, NC, USA). A value of two-sided $p < 0.05$ was considered statistically significant.

Supplementary Materials: The following are available online at http://www.mdpi.com/1422-0067/21/17/5966/s1, Figure S1. The effect of trichostatin A (TSA) on the activation of renal fibroblasts.

Author Contributions: Conceptualization, W.-C.T.; data curation, M.-T.T.; formal analysis, W.-C.T. and M.-T.T.; funding acquisition, W.-C.T. and D.-C.T.; investigation, W.-C.T.; methodology, W.-C.T.; project administration, D.-C.T.; resources, D.-C.T.; supervision, N.-J.C. and D.-C.T.; validation, M.-T.T.; writing—original draft, W.-C.T. and writing—review and editing, M.-T.T., N.-J.C. and D.-C.T. All authors have read and agreed to the published version of the manuscript.

Funding: This work was supported in part by the Ministry of Science and Technology (grant numbers MOST 102-2314-B-010-004-MY3, MOST 105-2314-B-010-016, MOST 106-2314-B-010-039-MY3 and MOST 107-2314-B-075-064-MY3); the Taipei Veterans General Hospital (grant numbers V105C-013, V106C-147, V107C-127, V107-B-037, V108-C-175 and V108-C-103); the Department of Health, Taipei City Government (grant numbers 10401-62-010 and 10501-62-006); the Taipei City Hospital (grant numbers TPCH-105-031 and TPCH-106-034); Foundation for Poison Control; the Ministry of Education's Aim for the Top University Plan in the National Yang-Ming University, Taiwan and the Center For Intelligent Drug Systems and Smart Bio-devices (IDS^{2}B) from the Featured Areas Research Center Program within the framework of the Higher Education Sprout Project by the Ministry of Education (MOE) in Taiwan.

Acknowledgments: The authors thank the Division of Experimental Surgery, Department of Surgery and Department of Pathology, Taipei Veterans General Hospital for technical assistance. They also thank the Clinical Research Core Laboratory and the Medical Science & Technology Building of Taipei Veterans General Hospital for providing experimental space and facilities.

Conflicts of Interest: The funding sources had no role in the study design, conduct or reporting. The authors declare that they have no conflicts of interest.

References

1. Wen, C.P.; Cheng, T.Y.; Tsai, M.K.; Chang, Y.C.; Chan, H.T.; Tsai, S.P.; Chiang, P.H.; Hsu, C.C.; Sung, P.K.; Hsu, Y.H.; et al. All-cause mortality attributable to chronic kidney disease: A prospective cohort study based on 462 293 adults in Taiwan. *Lancet* **2008**, *371*, 2173–2182. [CrossRef]
2. Zeisberg, M.; Neilson, E.G. Mechanisms of tubulointerstitial fibrosis. *J. Am. Soc. Nephrol.* **2010**, *21*, 1819–1834. [CrossRef] [PubMed]
3. Go, A.S.; Chertow, G.M.; Fan, D.; McCulloch, C.E.; Hsu, C.Y. Chronic kidney disease and the risks of death, cardiovascular events, and hospitalization. *N. Engl. J. Med.* **2004**, *351*, 1296–1305. [CrossRef] [PubMed]
4. Sud, M.; Tangri, N.; Pintilie, M.; Levey, A.S.; Naimark, D. Risk of end-stage renal disease and death after cardiovascular events in chronic kidney disease. *Circulation* **2014**, *130*, 458–465. [CrossRef] [PubMed]
5. Braun, L.; Sood, V.; Hogue, S.; Lieberman, B.; Copley-Merriman, C. High burden and unmet patient needs in chronic kidney disease. *Int. J. Nephrol. Renovasc. Dis.* **2012**, *5*, 151–163. [PubMed]
6. Ricardo, S.D.; van Goor, H.; Eddy, A.A. Macrophage diversity in renal injury and repair. *J. Clin. Investig.* **2008**, *118*, 3522–3530. [CrossRef]
7. Anders, H.J.; Ryu, M. Renal microenvironments and macrophage phenotypes determine progression or resolution of renal inflammation and fibrosis. *Kidney Int.* **2011**, *80*, 915–925. [CrossRef]
8. Wermuth, P.J.; Jimenez, S.A. The significance of macrophage polarization subtypes for animal models of tissue fibrosis and human fibrotic diseases. *Clin. Transl. Med.* **2015**, *4*, 2. [CrossRef]
9. Braga, T.T.; Agudelo, J.S.; Camara, N.O. Macrophages during the Fibrotic Process: M2 as Friend and Foe. *Front. Immunol.* **2015**, *6*, 602. [CrossRef]
10. Nikolic-Paterson, D.J.; Wang, S.; Lan, H.Y. Macrophages promote renal fibrosis through direct and indirect mechanisms. *Kidney Int. Suppl.* **2014**, *4*, 34–38. [CrossRef]
11. Ma, F.Y.; Liu, J.; Kitching, A.R.; Manthey, C.L.; Nikolic-Paterson, D.J. Targeting renal macrophage accumulation via c-fms kinase reduces tubular apoptosis but fails to modify progressive fibrosis in the obstructed rat kidney. *Am. J. Physiol. Renal Physiol.* **2009**, *296*, F177–F185. [CrossRef] [PubMed]
12. Lu, J.; Cao, Q.; Zheng, D.; Sun, Y.; Wang, C.; Yu, X.; Wang, Y.; Lee, V.W.; Zheng, G.; Tan, T.K.; et al. Discrete functions of M2a and M2c macrophage subsets determine their relative efficacy in treating chronic kidney disease. *Kidney Int.* **2013**, *84*, 745–755. [CrossRef] [PubMed]
13. Duan, J.; Liu, X.; Wang, H.; Guo, S.W. The M2a macrophage subset may be critically involved in the fibrogenesis of endometriosis in mice. *Reprod. Biomed. Online* **2018**, *37*, 254–268. [CrossRef] [PubMed]

14. Wang, Y.; Wehling-Henricks, M.; Samengo, G.; Tidball, J.G. Increases of M2a macrophages and fibrosis in aging muscle are influenced by bone marrow aging and negatively regulated by muscle-derived nitric oxide. *Aging Cell* **2015**, *14*, 678–688. [CrossRef] [PubMed]
15. Ivashkiv, L.B. Epigenetic regulation of macrophage polarization and function. *Trends Immunol.* **2013**, *34*, 216–223. [CrossRef] [PubMed]
16. Wanner, N.; Bechtel-Walz, W. Epigenetics of kidney disease. *Cell Tissue Res.* **2017**, *369*, 75–92. [CrossRef]
17. Tampe, B.; Zeisberg, M. Evidence for the involvement of epigenetics in the progression of renal fibrogenesis. *Nephrol. Dial. Transplant.* **2014**, *29* (Suppl. 1), i1–i8. [CrossRef]
18. Beckerman, P.; Ko, Y.A.; Susztak, K. Epigenetics: A new way to look at kidney diseases. *Nephrol. Dial. Transplant.* **2014**, *29*, 1821–1827. [CrossRef]
19. Cianciolo Cosentino, C.; Skrypnyk, N.I.; Brilli, L.L.; Chiba, T.; Novitskaya, T.; Woods, C.; West, J.; Korotchenko, V.N.; McDermott, L.; Day, B.W.; et al. Histone deacetylase inhibitor enhances recovery after AKI. *J. Am. Soc. Nephrol.* **2013**, *24*, 943–953. [CrossRef]
20. Gilbert, R.E.; Huang, Q.; Thai, K.; Advani, S.L.; Lee, K.; Yuen, D.A.; Connelly, K.A.; Advani, A. Histone deacetylase inhibition attenuates diabetes-associated kidney growth: Potential role for epigenetic modification of the epidermal growth factor receptor. *Kidney Int.* **2011**, *79*, 1312–1321. [CrossRef]
21. Van Beneden, K.; Geers, C.; Pauwels, M.; Mannaerts, I.; Verbeelen, D.; van Grunsven, L.A.; Van den Branden, C. Valproic acid attenuates proteinuria and kidney injury. *J. Am. Soc. Nephrol.* **2011**, *22*, 1863–1875. [CrossRef] [PubMed]
22. Marumo, T.; Hishikawa, K.; Yoshikawa, M.; Hirahashi, J.; Kawachi, S.; Fujita, T. Histone deacetylase modulates the proinflammatory and -fibrotic changes in tubulointerstitial injury. *Am. J. Physiol. Renal Physiol.* **2010**, *298*, F133–F141. [CrossRef] [PubMed]
23. Chevalier, R.L.; Forbes, M.S.; Thornhill, B.A. Ureteral obstruction as a model of renal interstitial fibrosis and obstructive nephropathy. *Kidney Int.* **2009**, *75*, 1145–1152. [CrossRef] [PubMed]
24. Huen, S.C.; Cantley, L.G. Macrophages in Renal Injury and Repair. *Annu. Rev. Physiol.* **2017**, *79*, 449–469. [CrossRef] [PubMed]
25. Pang, M.; Kothapally, J.; Mao, H.; Tolbert, E.; Ponnusamy, M.; Chin, Y.E.; Zhuang, S. Inhibition of histone deacetylase activity attenuates renal fibroblast activation and interstitial fibrosis in obstructive nephropathy. *Am. J. Physiol. Renal Physiol.* **2009**, *297*, F996–F1005. [CrossRef] [PubMed]
26. Lo, T.H.; Tseng, K.Y.; Tsao, W.S.; Yang, C.Y.; Hsieh, S.L.; Chiu, A.W.; Takai, T.; Mak, T.W.; Tarng, D.C.; Chen, N.J. TREM-1 regulates macrophage polarization in ureteral obstruction. *Kidney Int.* **2014**, *86*, 1174–1186. [CrossRef]
27. Tseng, W.C.; Yang, W.C.; Yang, A.H.; Hsieh, S.L.; Tarng, D.C. Expression of TNFRSF6B in kidneys is a novel predictor for progression of chronic kidney disease. *Mod. Pathol.* **2013**, *26*, 984–994. [CrossRef]
28. Tseng, W.C.; Chuang, C.W.; Yang, M.H.; Pan, C.C.; Tarng, D.C. Kruppel-like factor 4 is a novel prognostic predictor for urothelial carcinoma of bladder and it regulates TWIST1-mediated epithelial-mesenchymal transition. *Urol. Oncol.* **2016**, *34*, 485.e15–485.e24. [CrossRef]

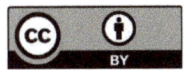

© 2020 by the authors. Licensee MDPI, Basel, Switzerland. This article is an open access article distributed under the terms and conditions of the Creative Commons Attribution (CC BY) license (http://creativecommons.org/licenses/by/4.0/).

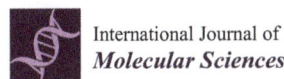

Review

Contribution of Predictive and Prognostic Biomarkers to Clinical Research on Chronic Kidney Disease

Michele Provenzano [1,*], Salvatore Rotundo [2], Paolo Chiodini [3], Ida Gagliardi [1], Ashour Michael [1], Elvira Angotti [4], Silvio Borrelli [5], Raffaele Serra [6], Daniela Foti [2], Giovambattista De Sarro [7] and Michele Andreucci [1,*]

1. Renal Unit, Department of Health Sciences, "Magna Graecia" University of Catanzaro, I-88100 Catanzaro, Italy; ida_88@libero.it (I.G.); ashourmichael@yahoo.com (A.M.)
2. Department of Health Sciences, "Magna Graecia" University of Catanzaro, I-88100 Catanzaro, Italy; srotundo91@gmail.com (S.R.); foti@unicz.it (D.F.)
3. Medical Statistics Unit, University of Campania Luigi Vanvitelli, I-80138 Naples, Italy; paolo.chiodini@unicampania.it
4. Clinical Biochemistry Unit, Azienda Ospedaliera Universitaria Mater Domini Hospital, I-88100 Catanzaro, Italy; e.angotti@materdominiaou.it
5. Renal Unit, University of Campania "Luigi Vanvitelli", I-80138 Naples, Italy; dott.silvioborrelli@gmail.com
6. Interuniversity Center of Phlebolymphology (CIFL), "Magna Graecia" University of Catanzaro, I-88100 Catanzaro, Italy; rserra@unicz.it
7. Pharmacology Unit, Department of Health Sciences, School of Medicine, "Magna Graecia" University of Catanzaro, I-88100 Catanzaro, Italy; desarro@unicz.it
* Correspondence: michiprov@hotmail.it (M.P.); andreucci@unicz.it (M.A.); Tel.: +39-3407544146 (M.P.); +39-3396814750 (M.A.)

Received: 29 June 2020; Accepted: 12 August 2020; Published: 14 August 2020

Abstract: Chronic kidney disease (CKD), defined as the presence of albuminuria and/or reduction in estimated glomerular filtration rate (eGFR) < 60 mL/min/1.73 m^2, is considered a growing public health problem, with its prevalence and incidence having almost doubled in the past three decades. The implementation of novel biomarkers in clinical practice is crucial, since it could allow earlier diagnosis and lead to an improvement in CKD outcomes. Nevertheless, a clear guidance on how to develop biomarkers in the setting of CKD is not yet available. The aim of this review is to report the framework for implementing biomarkers in observational and intervention studies. Biomarkers are classified as either prognostic or predictive; the first type is used to identify the likelihood of a patient to develop an endpoint regardless of treatment, whereas the second type is used to determine whether the patient is likely to benefit from a specific treatment. Many single assays and complex biomarkers were shown to improve the prediction of cardiovascular and kidney outcomes in CKD patients on top of the traditional risk factors. Biomarkers were also shown to improve clinical trial designs. Understanding the correct ways to validate and implement novel biomarkers in CKD will help to mitigate the global burden of CKD and to improve the individual prognosis of these high-risk patients.

Keywords: end-stage kidney disease (ESKD); cardiovascular disease; epidemiology; CKD; biomarkers

1. Introduction

A biomarker is defined, by a collaborative working group involved with both the United States National Institutes of Health (NIH) and the Food and Drug Administration (FDA), as "a characteristic that is measured as an indicator of normal biological processes, pathogenic processes, or responses to an exposure or intervention, including therapeutic interventions" [1]. This working group definition was formed on the initiative of the NIH with the aim of accelerating the development and clinical application of reliable biomarkers based on shared definitions. Indeed, an "ideal" biomarker is defined with the presence of some analytic features: (1) it should be measured and readily available in biological samples, such as blood or urine; (2) it should be reproducible, non-invasive, and not expensive [2]. In addition, several clinical features should also be provided to complete the biomarker's definition; it needs to allow for an early detection of a disease status, while it also needs to have high sensitivity and specificity, i.e., the biomarker needs to differentiate the pathologic status from the normal one and from other clinical conditions, as accurately as possible [3]. The effort made by the NIH–FDA working group is considerable ever since it forecasted and tried to solve the problems of biomarker development, from discovery to clinical application. Indeed, once a biomarker is found to be involved in one or more pathophysiological mechanisms of a disease, it may be introduced into clinical practice to see whether it offers advantages in clinical management and after completion of the validation phase that is considered a crucial step [4]. An important example of the pitfalls of biomarker development is illustrated in the chronic kidney disease (CKD) scenario. CKD is a chronic disease characterized by a poor prognosis, due to the strong association with the development of cardiovascular events, all-cause mortality, and renal events such as renal replacement therapies (RRT, i.e., dialysis or kidney transplantation) [5,6]. The Kidney Disease Improving Global Outcomes Work Group (KDIGO), in 2012, defined CKD with the presence of either decreased kidney function (estimated glomerular filtration rate (eGFR) < 60 mL/min/1.73 m^2) and/or albuminuria, namely, an abnormal amount of protein excretion with urine, for at least three months [7]. The global dimension of the disease is so important that CKD started to be considered a relevant public health problem. Indeed, according to the Global Burden of Kidney Disease, the CKD incidence and prevalence increased by 88.76% and 86.95%, respectively, from 1990 to 2016 [8]. Moreover, the mortality attributed to CKD increased by 41.5% between 1990 and 2017, a percentage that exceeded the mortality due to several neoplasms or cardiovascular (CV) disease [9]. Hence, great effort is advocated toward improving clinical decision-making and reinforcing treatment and prevention of CKD. The KDIGO working group proposed a classification called "CGA" that incorporates the cause (C) of kidney disease, as well as the eGFR (G) and albuminuria (A) levels, to stratify risk in patients with CKD and to better address the importance of the underlying disease. However, considering eGFR and albuminuria levels in cross-tabs, like those reported in KDIGO guidelines, does not take into consideration the complex mechanisms of CKD. In fact, all patients are stratified on the basis of eGFR and albuminuria and allocated in risk categories for prognostic estimations. This approach was also defined as "reductionist", since it does not consider the different etiologies of CKD and many other parameters, including serum or urine biomarkers, which could help clinical management of CKD [10]. Moreover, although the KDIGO also suggested considering the causes of kidney disease to predict poor outcomes in CKD patients, how to incorporate these parameters remains unclear [11]. Few studies included renal diagnoses in risk prediction models and, when diagnoses are present, they are classified in different ways (i.e., four, five, or even six categories) with large heterogeneity between studies, thus making an univocal interpretation difficult [12,13]. There is also a growing debate regarding the question whether an eGFR reduction below the threshold of 60 mL/min/1.73 m^2 represents the consequence of a physiologic senescence or a marker of renal pathology [14,15]. In fact, despite the evidence that eGFR reduction foresees both the onset of end-stage kidney disease (ESKD) and the all-cause death regardless of age, in large general and high-risk populations, other human studies showed that kidneys undergo structural and functional change with aging such as nephrosclerosis and a reduction in measured GFR [14,16]. At the same time, these changes are not associated with a reduction in single-nephron GFR; this is the likely reason why, in the absence of albuminuria, the GFR reduction alone determines only a small increased risk for age-standardized mortality and ESKD [16]. Owing to these important controversies and in an attempt to improve risk stratification and care of CKD patients, as well as to share clinical findings with the nephrology community, the International Society of Nephrology (ISN) started an international project called "closing the gaps", which encompasses a set of activities that have to be performed to improve the prognosis of CKD patients [17]. The core of this project is about the development, implementation, and clinical application of novel biomarkers in CKD patients. It indeed emerged that, with the exception of cystatin C, which is a filtration marker useful to estimate the eGFR and to improve risk prediction in CKD, the vast majority of previously tested biomarkers in CKD did not reach any clinical application [18]. The aim of this review is to report the principal pieces of evidence regarding biomarker development in CKD, the contribution of these biomarkers to both observational and interventional (i.e., randomized controlled trials) studies, and the possible strategies that could be followed to ameliorate this important branch of clinical research.

2. General Classification of Biomarkers

Depending on the intended use, biomarkers are classified as diagnostic, pharmacodynamic/response, monitoring, prognostic, or predictive [19]. We focus, in the present review article, on prognostic and predictive biomarkers, as they represent the most developed biomarkers in CKD patients, while they also incorporate characteristics from other categories of biomarkers. A prognostic biomarker is used to identify the probability of a clinical outcome in patients who are already suffering from the disease of interest [1,20]. Furthermore, prognostic biomarkers measure the association between the disease and clinical outcome in the absence of therapy or with standard therapy that all patients are likely to receive. On the other hand, predictive biomarkers are used to determine whether a patient is likely to benefit from a particular therapy. The clinical benefit could be either a good response to a drug if the biomarker is positive or, alternatively, a lack of benefit from the same drug, which can save a patient from drug toxicity or unnecessary side effects [1].

3. Prognostic Biomarkers in CKD

The importance of prognostic biomarkers in the CKD setting is crucial. Indeed, CKD is a multifactorial disease in which risk factors play different roles in different individuals and in different stages of the disease. It was demonstrated, for example, that the presence of type 2 diabetes leads to the development of CKD in up to 30% of subjects. This means that, in these patients, the deleterious pathogenetic mechanisms of diabetes mellitus are sufficient to damage the kidneys with the onset of typical diabetic glomerulosclerosis. Conversely, it is also possible that, in a portion of diabetic patients, the kidneys are injured by the co-existence of arterial hypertension, which causes different lesions (mainly injuring the kidney vessels), with a completely different prognosis.

3.1. Kidney Biomarkers

The assessment of correct risk stratification, i.e., the allocation of CKD patients to the true risk-of-event categories, always represents a difficult challenge for nephrologists and researchers, due to the large variability in etiology and prognosis of CKD [21,22]. In order to accomplish this aim, a growing number of risk prediction models in CKD patients were developed over the past several years. They show how kidney measures, such as albuminuria (or proteinuria) and eGFR, are strong prognostic biomarkers. Indeed, an eGFR reduction to levels below 60 mL/min/1.73 m^2 or even a small increase in albuminuria levels is associated with a significantly increased risk for CV events (CV mortality, coronary heart disease, stroke, heart failure), all-cause mortality, and ESKD (the most advanced stage of CKD that requires referral to renal replacement therapies such as hemodialysis), both in the general population and in patients with an already established CKD (Figure 1) [23–25].

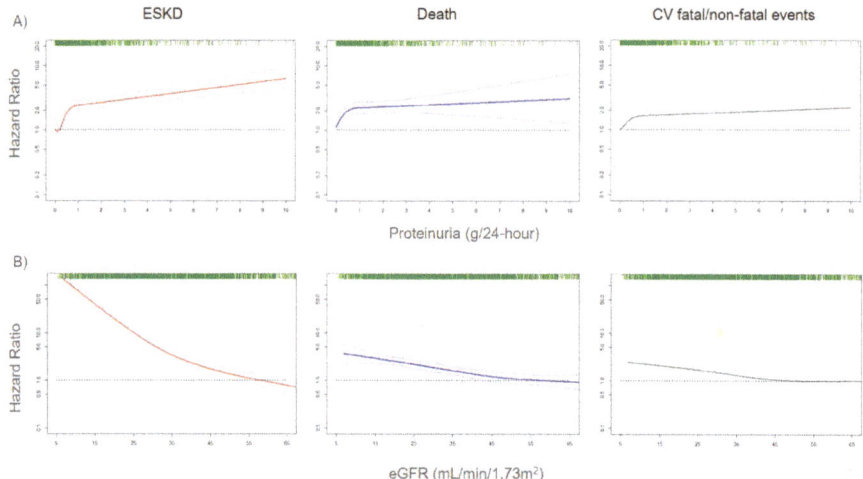

Figure 1. Adjusted risks for end-stage kidney disease (ESKD), death, and cardiovascular (CV) fatal and non-fatal events, by 24-h proteinuria (panel **A**) or estimated glomerular filtration rate (eGFR) (panel **B**) levels. Solid lines represent hazard ratios, whereas dashed lines the 95% confidence intervals. Hazard ratios were modeled by means of restricted cubic spline (RCS) due to the non-linear association with the endpoints. Knots are located at the zeroth, 25th, 50th, and 75th percentiles for proteinuria and 15, 30, 45, 60 mL/min/1.73 m^2 for eGFR. Risks are adjusted for the four-variable Tangri equation [26]: age, gender, eGFR, and proteinuria. Rug plots on the x-axis at the top (colored green) represent the distribution of observations. Data source: pooled analysis of six cohorts of CKD patients referred to Italian nephrology clinics [27].

Albuminuria and eGFR were also recently used to develop individual risk prediction models for both CV and renal risk in CKD patients. These models employ statistical measures (such as calibration, discrimination, and validation) that represent an essential step before applying risk estimates at the individual level [25,26,28,29]. Moreover, risk prediction models are available for patients with early, moderate, and severe stages of CKD. The addition of albuminuria and eGFR to traditional risk factors included in the model (such as age, gender, presence of diabetes, blood pressure, serum cholesterol) was associated with a significant improvement in risk prediction. Even more importantly, the contribution of albuminuria and eGFR to the prediction of CV events (CV mortality, coronary heart disease, stroke, and heart failure) was found to be greater than traditional CV risk factors [24]. This notwithstanding, a main limitation of available risk score is the insufficient, even absent, consideration of underlying causes of renal disease, which is a crucial point when considering that CKD is a set of multiple etiologies rather than a single disease [12,13]. However, these first prediction models established that measuring albuminuria and eGFR is a central step for assessing risk stratification in CKD patients. Mechanisms of damage of albuminuria and eGFR were partially explained. Albuminuria was shown to exert a direct harmful effect on renal glomeruli and tubules [30]. Moreover, it can also be considered as a systemic marker of endothelial dysfunction, and this explains the reason for which the presence of proteinuria strictly forecasts the onset of CV events in the general population, as well as CKD patients [31]. Similarly, eGFR reduction is linked to an increase of uremic toxins that are responsible for kidney and systemic damage. A drop in eGFR was also associated with the development of coronary atherosclerosis, regardless of the presence of diabetes mellitus, dyslipidemia, previous CV disease, and other comorbidities [32]. Several studies showed that an eGFR decrease is associated with the onset of sudden cardiac death (SCD), with the data being confirmed from the early stage of CKD, i.e., from eGFR < 60 mL/min/1.73 m^2 [33–35]. For each 10 mL/min decrement in eGFR, SCD risk increased by 11% [33]. SCD accounts for the vast majority of deaths in CKD patients and is also mediated by metabolic and electrophysiological abnormalities [36]. However, both eGFR and albuminuria have limitations in risk prediction. Albuminuria is not specific for any kidney disease, occurring in ischemic, diabetic, and tubulointerstitial nephropathies, as well as in the vast majority of glomerulonephritis and autoimmune diseases [13]. Albuminuria also presents a random variability, since urine protein excretion follows a circadian rhythm that is influenced by posture, exercise, or dietary factors [37]. The eGFR, albeit associated with a poor prognosis, could also be altered by temporary or reversible clinical conditions, such as volume depletions or sub-acute tubulointerstitial diseases [11]. Taken together, proteinuria and eGFR share the limitation of detecting kidney damage often when it is already established and is, thus, not reversible [15]. Furthermore, urine protein excretion is strictly dependent on eGFR levels, which are an expression of the number of functional nephrons in the kidney. In fact, we recently demonstrated that, in a model in which proteinuria is replaced by F-Uprot (proteinuria/eGFR × 100), an expression of the combination of the two biomarkers, the latter allowed refining risk stratification for ESKD outcome in all CKD stages, even in more advanced CKD [27]. Albuminuria levels are strictly dependent and, thus, modified by both systolic and diastolic blood pressure (BP). As long as the eGFR decreases, a given increase in BP is accompanied by an increase in urine protein excretion. This phenomenon was observed in both animal and human studies and is caused by the "remnant nephron effect", namely, the transmission of systemic hydrostatic pressure to the glomerular microcirculation [38,39]. Moreover, BP is a clinical parameter characterized per se by high variability, which is also detectable during 24-h ambulatory BP measurements (short-term variability) [40]. It was demonstrated that both systolic and diastolic BP variability influence albuminuria levels [41]. Hence, a number of variables were shown to influence albuminuria levels, and this could lead to biased risk estimation, particularly if the risk prediction is based on a single measurement of albuminuria. The ISN indeed highlighted that a consensus needs to be found on how often albuminuria should be measured to warrant a true prediction of cardiovascular and renal endpoints, as well as to monitor the course of CKD [18]. Owing to the evidence that eGFR and albuminuria are able to provide a strong but incomplete prediction of cardiorenal endpoints in CKD patients, the next step of prognostic research focused on the development and assessment of biomarkers that provide useful prognostic information beyond proteinuria and eGFR. A number of markers of inflammation, oxidative stress, or tissue remodeling aroused interest in improving CV and renal risk prediction in CKD patients.

3.2. Markers of Oxidative Stress, Tissue Remodeling, and Metabolism

Myeloperoxidase (MPO) is a biomarker of oxidative stress that fosters nitic oxide consumption and which is associated with the development of atherosclerotic lesions, CV disease, and eGFR decline in CKD [42,43]. A recent observational analysis of the Chronic Renal Insufficiency Cohort (CRIC), which enrolled approximately 4000 patients with CKD in the United States (US), showed that serum MPO levels were associated with the risk of renal outcome, defined as initiation of RRT, 50% eGFR decline, or eGFR ≤ 15 mL/min/1.73 m^2 [44]. The key element of this analysis was that the effect of MPO was significant even after adjustment for main confounders, such as baseline eGFR and proteinuria levels. Matrix metalloproteinases (MMPs), endopeptidases involved in tissue development, and homeostasis through the regulation of cell differentiation, apoptosis, and angiogenesis were shown to intervene in inflammatory and fibrotic processes across the kidneys [45,46]. Blood and urine levels of MMPs were linked to renal and CV disease in previous clinical studies in humans. Serum and urine MMP-2, -8, and -9 levels are increased in patients with diabetic CKD, with MMP-9 being significantly associated with the severity of albuminuria [47,48]. Increased plasma levels of TIMP-1 (tissue inhibitor of metalloproteinases-1) predicted the incidence of CKD regardless of inflammatory markers such as C-reactive protein [49]. MMPs and TIMPs also play a role in accelerating the atherosclerotic process by increasing cell migration to the plaque fibrous cap that in turn determines plaque inflammation and rupture [50]. Indeed, the levels of several MMPs (MMP-1, -2, -8, -9) and TIMP-1 were found to be increased in patients with peripheral arterial disease, including those with aneurysms of the arterial wall [51]. Fibroblast growth factor-23 (FGF-23), a hormone involved in phosphorus metabolism that increases progressively as kidney function declines, was significantly associated with mortality, atherosclerotic events, heart failure (HF), and ESKD in CKD patients [52,53].

3.3. Cardiac Biomarkers

Several cardiac biomarkers were investigated, mainly for establishing their role in CV and renal risk prediction in CKD patients. Cardiac troponins (high-sensitivity cardiac troponin (hs-cTnT)) and natriuretic peptides (N-terminal pro-B-type natriuretic peptide (NT-proBNP)) are largely used in CV medicine to diagnose coronary artery disease (CAD) and heart failure (HF), respectively. Both these biomarkers are, thus, an expression of subclinical abnormalities in the heart [54,55]. However, one major problem that makes their introduction in individual risk prediction difficult is that cardiac markers are an expression of both cardiac and kidney dysfunction and cannot discern these two conditions. Natriuretic peptides act by promoting the tubular natriuresis across the kidney and counteracting the effects of renin–angiotensin–aldosterone system, which is triggered by heart failure, as well as renal dysfunction [56]. Concerns about the interpretation of hs-cTnT and natriuretic peptides also derive from the evidence that these marker concentrations are influenced by kidney function levels [56,57]. So far, cardiac markers found more application in the context of prognostic estimation of cardiorenal syndromes (CRS), clinical disorders where an acute or chronic dysfunction of one organ may lead to an acute or chronic dysfunction of the other, thus testifying the strict relationship between the heart and the kidney [58]. In the general population, hs-cTnT and NT-proBNP were shown to be strong predictors for incident HF over time [59,60]. In the setting of CKD, an attempt to evaluate, with appropriate statistical tools, the contribution of cardiac markers to the development of CV events was made using the Atherosclerosis Risk in Communities study (ARIC) population. In this study, examining 7682 non-CKD and 970 patients with CKD stage 1–5, hs-cTnT and NT-proBNP were associated with the development of CV events (defined as the composite of coronary heart disease, stroke, and HF) independently of kidney measures (eGFR and albuminuria) [61]. The finding was confirmed for both CKD and non-CKD patients, as well as for patients with or without previous CV disease. However, the interpretation of these results should be done with caution since the ARIC cohort was stratified, for this analysis, by the presence/absence of CKD, thus limiting the influence of kidney measures on CV risk prediction [61]. Results of the association between cardiac markers and renal outcomes in CKD patients are even more conflicting. The CRIC investigators found, in a cohort of over 3000 CKD patients, that increased plasma levels of growth differentiation factor-15 (GDF-15, a member of the transforming growth factor (TGF)-β cytokine family), hs-cTnT, and NT-proBNP were associated with CKD progression. defined as the onset of ESKD or 50% eGFR decline [62]. However, when all these parameters were added to the prediction model including traditional CV risk factors, the model discrimination (i.e., the ability of the model to separate individuals who develop events from those who do not; see more details in Section 5) did not improve, meaning that their clinical utility was scarce. Moreover, in the Framingham cohort, hs-cTnT was not associated with a faster eGFR decline or with incident CKD [63]. There is, overall, a need for future work to assess the role of cardiac markers in CV and renal risk prediction [61–63].

3.4. Filtration and Urinary Biomarkers

Filtration biomarkers and urinary markers were also investigated. The use of cystatin C to estimate GFR (eGFR$_{cys}$) improved the risk stratification for death, death from CV causes, and ESKD with a large proportion (23%) of patients being reclassified toward true risk estimates when compared with eGFR estimated from serum creatinine (eGFR$_{crea}$) [64]. eGFR$_{cys}$ was also shown to predict the onset of SCD in elderly CKD patients [35]. The combination of serum creatinine and cystatin C for estimating eGFR (eGFR$_{cys-crea}$) allowed clinicians to anticipate the risk prediction of worse outcomes at 85 mL/min, which is well above the 60 mL/min threshold defined by eGFR$_{crea}$. β2-microglobulin, another filtration marker, showed a statistical power similar to cystatin C in improving prediction of ESKD, all-cause mortality, and new onset of CV disease beyond eGFR$_{crea}$ [65]. With respect to urinary markers, some evidence, albeit controversial, was provided for the association of urinary markers of tubule damage (interleukin (IL)-18, kidney injury molecule-1 (KIM-1), neutrophil gelatinase-associated lipocalin (NGAL)), repair (human cartilage glycoprotein-40 (YKL-40)), and inflammation (monocyte chemoattractant protein-1 (MCP-1)) with the risk of ESKD [66,67]. In fact, when risk prediction models were adjusted for baseline eGFR and albuminuria, the associations of these biomarkers with clinical outcome were consistently attenuated. However, the highest values of KIM-1, MCP-1, and YKL-40 also provided useful risk estimation beyond eGFR and albuminuria in a post hoc analysis of the Systolic Blood Pressure Intervention Trial SPRINT trial [68]. Interestingly, urinary IL-18 and NGAL levels were shown to predict linear eGFR decline over time, an endpoint of growing interest in clinical research [68].

3.5. Prognostic Role of Proteomics, Metabolomics, and Genomics

Proteomics metabolomics and genomics recently provided great input to the implementation of novel biomarkers [69–71]. The advantage of these "omics" techniques is to provide a combination of informative peptides/metabolites that are able to classify patients (hence, the appellation of classifiers) into significant clinical or risk categories. A well-depicted classifier in CKD patients is the CKD273, a panel of 273 urine peptides shown to predict, in long-term follow-up cohort studies, eGFR decline with a strong and independent effect to the onset of albuminuria, particularly in diabetic patients [72–74]. In further risk prediction models, CKD273 was also able to reclassify about 30% of patients compared with the standard equation that considers eGFR and albuminuria, for the risk of CKD progression [75]. The CRIC investigators described, in a recent manuscript, the association between a panel of 13 urine metabolites and CKD progression [76]. Results of this analysis are encouraging since the levels of four metabolites, namely, 3-hydroxyisobutyrate (3-HIBA), 3-methylcrotonylglycine, citric acid, and aconitic acid, were associated with eGFR decline, with 3-HIBA and aconitic acid levels also significantly associated with the hard endpoint ESKD. Of particular interest is the prognostic role of the genetic causes of CKD. Of all CKD cases diagnosed at a young age (<25 years), an actual 30% are determined by monogenic disorders, and inherited CKD is globally more prevalent (prevalence ranged between 30% and 75%) than previously thought, particularly in the presence of a family history of CKD [77,78]. More importantly, the advent of genome-wide association studies (GWAS) allowed the discovery of several single-nucleotide polymorphisms (SNPs) associated with an increased risk for CKD or with a worse prognosis in patients already affected by CKD [78]. Polymorphisms in the Uromodulin (UMOD) gene region rs4293393, which codifies the most abundant urinary protein in healthy subjects, namely, uromodulin (also called Tamm–Horsfall protein), are associated with an increased risk of incident CKD [79]. A similar role in predicting the onset of CKD was exerted by other SNPs such as Protein Kinase AMP-Activated Non-Catalytic Subunit Gamma 2 (PRKAG2), Longevity Assurance Gene Homologs (LASS2), Disabled Homolog 2 (alias DAB Adaptor Protein 2, DAB2), Dachshund Family Transcription Factor 1 (DACH1), and Stanniocalcin 1 (STC1) [80]. Apolipoprotein L1 (APOL1) gene variants were also studied in CKD patients. APOL1 encodes apolipoprotein L1, which is involved in the lysis of *Trypanosoma brucei* and other trypanosomes [81]. The G1 and G2 variants of APOL1 were associated with an increased risk of eGFR decline and disease progression to ESKD in CKD populations [82]. Interestingly, information derived from the SNPs were recently combined into a genetic risk score [78]. This score was shown to be associated with eGFR decline and kidney outcome regardless of albuminuria and other renal risk factors encompassing diabetes, history of CV disease, and hypertension. A number of studies assessing the associations between SNPs and kidney measures were carried-out by the United Kingdom (UK) biobank, a large cohort of over 500,000 participants enrolled in 2006–2010, from which genotypic information was widely collected [83]. Analyses of the UK biobank provided a great contribution to the prognostic research in CKD. For example, genetically predicted testosterone and fasting insulin, with the latter being an expression of insulin resistance, were found to be associated with CKD and worse kidney function in men, thus highlighting the possible reasons for discrepancy in CKD prevalence and CKD progression among men and women [84,85]. Intriguingly, a genome-wide association study of UK biobank showed that albumin-to-creatinine ratio (ACR) is dependent on multiple pathways and that an ACR genetic risk score may improve the prediction of hypertension and stroke [86].

4. Predictive Biomarkers in CKD

Predictive biomarkers are used in disparate fields of medicine to assess the likelihood of response to treatments and the individual pathophysiology of the disease. One major example of this strategy is represented by the large use of predictive biomarkers in oncology. Causative mutations of the breast cancer genes 1 and 2 (BRCA1/2) were found to be predictive biomarkers for identifying the response to poly(ADP-ribose) polymerase (PARP) inhibitors [87]. Such a discovery is crucial as BRCA1/2 provide information on the best drug for the individual patient in order to improve their prognosis. While, in oncology, a set of pathophysiological mechanisms is crucial for tumor development, what complicates the application of predictive biomarkers in chronic diseases is that different mechanisms are active in different stages of the disease itself and in different patients [88]. This means that, if a treatment is started on the basis of a blood/urine biomarker level, the individual prognosis may remain unchanged or even worsen, due to the presence of other active mechanisms of damage, as well as, most importantly, different disease entities that cause the chronic decline of renal function through diverse pathophysiological pathways. Notwithstanding, in chronic disease, great research effort was also started with the aim of personalizing treatments following the methodological concept of "the right drug for the right patient". Hence, the implementation of predictive biomarkers represents a topic of increasing importance.

4.1. Kidney Biomarkers

In nephrology, the most used predictive biomarkers are eGFR and albuminuria. Both these biomarkers can be considered as "dynamic" predictive biomarkers. In fact, their levels change over time with the effects of treatment, such that they can be efficiently used for monitoring the course of CKD and the appropriateness of the therapy followed by the patient. In the past few decades, several interventional studies were carried out testing the effect of nephroprotective drugs on hard endpoints such as mortality, CV events, and ESKD in patients with CKD [89–96]. Although interventions differed between studies, with principally antihypertensive drugs and albuminuria-lowering agents being tested, all these trials pointed out that the CV, mortality, and ESKD risk reductions were strictly associated with a reduction in albuminuria after the start of treatment. Moreover, the magnitude of treatment effect was greater in patients with higher albuminuria levels at the time of the initial visit [95,96]. These findings are reinforced by the evidence that albuminuria changes also played a potentially beneficial role in negative clinical trials. In the Aliskiren Trial in Type 2 Diabetes Using Cardiorenal Endpoints (ALTITUDE), which failed in demonstrating the advantage of adding Aliskiren to an angiotensin-converting enzyme inhibitor (ACEi) or an angiotensin-receptor blocker (ARB) on CV and renal outcomes, patients who showed an albuminuria reduction in the Aliskiren arm (37%) were largely protected against CKD progression compared with those who did not show a reduction in albuminuria levels [97]. All these pieces of evidence testified that albuminuria has great predictive and prognostic power in CKD patients and, although further studies are needed to find the correct threshold of albuminuria reduction that can confer CV and renal risk protection after an appropriate treatment, there is a general consensus that a 30% reduction in its levels from baseline to six months could be acceptable [98]. With respect to eGFR, it was demonstrated that a doubling of serum creatinine level, which corresponds approximately to a 57% eGFR decline, was able to predict CKD progression in previous clinical trials in diabetic CKD patients [99]. The importance of that evidence is highlighted by the fact that, in these previous trials, eGFR decline correlated with renal outcomes after exposure to nephroprotective treatments, thus affirming its role as a predictive biomarker, in addition to a prognostic biomarker [100]. Since then, the association of lesser eGFR declines with CKD outcomes was tested. A post hoc analysis of the Reduction of End Points in Non-Insulin-Dependent Diabetes with the Angiotensin II Antagonist Losartan (RENAAL) and Irbesartan Diabetic Nephropathy Trial

(IDNT) clinical trials, two studies that evaluated the efficacy of ARB treatment in patients with diabetes mellitus and nephropathy, showed that 30% and 40% eGFR declines may improve the power of clinical trials if the drug investigated does not determine an acute (within three months of the start of treatment) drop in eGFR [101]. A larger meta-analysis of 37 clinical trials in CKD patients documented a strong association between 30% and 40% eGFR decline in the first 12 months of treatment and the onset of kidney disease progression [100].

4.2. Biomarkers of Tissue Remodeling

In addition to proteinuria and eGFR, other promising predictive biomarkers in CKD were described. A change in serum levels of MMPs after exposure to BB-1101, a synthetic hydroxamic acid-based inhibitor of MMP, was associated with a reduction in proteinuria in experimental models of glomerular damage [102]. A similar effect was observed in diabetic CKD patients who underwent treatment with doxycycline, an antibiotic from the tetracycline family, and who were already treated with renin–angiotensin–aldosterone inhibitors (RAAS-i) [103]. Moreover, MMPs are also involved in the mechanism that leads to CV risk reduction exerted by sodium–glucose cotransporter 2 inhibitors (SGLT2-i) through the activation of RECK (reversion-inducing cysteine-rich protein with kazal motifs), an endogenous inhibitor of MMPs [104]. That mechanism appeared to be independent of proteinuria levels and could also be useful for selecting high-risk normoalbuminuric CKD patients to be enrolled in future clinical trials, who represent a non-trivial proportion of the CKD cohort [21].

4.3. Ultrasound Biomarkers

Evidence is also emerging for a possible role of the renal resistive index (RRI) as a dynamic predictive biomarker. RRI is a Doppler ultrasonographic index, whose increase reflects both renal and systemic vascular impairment [105]. RRI was also found to predict the onset of CV and kidney outcomes in patients with CKD or essential hypertension [106,107]. RRI values are changed over time by different drug classes, such as RAAS-i and SGLT2-i; novel studies will hopefully reveal in the future if these treatment-induced modifications could also predict hard CV and renal endpoints [108,109].

4.4. Predictive Role of Proteomics, Metabolomics, and Genomics

A polymorphism of the angiotensin-converting enzyme gene caused by an insertion/deletion (ACE/ID) modifies the systemic and renal activity of the RAAS, which was recognized to be a trigger of kidney damage [110]. The ACE/DD–ACE/ID polymorphism was able to predict the response to losartan in type 2 diabetic patients enrolled in the RENAAL trial, that is, patients with worse prognosis (D allele carriers) had the best response to losartan [111]. Complex biomarkers and classifiers have a predictive role, in addition to a prognostic role. A set of 21 serum metabolites were selected from a larger panel through a penalized regression analysis, and they were shown to correctly predict the albuminuria response to ARB treatment in type 2 diabetic patients [112]. This classifier revealed that the enzyme nitric oxide synthase 3 (NOS3) is crucial to forecast the response to ARB therapy in diabetic CKD, since it is involved in the molecular mechanism of action of these drugs. A proteomic predictive classifier was developed from the Prevention of REnal and Vascular ENd-stage Disease (PREVEND) study, using plasma proteomics profiles of fibrosis and kidney damage that allowed predicting the albuminuria change in patients treated with RAAS-i [113]. The principal characteristics of prognostic and predictive biomarkers are depicted in Table 1.

Table 1. Summary of the principal prognostic and predictive biomarkers in chronic kidney disease patients.

Biomarkers	Characteristics	Prognostic/Predictive values
Cystatin C	Low-molecular-weight protein, produced by all types of nucleated cells, which acts as a cysteine protease inhibitor. It is freely filtered by the renal glomeruli, then 99% reabsorbed and metabolized in the renal proximal tubule; it is not secreted.	Cystatin C improves the estimation of eGFR and risk prediction of CV and renal events. It also allows a more precise stratification of patients according to their CV and renal risk [64].
β2-microglobulin	Protein present on the surface of immune cells, as a constant subunit of class I histocompatibility antigens. It is also found in blood and other biological fluids, as an expression of cell turnover. It is filtered by the renal glomerulus and reabsorbed at the tubular level.	It improves the prediction of ESKD, all-cause mortality, and new onset of CV disease [65].
hs-cTnT	Cardiac troponins are enzymes present in both skeletal and cardiac muscles. They regulate muscle contraction by controlling the calcium-mediated interaction of actin and myosin.	It improves the risk prediction of CV events, particularly heart failure regardless of the level of kidney function [55,57,114,115], as well as the risk prediction of microvascular events (nephropathy or retinopathy) in diabetic patients and the risk prediction of CKD progression.
NT-proBNP	Amino terminal fragment of the natriuretic type B peptide, normally produced in the heart and released in the case of cardiac stresses consequent to water overload conditions.	It improves the risk prediction of CV events, particularly heart failure regardless of the level of kidney function [55,57,114,115], as well as microvascular events (nephropathy or retinopathy) in diabetic patients and CKD progression. In the SONAR trial, it was used as a predictive biomarker in order to exclude patients with sodium retention after treatment with atrasentan [94].
sST2	A soluble form of the ST2 protein. It is a member of the interleukin 1 receptor family. In the case of myocardial stress, there is an upregulation of the ST2 gene and an increase in sST2 levels; by interacting with IL-33 (ligand for ST2), it counteracts the cardioprotective effect deriving from the ST2-IL 33 bond.	It showed an incremental prediction ability (over NT-proBNP) of death and hospitalizations due to HF in CKD patients [62,116]. It does not predict the risk of CKD progression.
GDF-15	Member of TGF-β cytokine family that is released in response to cellular stress. It appears to have a role in regulating inflammatory processes, apoptosis, cell repair, and cell growth.	It improves the risk prediction of both CV and microvascular events [62,116].
FGF-23	A protein belonging to the family of fibroblast growth factors, involved in the metabolism of phosphates. It is secreted in response to increased serum phosphate or calciprotein particles (colloidal nanoparticles of calcium phosphate dispersed in the blood), from osteocytes/osteoblasts. It acts on the kidneys by reducing the expression of a sodium phosphate transporter located in the renal proximal tubule, thus increasing the urinary excretion of phosphates.	It was significantly associated with mortality, atherosclerotic events, HF, and ESKD in CKD patients [52,53].
MMPs	Calcium-dependent endopeptidases that contain zinc and that are involved in the various processes of tissue development and cellular homeostasis.	Serum MMP-2, -8, and -9 and TIMP-1 are associated with atherogenesis, the severity of kidney damage, and the onset of left-ventricular hypertrophy and peripheral vascular disease [45–51]. MMPs levels are modified by selective and nonselective drugs. Changes in MMP levels are associated with a reduction of CV risk [102–104].

Table 1. Cont.

Biomarkers	Characteristics	Prognostic/Predictive values
Urinary markers	Urinary markers of tubule damage (IL-18, KIM-1, NGAL), repair (YKL-40), and inflammation (MCP-1).	Increased urinary concentrations of these biomarkers predict a linear decline in eGFR over time [65–67].
eGFR$_{crea}$	eGFR$_{crea}$ is an estimation of the kidney function level, based on serum creatinine levels, age, gender, and race.	A reduction of eGFR is a potent predictor of CV and renal endpoints [21–23]. A treatment-induced reduction of eGFR (30% and 40% reduction) is considered to be a surrogate endpoint of ESKD [73–75].
Proteinuria	Presence of an abnormal quantity of proteins in urine. It is considered the principal marker of kidney damage.	The increase in proteinuria levels is strongly associated with the onset of fatal and non-fatal CV events [23–25]. In clinical trials, patients who developed a significant reduction in proteinuria levels, during the first months after treatment, were protected against CV and renal events over time [89–97].
F-Uprot	It combines the prognostic/predictive power of two biomarkers (proteinuria and eGFR). Proteinuria/eGFR × 100.	It improves risk stratification for ESKD outcomes at all the stages of CKD [27].
MPO	It is an enzyme belonging to the class of oxide reductase, with bactericidal and pro-inflammatory action.	It is a prognostic marker of cardiovascular risk, and it is associated with the risk of renal outcome (RRI, 50% eGFR decline, eGFR ≤ 15 mL/min/1.73 m^2) [42–44].
RRI	Renal resistive index (RRI) is an ultrasonographic index of intrarenal arteries, defined as (peak systolic velocity − end diastolic velocity)/peak systolic velocity.	Raised RI levels above have been shown to reflect renal and systemic vascular impairment and predict CV events in hypertensive and CKD patients [105–107]. Medications as RAAS inhibitors and SGLT2-i reduce RRI levels over time and improve vascular damage [108,109].
ACE ID/DD	Insertion (I)/deletion (D) polymorphism of the angiotensin-converting enzyme (ACE) gene influences the circulating and renal activity of RAAS.	The D allele patients showed a poor CV prognosis in the RENAAL trial [110,111]. Patients with the DD genotype, despite being at a high risk of CV events, showed the better response to losartan in the RENAAL study [110,111].
Classifiers	A classifier is a combination of the informative markers able to classify patients according to their risk of developing an outcome or likelihood of response to a treatment.	13 metabolites predicted CKD progression in the CRIC cohort [76]. A panel of 21 metabolites was shown to predict the proteinuric response to ARBs [112].
CKD273	It is the combination of 273 urinary peptides identified as early indicators of molecular changes that predict the development or progression of CKD. The main components of CKD273 are collagen fragments and protein fragments, including proteins involved in inflammation.	It predicts the risk of development or progression of CKD, allowing the implementation of preventive attitudes. It is used in clinical trials to predict the development of CKD in response to a therapeutic approach [72–75].

eGFR, estimated Glomerular Filtration Rate; CV, Cardiovascular; ESKD, End-Stage-Kidney-Disease; hs-cTnT, high-sensitivity cardiac troponin; CKD, Chronic Kidney Disease; NT-proBNP, N-terminal pro-B-type natriuretic peptide; SONAR, study of diabetic nephropathy with the endothelin receptor antagonist atrasentan; sST2, soluble form of ST2; IL, interleukin; HF, Heart Failure; GDF-15, growth differentiation factor-15; TGF-β, transforming growth factor β; FGF-23, Fibroblast Growth Factor 23; MMP, Matrix metalloproteinases; TIMP, tissue inhibitor of metalloproteinases; KIM-1, Kidney Injury Molecule-1; NGAL, neutrophil gelatinase-associated lipocalin; YKL-40, repair human cartilage glycoprotein-40; MCP-1, monocyte chemoattractant protein-1; MPO, Myeloperoxidase; RRT, Renal Replacement Therapies; RAAS, Renin–Angiotensin–Aldosterone System; SGLT2-i, sodium–glucose cotransporter 2 inhibitors; RENAAL, Reduction of End Points in Non-Insulin-Dependent Diabetes with the Angiotensin II Antagonist Losartan; CRIC, Chronic Renal Insufficiency Cohort; ARBs angiotensin-receptor blockers.

5. Implementation of Biomarkers in Observational Studies

Owing to the importance of improving risk stratification beyond traditional kidney measures and to help clinical decision-making in CKD patients, the evaluation of novel biomarkers acquired great emphasis in clinical research, as witnessed by the growing number of publications on this topic [114]. However, before a biomarker can find full application in clinical practice, several steps need to be satisfied and reported. The first questions that should be addressed are the following: What will be the clinical intended use of the biomarker? Is the assay analytic performance acceptable for the intended use? To answer these important questions, the development process should start with assessing the analytic and clinical validity of the biomarker. Analytic validity refers to evaluating whether the characteristics of the measured biomarker are acceptable in term of precision, accuracy, and reproducibility [115]. It is indeed important to be aware that biomarker levels may vary in clinical practice due to factors not linked to the disease of interest being classified as pre-analytical and analytical factors [116]. Pre-analytical variation depends on several factors that include lifestyle (exercise, smoking habit, obesity), age, race, influence of gender, specimen collections (fasting, time, and temperature of storage) [117]. For instance, albuminuria, measured with the available methods, such as 24-h urine collection or albumin-to-creatinine ratio, is extremely influenced by physical exercise and other conditions that determine a day-by-day variation, defined as random variation [37]. Urinary NGAL concentration is stable in urine for up to seven days, but it is increased by the presence of white blood cells that are an important confounder [118]. Analytic variation is mainly defined by two parameters, which are bias and precision [119]. Bias is the amount by which an average of many repeated measurements made using the assay systematically over- or underestimates the true value. Precision represents the repeatability of measurements under unchanged assay conditions in a laboratory. While analytic validation is often discussed, it is seldom handled in a proper fashion. It was suggested to deepen analytic validation, while developing a biomarker, and to report metrics, such as precision, reproducibility, accuracy, analytic sensitivity, limits of detection and quantification, linearity, and analytic specificity [120]. A descriptive summary of these measures is reported in Table 2.

Table 2. Principal tools used to assess analytic validation.

Features	Definition	Statistical Metric
Precision	Intra-assay agreement of a set of results among themselves. It could be expressed by coefficient of variation (CV).	$CV_{(\%)} = (\text{Standard deviation}_{samples}/\text{Mean}_{samples}) \times 100$
Reproducibility	Concordance between various measurements carried out in different laboratories and experimental conditions on the same sample.	
Accuracy	Closeness of the agreement between result of a single measurement and true value obtained using a reference standard method.	
Trueness	Concordance between a series of assays and the real value of analyte concentration.	
Bias	Systematic difference of the series of measurements with true value.	$Bias_{(\%)} = (\text{Mean}_{sample} - \text{True value}) \times 100$
Limit of blank	Highest apparent analyte concentration founded by testing specimens without analyte.	$LoB = \text{Mean}_{blank} + 1.645(SD_{blank})$
Limit of detection	Average of lowest concentration of analyte which can be distinguished from a blank sample.	$LoD = LoB + 1645(SD_{samples})$
Limit of quantification	Smallest concentration of analyte with an acceptable accuracy and precision.	
Linearity	Proportionality between a set of measured values and true concentration of analyte.	
Analytic specificity	Ability to measure only and exclusively the analyte of interest.	
Analytic sensibility	Ability to measure lowest concentration of analyte.	

Clinical validity is the next important step and consists of demonstrating that biomarker measurement is associated with a clinical characteristic of interest [115]. The first steps of clinical validation are the proof of concept and prospective validation [114]. Proof of concept means to assess whether biomarker levels differ between subjects who develop the event of interest vs. non-events. This phase is essential since it allows understanding if the biomarker can play a role in the context of disease, and continuing its development is convenient. To this aim, a cross-sectional design could be sufficient [121]. Next, it is necessary, in prognostic validation, to evaluate if the biomarker is significantly associated with the event of interest, with a prospective analysis. Moreover, it is important that the magnitude of this association is not attenuated when the analysis is adjusted for traditional risk factors, such as age, gender, and proteinuria and eGFR levels in CKD patients. This step provides other useful information such as the distribution of the biomarker and, therefore, how to incorporate the biomarker levels in multivariable analyses. It is suggested to start by adding to the model the biomarker variable as a continuous variable, before applying a categorization (e.g., tertiles or quartiles) [122]. For instance, proteinuria has a skewed distribution and is often added as a log-transformed variable or restricted cubic spline in CKD prognostic models [27]. The prospective validation step is also important for selecting variables to be included in the model. This can be done by using a knowledge-driven (or a priori) method, based on the already known biological association of the variables with the outcome, or data-driven methods, which are automated tools that select a small set of variables from a larger one, in order to maximize the model fit [123]. In the case of a large number of predictors, as often happens during the development of proteomic/metabolomic classifiers, regularization or dimension reduction methods can be used [124]. The metabolomic classifier for the prediction of response to ARB treatment, which we described in Section 4, was developed by means of least absolute shrinkage and selection operator (LASSO), a regularization technique that shrinks the variables regression coefficients through a tuning parameter and retains the best predictors in the model. LASSO was also shown to work very well with small sample sizes [112]. The third phase of clinical validation is focused on the incremental value of the biomarker on the previous assessed risk models. In nephrology, what is essentially required in biomarker research is to demonstrate that a biomarker adds information, in the prediction of a defined endpoint, on top of already assessed risk factors. This process needs a hierarchical assessment, since a likelihood ratio test (LR test) should be firstly reported to determine if the biomarker remains associated with the endpoint after controlling for previously established risk factors. Next, three measures of performance should be reported: discrimination, calibration, and reclassification [125]. These three domains are important to warrant the applicability of the biomarker predictive performance to the individual patient. Discrimination refers to the ability of the model to attribute a high risk to patients who develop the outcome of interest and, accordingly, a low risk to those who do not [126]. A measure that depicts sensitivity and specificity for all possible thresholds of a biomarker is the receiver operating characteristic (ROC) curve. To evaluate discrimination, it is, thus, suggested to present the ROC derived from the model together with the area under the curve (AUC), also labeled the *c*-statistic [127]. The difference in *c*-statistic between models with and without the biomarker should also be presented. Calibration is the degree of agreement between observed and predicted outcomes. It is suggested to depict calibration graphically by plotting the mean predicted versus mean observed outcome probability for intervals (usually deciles) of risk in a predictiveness curve or by representing observed event rates versus mean predicted risk, thus creating a calibration plot, with points that should lie along a 45° line if the model is well calibrated [126]. Reclassification metrics provide useful information on the proportion (%) of patients that are reclassified in the true risk category (lower or higher risk), whether or not the new biomarker is added to a traditional risk prediction model. The most used reclassification metrics are the net reclassification improvement (NRI), the integrated discrimination index (IDI), and reclassification tables which directly depict the movement of patients between risk categories based on the risk predicted by models with and without the biomarker [127]. After showing measures of performance, it would be necessary to internally or externally validate the model. External validation implies that the risk prediction model, including the biomarker, is re-run within an external cohort of patients with similar characteristics (e.g., CKD patients) to confirm predictive accuracy in all sequences. Alternatively, several methods of internal validation, such as bootstrapping or cross-validation, can be computed [128]. The appropriateness of methodology used to develop a biomarker is a key element to obtain useful clinical results. This is particularly true if we consider that only a few prediction models in nephrology reported these measures appropriately [129]. However, this is not the only limitation. Most of the proposed biomarkers are yet to complete the sequence from discovery to clinical application, because they were developed in studies with a small sample size without validation, thus providing heterogeneous results. The ISN prompted that biomarker research would take advantage from the setting up of large, observational cohort studies and possibly a long-term follow-up in which biomarker development and validation could be strengthened and provide robust evidence for clinicians [18]. This also requires the standardization of data collection, storage, and database structure across countries, as well as a collaboration among academia, industry, and regulatory authorities in order to warrant a correct dissemination of results.

6. Biomarkers in Intervention Studies

Projecting clinical trials, which test the effect of novel pharmacological treatments on prognosis of CKD patients, is always an important challenge. In the past few decades, all nephrology communities expressed the need for clinicians to have more therapeutic tools, with each one specific for a particular etiology of CKD, in order to improve the care of patients with CKD and to deal promptly with the complexity of kidney disease, abandoning the "reductionist" approach [10,130]. The milestone of intervention studies in nephrology dates back to the years 1990–2000 when the Collaborative Study Group, the RENAAL, and the IDNT trials showed the efficacy of RAAS-i (ACEi and ARBs) in reducing CV and renal risk in patients with diabetes and CKD [76,131,132]. Since then, a number of clinical trials were carried out with an attempt to reduce the high residual risk in CKD patients, but they missed the target [133]. The reasons for this breakdown are several and include the enrolment, in clinical trials, of a large number of CKD patients with heterogeneous etiologies and the add-on strategy. The add-on strategy consists of adding a pharmacological agent to patients who are already being treated with a drug belonging to the same class. This was adopted, for example, in the Veterans Affairs Nephropathy in Diabetes (VA-NEPHRON-D) clinical trial, which tested the effect of dual RAAS blockade ACEi + ARB, or in the ALTITUDE trial, with the addition of Aliskiren, a renin inhibitor, to RAAS-i [134,135]. In these studies, the intensification of RAAS blockade did not result in further CV or renal risk protection and even increased the risk of these endpoints. Hence, a series of initiatives were started to improve clinical trial designs. The focus is indeed to move from large trials to smaller studies that enroll similar patients so that the treatment effect can be adequately measured [26]. Biomarkers play a central role in this context (Figure 2), being useful to enrich clinical trial CKD populations through at least three important ways called biomarker-based approaches: (1) by identifying patients at increased risk for developing an event (risk-based enrichment); (2) by selecting a population based on the response to a drug of interest (predictive response enrichment or adaptive enrichment); (3) by detecting subgroup of similar patients within a master trial protocol [136].

Risk-based enrichment was used in the proteomic prediction and renin angiotensin aldosterone system inhibition prevention of early diabetic nephropathy in type 2 diabetic patients with normoalbuminuria (PRIORITY) study. The PRIORITY study enrolled patients with diabetes mellitus and normal albuminuria at increased risk for developing albuminuria [137]. High or low risk was established based on urine CKD273 levels, and only high-risk patients were then randomized to receive spironolactone or placebo. Although the trials did not show a significant effect of spironolactone on preventing the development of albuminuria, high-risk patients identified with CKD273 were at increased risk of CKD progression vs. low risk patients ($p < 0.001$). PRIORITY was an innovative design, since it anticipated the treatment of albuminuria in patients who were only likely to develop albuminuria, but not yet with albuminuria. The adaptive enrichment design consists of exposing all patients to a short-term period (usually called run-in) of treatment with the drug of interest before randomization. In this case, biomarkers could inform on the response/non-response to treatment. Such a design was adopted in previous trials like the Study of Heart and Renal Protection (SHARP) study and more recently in the study of diabetic nephropathy with the endothelin receptor antagonist atrasentan (SONAR) trial [94,138]. Patients enrolled in SONAR underwent a six-month treatment period with atrasentan, and only patients who manifested a 30% reduction in albuminuria levels (measured as albumin-to-creatinine ratio) were then randomized. Hence, albuminuria worked as a biomarker for the prediction of response to treatment. Moreover, the SONAR trial included the assessment of "secondary" risk markers, such as the B-type natriuretic peptide levels. Patients who showed a significant increase in this marker during run-in were excluded from the study. This strategy allows assessing the individual response to treatment, including the effect of a drug on primary and secondary markers and, thus, to capture in a reliable manner the effect of treatment after randomization. An extension of the adaptive enrichment trial is given by the master trial protocol [139]. Master protocols can be planned to test the efficacy of multiple interventions, each targeting a subgroup of patients defined by a biomarker. Master protocols encompass umbrella, basket, and platform trials. Platform trials aroused the interest of the nephrology community [136]. The platform is an experimental cohort of patients followed periodically to assess laboratory and clinical measurements. Within the platform, multiple treatments can be started or withdrawn and, if a defined treatment shows benefits in a defined subgroup of the platform, it can be introduced in clinical practice [140]. This approach allows the acceleration of the experimental phase of drug development, to improve the application of biomarkers and to save time and financial sources. Future perspectives around the implementation of available biomarkers are depicted in Table 3.

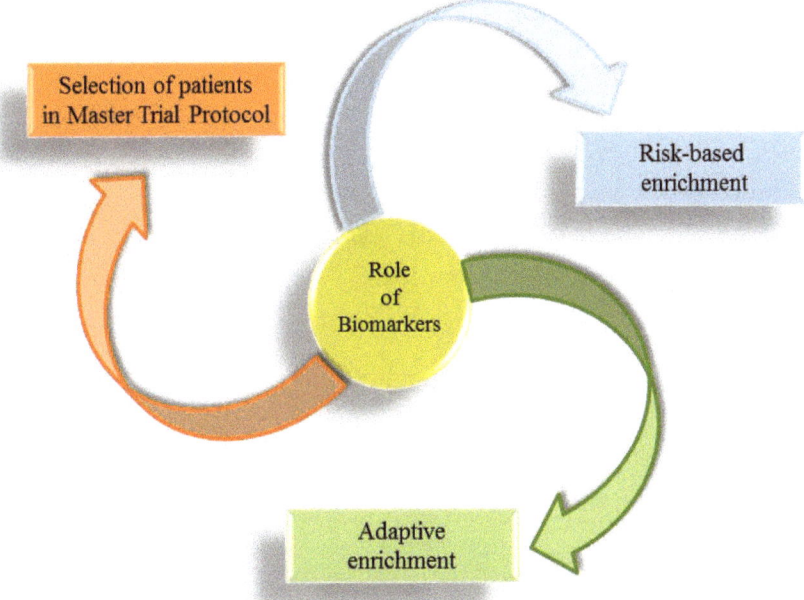

Figure 2. Biomarker-based approaches for patient selection in clinical trials.

Table 3. Validation score and future perspectives in the development of biomarkers in CKD patients.

Biomarkers	Validation Criteria	Future Perspectives
Proteinuria	Analytic validation: +/− Clinical proof of concept: + Clinical prospective validation: + Incremental value of the biomarker: + Introduction in clinical trials: +	Further studies are needed to establish (1) how this marker should be used for monitoring disease progression considering, among all factors, its variability, and (2) what are the true cut-offs for response to treatments. Inclusion of proteinuria in risk prediction models that include the presence of renal diagnoses is also needed.
eGFR$_{crea}$	Analytic validation: + Clinical proof of concept: + Clinical prospective validation: + Incremental value of the biomarker: + Introduction in clinical trials: +/−	eGFR$_{crea}$ is an important marker used to stratify risk in CKD patients. Further studies could refine the assessment of eGFR$_{crea}$ as a biomarker of response to nephroprotective treatments in clinical trials. Inclusion of eGFR$_{crea}$ in risk prediction models that include the presence of renal diagnoses is also needed.
Markers of oxidative stress, tissue remodeling, and metabolism	Analytic validation: + Clinical proof of concept: + Clinical prospective validation: +/− Incremental value of the biomarker: − Introduction in clinical trials: +/−	The prognostic role of these markers should be evaluated in larger cohort studies. Individual prognostic measures should be provided. Although pilot experimental trials showed promising results, stronger evidence in CKD patients around the changes in these markers after treatment initiation is needed.
Cardiac markers	Analytic validation: +/− Clinical proof of concept: + Clinical prospective validation: +/− Incremental value of the biomarker: +/− Introduction in clinical trials: −	Although cardiac markers levels are associated with the severity of CKD, their assessment is confounded by the coexistence of CV disease, as well as by the eGFR levels. Further studies are needed to establish the true role of these markers in CKD patients.
Filtration and urinary markers	Analytic validation: +/− Clinical proof of concept: + Clinical prospective validation: + Incremental value of the biomarker: − Introduction in clinical trials: −	The prognostic role of these markers should be evaluated in larger studies. Individual risk prediction models that include these parameters and intervention studies assessing their changes over time should be implemented.
Ultrasound markers	Analytic validation: + Clinical proof of concept: + Clinical prospective validation: + Incremental value of the biomarker: +/− Introduction in clinical trials: +/−	RRI was found to be associated with CV and renal events in CKD patients, being a promising marker. However, larger clinical trials evaluating the association between changes (treatment-induced) in RRI and clinical outcomes should be performed in the future.
Proteomics, metabolomics, and genomics	Analytic validation: + Clinical proof of concept: + Clinical prospective validation: + Incremental value of the biomarker: + Introduction in clinical trials: +/−	Omics approaches show useful prognostic and predictive information in addition to traditional risk factors. Improving the inclusion of these markers in clinical trials may inform on their clinical applicability.

+, fully present; +/−, partially present; −, absent. CKD, chronic kidney disease; eGFR, estimated glomerular filtration rate; RRI, renal resistive index; CV, cardiovascular.

7. Conclusions

CKD is a growing public health problem with high morbidity and mortality. The current classification considers the eGFR and albuminuria levels to classify patients in prognostic categories. Novel biomarkers were also developed to improve risk stratification and clinical decision-making, as well as guide CKD patient enrichment in clinical trials. Despite the great efforts made, only a few biomarkers found a large clinical application to date. More emphasis should be placed on the development process of biomarkers, which needs to be methodologically rigorous, well validated, and correctly diffused. A "real-world" assessment of biomarkers that can be performed by analyzing large databases with long-term follow-up may substantially contribute to understanding whether a definite biomarker can find clinical application. The implementation of biomarkers in CKD is highly expected in the future, since they provide information on the mechanisms of kidney disease, improve clinical practice, and, in most cases, are able to forecast both CV and renal endpoints, which represent the most frequent events in CKD patients.

Author Contributions: Conceptualization, M.P., S.R., I.G., and M.A.; methodology, M.P., S.R., P.C. and M.A.; validation, M.P., S.R., I.G., A.M., E.A., S.B., R.S., D.F., G.D.S., and M.A.; writing—original draft preparation, M.P., S.R., I.G., A.M., G.D.S., and M.A.; writing—review and editing, M.P., S.R., P.C., I.G., A.M., G.D.S., and M.A.; visualization, M.P., S.R., P.C., I.G., A.M., E.A., S.B., R.S., D.F., G.D.S., and M.A.; supervision, M.P. and M.A. All authors have read and agreed to the published version of the manuscript.

Funding: This research received no external funding.

Acknowledgments: We thank all the investigators of the "Magna Graecia" University of Catanzaro and the University of Campania "L. Vanvitelli", who collaborated on the manuscript, for their insight.

Conflicts of Interest: The authors declare no conflict of interest.

References

1. FDA-NIH Biomarker Working Group. *BEST (Biomarkers, Endpoints, and other Tools) Resource*; Food and Drug Administration (US): Silver Spring, MD, USA; National Institutes of Health (US): Bethesda, MD, USA, 2020. Available online: www.ncbi.nlm.nih.gov/books/NBK326791 (accessed on 25 June 2020).
2. Pepe, M.; Janes, H. Methods for Evaluating Prediction Performance of Biomarkers and Tests. In *Risk Assessment and Evaluation of Predictions*; Lecture Notes in Statistics; Lee, M.L., Gail, M., Pfeiffer, R., Satten, G., Cai, T., Gandy, A., Eds.; Springer: New York, NY, USA, 2013; Volume 215. [CrossRef]
3. Devarajan, P.; Williams, L.M. Proteomics for biomarker discovery in acute kidney injury. *Semin. Nephrol.* **2007**, *27*, 637–651. [CrossRef] [PubMed]
4. Simon, R. Development and validation of biomarker classifiers for treatment selection. *J. Stat. Plan. Inference* **2008**, *138*, 308–320. [CrossRef] [PubMed]
5. Provenzano, M.; Coppolino, G.; De Nicola, L.; Serra, R.; Garofalo, C.; Andreucci, M.; Bolignano, D. Unraveling cardiovascular risk in renal patients: A new take on old tale. *Front. Cell Dev. Biol.* **2019**, *7*, 314. [CrossRef] [PubMed]
6. Provenzano, M.; Coppolino, G.; Faga, T.; Garofalo, C.; Serra, R.; Andreucci, M. Epidemiology of cardiovascular risk in chronic kidney disease patients: The real silent killer. *Rev. Cardiovasc. Med.* **2019**, *20*, 209–220. [CrossRef]
7. Kidney Disease Improving Global Outcomes Work Group. CVD, medication dosage, patient safety, infections, hospitalizations, and caveats for investigating complications of CKD. *Kidney Int. Suppl.* **2013**, *3*, 91–111. [CrossRef]
8. Xie, Y.; Bowe, B.; Mokdad, A.H.; Xian, H.; Yan, Y.; Li, T.; Maddukuri, G.; Tsai, C.-Y.; Floyd, T.; Al Aly, Z. Analysis of the Global Burden of Disease study highlights the global, regional, and national trends of chronic kidney disease epidemiology from 1990 to 2016. *Kidney Int.* **2018**, *94*, 567–581. [CrossRef]
9. Bikbov, B.T.; A Purcell, C.; Levey, A.S.; Smith, M.; Abdoli, A.; Abebe, M.; Adebayo, O.M.; Afarideh, M.; Agarwal, S.K.; Agudelo-Botero, M.; et al. Global, regional, and national burden of chronic kidney disease, 1990–2017: A systematic analysis for the Global Burden of Disease Study 2017. *Lancet* **2020**, *395*, 709–733. [CrossRef]

10. Hall, Y.N.; Himmelfarb, J. The CKD classification system in the precision medicine era. *Clin. J. Am. Soc. Nephrol.* **2016**, *12*, 346–348. [CrossRef]
11. Inker, L.A.; Astor, B.C.; Fox, C.H.; Isakova, T.; Lash, J.P.; Peralta, C.A.; Tamura, M.K.; Feldman, H.I. KDOQI US commentary on the 2012 KDIGO Clinical Practice Guideline for the Evaluation and Management of CKD. *Am. J. Kidney Dis.* **2014**, *63*, 713–735. [CrossRef]
12. De Nicola, L.; Provenzano, M.; Chiodini, P.; Borrelli, S.; Garofalo, C.; Pacilio, M.; Liberti, M.E.; Sagliocca, A.; Conte, G.; Minutolo, R. Independent role of underlying kidney disease on renal prognosis of patients with chronic kidney disease under nephrology care. *PLoS ONE* **2015**, *10*, e0127071. [CrossRef]
13. Haynes, R.; Staplin, N.; Emberson, J.R.; Herrington, W.G.; Tomson, C.; Agodoa, L.; Tesař, V.; Levin, A.; Lewis, D.; Reith, C.; et al. Evaluating the contribution of the cause of kidney disease to prognosis in CKD: Results from the Study of Heart and Renal Protection (SHARP). *Am. J. Kidney Dis.* **2014**, *64*, 40–48. [CrossRef] [PubMed]
14. Conte, G.; Minutolo, R.; De Nicola, L.; Hallan, S.I.; Gansevoort, R.T. Pro: Thresholds to define chronic kidney disease should not be age-dependent. *Nephrol. Dial. Transplant.* **2014**, *29*, 770–774. [CrossRef] [PubMed]
15. Glassock, R.J. Con: Thresholds to define chronic kidney disease should not be age dependent. *Nephrol. Dial. Transplant.* **2014**, *29*, 774–779. [CrossRef] [PubMed]
16. Hommos, M.S.; Glassock, R.J.; Rule, A.D. Structural and functional changes in human kidneys with healthy aging. *J. Am. Soc. Nephrol.* **2017**, *28*, 2838–2844. [CrossRef] [PubMed]
17. Levin, A.; Tonelli, M.; Bonventre, J.; Coresh, J.; Donner, J.-A.; Fogo, A.B.; Fox, C.S.; Gansevoort, R.T.; Heerspink, H.J.; Jardine, M.; et al. Global kidney health 2017 and beyond: A roadmap for closing gaps in care, research, and policy. *Lancet* **2017**, *390*, 1888–1917. [CrossRef]
18. Pena, M.J.; Stenvinkel, P.; Kretzler, M.; Adu, D.; Agarwal, S.K.; Coresh, J.; Feldman, H.I.; Fogo, A.B.; Gansevoort, R.T.; Harris, D.C.; et al. Strategies to improve monitoring disease progression, assessing cardiovascular risk, and defining prognostic biomarkers in chronic kidney disease. *Kidney Int. Suppl.* **2017**, *7*, 107–113. [CrossRef]
19. IOM (Institute of Medicine). *Evaluation of Biomarkers and Surrogate Endpoints in Chronic Disease*; The National Academies Press: Washington, DC, USA, 2010.
20. Serra, R.; Ielapi, N.; Barbetta, A.; Andreucci, M.; De Franciscis, S. Novel biomarkers for cardiovascular risk. *Biomark. Med.* **2018**, *12*, 1015–1024. [CrossRef]
21. De Nicola, L.; Provenzano, M.; Chiodini, P.; Borrelli, S.; Russo, L.; Bellasi, A.; Santoro, D.; Conte, G.; Minutolo, R. Epidemiology of low-proteinuric chronic kidney disease in renal clinics. *PLoS ONE* **2017**, *12*, e0172241. [CrossRef]
22. Minutolo, R.; Gabbai, F.B.; Chiodini, P.; Garofalo, C.; Stanzione, G.; Liberti, M.E.; Pacilio, M.; Borrelli, S.; Provenzano, M.; Conte, G.; et al. Reassessment of Ambulatory blood pressure improves renal risk stratification in nondialysis chronic kidney disease. *Hypertension* **2015**, *66*, 557–562. [CrossRef]
23. Astor, B.C.; Matsushita, K.; Gansevoort, R.T.; Van Der Velde, M.; Woodward, M.; Levey, A.S.; De Jong, P.E.; Coresh, J. Lower estimated glomerular filtration rate and higher albuminuria are associated with mortality and end-stage renal disease. A collaborative meta-analysis of kidney disease population cohorts. *Kidney Int.* **2011**, *79*, 1331–1340. [CrossRef]
24. Gansevoort, R.T.; Matsushita, K.; Van Der Velde, M.; Astor, B.C.; Woodward, M.; Levey, A.S.; De Jong, P.E.; Coresh, J. Chronic kidney disease prognosis consortium lower estimated GFR and higher albuminuria are associated with adverse kidney outcomes. A collaborative meta-analysis of general and high-risk population cohorts. *Kidney Int.* **2011**, *80*, 93–104. [CrossRef] [PubMed]
25. Matsushita, K.; Coresh, J.; Sang, Y.; Chalmers, J.P.; Fox, C.; Guallar, E.; Jafar, T.; Jassal, S.K.; Landman, G.W.; Muntner, P.; et al. Estimated glomerular filtration rate and albuminuria for prediction of cardiovascular outcomes: A collaborative meta-analysis of individual participant data. *Lancet Diabetes Endocrinol.* **2015**, *3*, 514–525. [CrossRef]
26. Tangri, N.; Stevens, L.A.; Griffith, J.; Tighiouart, H.; Djurdjev, O.; Naimark, D.M.; Levin, A.; Levey, A.S. A predictive model for progression of chronic kidney disease to kidney failure. *JAMA* **2011**, *305*, 1553–1559. [CrossRef] [PubMed]

27. Provenzano, M.; Chiodini, P.; Minutolo, R.; Zoccali, C.; Bellizzi, V.; Conte, G.; Locatelli, F.; Tripepi, G.; Del Vecchio, L.; Mallamaci, F.; et al. Reclassification of chronic kidney disease patients for end-stage renal disease risk by proteinuria indexed to estimated glomerular filtration rate: Multicentre prospective study in nephrology clinics. *Nephrol. Dial. Transplant.* **2018**, *35*. [CrossRef]
28. Schroeder, E.B.; Yang, X.; Thorp, M.L.; Arnold, B.M.; Tabano, D.; Petrik, A.F.; Smith, D.H.; Platt, R.W.; Johnson, E.S. Predicting 5-Year Risk of RRT in Stage 3 or 4 CKD: Development and external validation. *Clin. J. Am. Soc. Nephrol.* **2016**, *12*, 87–94. [CrossRef]
29. Grams, M.E.; Sang, Y.; Ballew, S.H. Predicting timing of clinical outcomes in patients with chronic kidney disease and severely decreased glomerular filtration rate. *Kidney Int.* **2018**, *94*, 1025–1026. [CrossRef]
30. Abbate, M.; Zoja, C.; Remuzzi, G. How does proteinuria cause progressive renal damage? *J. Am. Soc. Nephrol.* **2006**, *17*, 2974–2984. [CrossRef]
31. Provenzano, M.; Garofalo, C.; Chiodini, P. Ruolo della proteinuria nella ricerca clinica: Per ogni vecchia risposta, una nuova domanda [Role of proteinuria in clinical research: For each old-answer, a new key-question]. *Recenti Prog Med.* **2020**, *111*, 74–81. [CrossRef]
32. Nakano, T.; Ninomiya, T.; Sumiyoshi, S.; Fujii, H.; Doi, Y.; Hirakata, H.; Tsuruya, K.; Iida, M.; Kiyohara, Y.; Sueishi, K. Association of kidney function with coronary atherosclerosis and calcification in autopsy samples from Japanese elders: The Hisayama study. *Am. J. Kidney Dis.* **2010**, *55*, 21–30. [CrossRef]
33. Pun, P.H.; Smarz, T.R.; Honeycutt, E.F.; Shaw, L.K.; Al-Khatib, S.M.; Middleton, J.P. Chronic kidney disease is associated with increased risk of sudden cardiac death among patients with coronary artery disease. *Kidney Int.* **2009**, *76*, 652–658. [CrossRef]
34. Deo, R.; Lin, F.; Vittinghoff, E.; Tseng, Z.H.; Hulley, S.B.; Shlipak, M.G. Kidney dysfunction and sudden cardiac death among women with coronary heart disease. *Hypertension* **2008**, *51*, 1578–1582. [CrossRef] [PubMed]
35. Deo, R.; Sotoodehnia, N.; Katz, R.; Sarnak, M.J.; Fried, L.F.; Chonchol, M.; Kestenbaum, B.; Psaty, B.M.; Siscovick, D.S.; Shlipak, M.G. Cystatin C and sudden cardiac death risk in the elderly. *Circ. Cardiovasc. Qual. Outcomes* **2010**, *3*, 159–164. [CrossRef] [PubMed]
36. Meier, P.; Vogt, P.; Blanc, E. Ventricular arrhythmias and sudden cardiac death in end-stage renaldisease patients on chronic hemodialysis. *Nephron* **2001**, *87*, 199–214. [CrossRef] [PubMed]
37. Van Acker, B.A.C.; Stroomer, M.K.J.; Gosselink, M.A.H.E.; Koomen, G.C.M.; Koopman, M.G.; Arisz, L. Urinary protein excretion in normal individuals: Diurnal changes, influence of orthostasis and relationship to the renin-angiotensin system. *Contrib. Nephrol.* **1993**, *101*, 143–150.
38. Fotheringham, J.; Odudu, A.; McKane, W.; Ellam, T. Modification of the relationship between blood pressure and renal albumin permeability by impaired excretory function and diabetes. *Hypertension* **2015**, *65*, 510–516. [CrossRef]
39. Willows, J.; Odudu, A.; Logan, I.; Sheerin, N.; Tomson, C.; Ellam, T. changing protein permeability with nephron loss: Evidence for a human remnant nephron effect. *Am. J. Nephrol.* **2019**, *50*, 152–159. [CrossRef]
40. Mallamaci, F.; Tripepi, G.; D'Arrigo, G.; Borrelli, S.; Garofalo, C.; Stanzione, G.; Provenzano, M.; De Nicola, L.; Conte, G.; Minutolo, R.; et al. Blood pressure variability, mortality, and cardiovascular outcomes in CKD patients. *Clin. J. Am. Soc. Nephrol.* **2019**, *14*, 233–240. [CrossRef]
41. Zhou, T.L.; Rensma, S.P.; Van Der Heide, F.C.; Henry, R.M.; Kroon, A.A.; Houben, A.J.; Jansen, J.F.; Backes, W.H.; Berendschot, T.T.; Schouten, J.S.; et al. Blood pressure variability and microvascular dysfunction. *J. Hypertens.* **2020**, *38*. [CrossRef]
42. Xu, G.; Luo, K.; Liu, H.; Huang, T.; Fang, X.; Tu, W. The progress of inflammation and oxidative stress in patients with chronic kidney disease. *Ren. Fail.* **2014**, *37*, 45–49. [CrossRef]
43. Ismael, F.O.; Proudfoot, J.M.; Brown, B.E.; Van Reyk, D.M.; Croft, K.D.; Davies, M.J.; Hawkins, C.L. Comparative reactivity of the myeloperoxidase-derived oxidants HOCl and HOSCN with low-density lipoprotein (LDL): Implications for foam cell formation in atherosclerosis. *Arch. Biochem. Biophys.* **2015**, *573*, 40–51. [CrossRef]
44. Correa, S.; Pena-Esparragoza, J.K.; Scovner, K.M.; Waikar, S.S.; Mc Causland, F.R. Myeloperoxidase and the risk of CKD Progression, cardiovascular disease, and death in the Chronic Renal Insufficiency Cohort (CRIC) Study. *Am. J. Kidney Dis.* **2020**, *76*, 32–41. [CrossRef] [PubMed]

45. Provenzano, M.; Andreucci, M.; Garofalo, C.; Faga, T.; Michael, A.; Ielapi, N.; Grande, R.; Sapienza, P.; De Franciscis, S.; Mastroroberto, P.; et al. The association of matrix metalloproteinases with chronic kidney disease and peripheral vascular disease: A light at the end of the tunnel? *Biomolecules* **2020**, *10*, 154. [CrossRef] [PubMed]
46. Butrico, L.; Barbetta, A.; Ciranni, S.; Andreucci, M.; Mastroroberto, P.; De Franciscis, S. Role of metalloproteinases and their inhibitors in the development of abdominal aortic aneurysm: Current insights and systematic review of the literature. *Chirurgia* **2017**, *30*, 151–159. [CrossRef]
47. Lauhio, A.; Sorsa, T.; Srinivas, R.; Stenman, M.; Tervahartiala, T.; Stenman, U.-H.; Grönhagen-Riska, C.; Honkanen, E. Urinary matrix metalloproteinase -8, -9, -14 and their regulators (TRY-1, TRY-2, TATI) in patients with diabetic nephropathy. *Ann. Med.* **2008**, *40*, 312–320. [CrossRef] [PubMed]
48. Tashiro, K.; Koyanagi, I.; Ohara, I.; Ito, T.; Saitoh, A.; Horikoshi, S.; Tomino, Y. Levels of urinary matrix metalloproteinase-9 (MMP-9) and renal injuries in patients with type 2 diabetic nephropathy. *J. Clin. Lab. Anal.* **2004**, *18*, 206–210. [CrossRef]
49. Lieb, W.; Song, R.J.; Xanthakis, V.; Vasan, R.S. Association of circulating tissue inhibitor of Metalloproteinases-1 and Procollagen type III Aminoterminal peptide levels with incident heart failure and chronic kidney disease. *J. Am. Hear. Assoc.* **2019**, *8*, e011426. [CrossRef]
50. Forough, R.; Koyama, N.; Hasenstab, D.; Lea, H.; Clowes, M.; Nikkari, S.T.; Clowes, A.W. Overexpression of tissue inhibitor of matrix metalloproteinase-1 inhibits vascular smooth muscle cell functions In Vitro and In Vivo. *Circ. Res.* **1996**, *79*, 812–820. [CrossRef]
51. Newman, K.M.; Jean-Claude, J.; Li, H.; Scholes, J.V.; Ogata, Y.; Nagase, H.; Tilson, M. Cellular localization of matrix metalloproteinases in the abdominal aortic aneurysm wall. *J. Vasc. Surg.* **1994**, *20*, 814–820. [CrossRef]
52. Scialla, J.J.; Xie, H.; Rahman, M.; Anderson, A.H.; Isakova, T.; Ojo, A.; Zhang, X.; Nessel, L.; Hamano, T.; Grunwald, J.E.; et al. Fibroblast Growth Factor-23 and cardiovascular events in CKD. *J. Am. Soc. Nephrol.* **2013**, *25*, 349–360. [CrossRef]
53. Isakova, T.; Xie, H.; Yang, W.; Xie, D.; Anderson, A.H.; Scialla, J.J.; Wahl, P.; Gutiérrez, O.M.; Steigerwalt, S.; He, J.; et al. Fibroblast Growth Factor 23 and risks of mortality and end-stage renal disease in patients with chronic kidney disease. *JAMA* **2011**, *305*, 2432–2439. [CrossRef]
54. Defilippi, C.R.; De Lemos, J.A.; Christenson, R.H.; Gottdiener, J.S.; Kop, W.J.; Zhan, M.; Seliger, S. Association of serial measures of cardiac troponin T using a sensitive assay with incident heart failure and cardiovascular mortality in older adults. *JAMA* **2010**, *304*, 2494–2502. [CrossRef] [PubMed]
55. Ballew, S.H.; Matsushita, K. Cardiovascular risk prediction in CKD. *Semin. Nephrol.* **2018**, *38*, 208–216. [CrossRef] [PubMed]
56. Srisawasdi, P.; Vanavanan, S.; Charoenpanichkit, C.; Kroll, M.H. The Effect of renal dysfunction on BNP, NT-proBNP, and their ratio. *Am. J. Clin. Pathol.* **2010**, *133*, 14–23. [CrossRef] [PubMed]
57. Matsushita, K.; Ballew, S.H.; Coresh, J. Cardiovascular risk prediction in people with chronic kidney disease. *Curr. Opin. Nephrol. Hypertens.* **2016**, *25*, 518–523. [CrossRef]
58. Rangaswami, J.; Bhalla, V.; Blair, J.E.; Chang, T.I.; Costa, S.; Lentine, K.L.; Lerma, E.V.; Mezue, K.; Molitch, M.; Mullens, W.; et al. Cardiorenal syndrome: Classification, pathophysiology, diagnosis, and treatment strategies: A scientific statement from the american heart association. *Circulation* **2019**, *139*, e840–e878. [CrossRef]
59. Saunders, J.T.; Nambi, V.; De Lemos, J.A.; Chambless, L.E.; Virani, S.S.; Boerwinkle, E.; Hoogeveen, R.C.; Liu, X.; Astor, B.C.; Mosley, T.H.; et al. Cardiac troponin T measured by a highly sensitive assay predicts coronary heart disease, heart failure, and mortality in the Atherosclerosis Risk in Communities study. *Circulation* **2011**, *123*, 1367–1376. [CrossRef]
60. Agarwal, S.K.; Chambless, L.E.; Ballantyne, C.M.; Astor, B.; Bertoni, A.G.; Chang, P.P.; Folsom, A.R.; He, M.; Hoogeveen, R.C.; Ni, H.; et al. Prediction of incident heart failure in general practice: The Atherosclerosis Risk in Communities (ARIC) study. *Circ. Hear. Fail.* **2012**, *5*, 422–429. [CrossRef]
61. Matsushita, K.; Sang, Y.; Ballew, S.H.; Astor, B.C.; Hoogeveen, R.C.; Solomon, S.D.; Ballantyne, C.M.; Woodward, M.; Coresh, J. Cardiac and kidney markers for cardiovascular prediction in individuals with chronic kidney disease. *Arter. Thromb. Vasc. Boil.* **2014**, *34*, 1770–1777. [CrossRef]
62. Bansal, N.; Zelnick, L.; Shlipak, M.G.; Anderson, A.; Christenson, R.; Deo, R.; Defilippi, C.; Feldman, H.; Lash, J.; He, J.; et al. Cardiac and stress biomarkers and chronic kidney disease progression: The CRIC study. *Clin. Chem.* **2019**, *65*, 1448–1457. [CrossRef]

63. Ho, J.E.; Hwang, S.-J.; Wollert, K.C.; Larson, M.G.; Cheng, S.; Kempf, T.; Vasan, R.S.; Januzzi, J.L.; Wang, T.J.; Fox, C.S. Biomarkers of cardiovascular stress and incident chronic kidney disease. *Clin. Chem.* **2013**, *59*, 1613–1620. [CrossRef]
64. Shlipak, M.G.; Matsushita, K.; Ärnlöv, J.; Inker, L.A.; Katz, R.; Polkinghorne, K.R.; Rothenbacher, D.; Sarnak, M.J.; Astor, B.C.; Coresh, J.; et al. Cystatin C versus creatinine in determining risk based on kidney function. *N. Engl. J. Med.* **2013**, *369*, 932–943. [CrossRef] [PubMed]
65. Foster, M.C.; Coresh, J.; Hsu, C.-Y.; Xie, D.; Levey, A.S.; Nelson, R.G.; Eckfeldt, J.H.; Vasan, R.S.; Kimmel, P.L.; Schelling, J.; et al. Serum β-trace protein and β2-microglobulin as predictors of ESRD, mortality, and cardiovascular disease in adults with CKD in the Chronic Renal Insufficiency Cohort (CRIC) study. *Am. J. Kidney Dis.* **2016**, *68*, 68–76. [CrossRef] [PubMed]
66. Ix, J.H.; Katz, R.; Bansal, N.; Foster, M.; Weiner, D.E.; Tracy, R.P.; Jotwani, V.; Hughes-Austin, J.; McKay, D.; Gabbai, F.; et al. Urine fibrosis markers and risk of allograft failure in kidney transplant recipients: A Case-Cohort Ancillary Study of the FAVORIT Trial. *Am. J. Kidney Dis.* **2017**, *69*, 410–419. [CrossRef] [PubMed]
67. Puthumana, J.; Hall, I.E.; Reese, P.P.; Schroppel, B.; Weng, F.L.; Thiessen-Philbrook, H.; Doshi, M.D.; Rao, V.; Lee, C.G.; Elias, J.A.; et al. YKL-40 associates with renal recovery in deceased donor kidney transplantation. *J. Am. Soc. Nephrol.* **2017**, *28*, 661–670. [CrossRef]
68. Malhotra, R.; Katz, R.; Jotwani, V.; Ambrosius, W.T.; Raphael, K.L.; Haley, W.; Rastogi, A.; Cheung, A.K.; Freedman, B.I.; Punzi, H.; et al. Urine markers of kidney tubule cell injury and kidney function decline in SPRINT Trial participants with CKD. *Clin. J. Am. Soc. Nephrol.* **2020**, *15*, 349–358. [CrossRef] [PubMed]
69. Sun, L.; Zou, L.-X.; Chen, M.-J. Make precision medicine work for chronic kidney disease. *Med Princ. Pr.* **2016**, *26*, 101–107. [CrossRef]
70. Serra, R.; Ssempijja, L.; Provenzano, M.; Andreucci, M. Genetic biomarkers in chronic venous disease. *Biomark Med.* **2020**, *14*, 75–80. [CrossRef]
71. Serra, R.; Ielapi, N.; Barbetta, A.; Buffone, G.; Bevacqua, E.; Andreucci, M. Biomarkers for precision medicine in phlebology and wound care: A systematic review. *Acta. Phlebol.* **2017**, *18*, 52–56. [CrossRef]
72. Good, D.M.; Zürbig, P.; Argilés, A.; Bauer, H.W.; Behrens, G.; Coon, J.J.; Dakna, M.; Decramer, S.; Delles, C.; Dominiczak, A.F.; et al. Naturally occurring human urinary peptides for use in diagnosis of chronic kidney disease. *Mol. Cell. Proteom.* **2010**, *9*, 2424–2437. [CrossRef]
73. Argiles, A.; Siwy, J.; Duranton, F.; Gayrard, N.; Dakna, M.; Lundin, U.; Osaba, L.; Delles, C.; Mourad, G.; Weinberger, K.M.; et al. A new proteomics classifier assessing CKD and its prognosis. *PLoS ONE* **2013**, *8*, e62837. [CrossRef]
74. Roscioni, S.S.; De Zeeuw, D.; Hellemons, M.E.; Mischak, H.; Zürbig, P.; Bakker, S.J.L.; Gansevoort, R.T.; Reinhard, H.; Persson, F.; Lajer, M.; et al. A urinary peptide biomarker set predicts worsening of albuminuria in type 2 diabetes mellitus. *Diabetologia* **2012**, *56*, 259–267. [CrossRef] [PubMed]
75. Schanstra, J.P. Diagnosis and prediction of progression of chronic kidney disease by assessment of urinary peptides. *J. Am. Soc. Nephrol.* **2014**, *26*, 1999–2010. [CrossRef] [PubMed]
76. Kwan, B.; Fuhrer, T.; Zhang, J.; Darshi, M.; Van Espen, B.; Montemayor, D.; De Boer, I.H.; Dobre, M.; Hsu, C.-Y.; Kelly, T.N.; et al. Metabolomic markers of kidney function decline in patients with diabetes: Evidence From the Chronic Renal Insufficiency Cohort (CRIC) study. *Am. J. Kidney Dis.* **2020**. [CrossRef] [PubMed]
77. Connaughton, D.M.; Hildebrandt, F. Personalized medicine in chronic kidney disease by detection of monogenic mutations. *Nephrol. Dial. Transplant.* **2019**, *35*, 390–397. [CrossRef] [PubMed]
78. Thio, C.H.; Van Der Most, P.J.; Nolte, I.M.; Van Der Harst, P.; Bültmann, U.; Gansevoort, R.T.; Snieder, H. Evaluation of a genetic risk score based on creatinine-estimated glomerular filtration rate and its association with kidney outcomes. *Nephrol. Dial. Transplant.* **2017**, *33*, 1757–1764. [CrossRef] [PubMed]
79. Köttgen, A.; Hwang, S.-J.; Larson, M.G.; Van Eyk, J.E.; Fu, Q.; Benjamin, E.J.; Dehghan, A.; Glazer, N.L.; Kao, W.L.; Harris, T.B.; et al. Uromodulin levels associate with a common UMOD variant and risk for incident CKD. *J. Am. Soc. Nephrol.* **2009**, *21*, 337–344. [CrossRef]
80. Böger, C.A.; Gorski, M.; Li, M.; Hoffmann, M.M.; Huang, C.; Yang, Q.; Teumer, A.; Krane, V.; O'Seaghdha, C.M.; Kutalik, Z.; et al. Association of eGFR-related loci identified by GWAS with incident CKD and ESRD. *PLoS Genet.* **2011**, *7*, e1002292. [CrossRef]
81. Pays, E.; Vanhollebeke, B. Human innate immunity against African trypanosomes. *Curr. Opin. Immunol.* **2009**, *21*, 493–498. [CrossRef]

82. Parsa, A.; Kao, W.L.; Xie, D.; Astor, B.C.; Li, M.; Hsu, C.-Y.; Feldman, H.I.; Parekh, R.S.; Kusek, J.W.; Greene, T.H.; et al. APOL1 risk variants, race, and progression of chronic kidney disease. *N. Engl. J. Med.* **2013**, *369*, 2183–2196. [CrossRef]
83. Sudlow, C.; Gallacher, J.; Allen, N.; Beral, V.; Burton, P.; Danesh, J.; Downey, P.; Elliott, P.; Green, J.; Landray, M.; et al. UK Biobank: An open access resource for identifying the causes of a wide range of complex diseases of middle and old age. *PLoS Med.* **2015**, *12*, e1001779. [CrossRef]
84. Zhao, J.; Schooling, C.M. Sex-specific associations of insulin resistance with chronic kidney disease and kidney function: A bi-directional Mendelian randomisation study. *Diabetologia* **2020**, *63*, 1–10. [CrossRef]
85. Zhao, J.; Schooling, C.M. The role of testosterone in chronic kidney disease and kidney function in men and women: A bi-directional Mendelian randomization study in the UK Biobank. *BMC Med.* **2020**, *18*, 122. [CrossRef] [PubMed]
86. Casanova, F.; Tyrrell, J.; Beaumont, R.N.; Ji, Y.; Jones, S.E.; Hattersley, A.T.; Weedon, M.N.; Murray, A.; Shore, A.C.; Frayling, T.M.; et al. A genome-wide association study implicates multiple mechanisms influencing raised urinary albumin–creatinine ratio. *Hum. Mol. Genet.* **2019**, *28*, 4197–4207. [CrossRef]
87. Ledermann, J.A.; Harter, P.; Gourley, C.; Friedlander, M.; Vergote, I.; Rustin, G.; Scott, C.; Meier, W.; Shapira-Frommer, R.; Safra, T.; et al. Olaparib maintenance therapy in platinum-sensitive relapsed ovarian cancer. *N. Engl. J. Med.* **2012**, *366*, 1382–1392. [CrossRef]
88. Perco, P.; Pena, M.; Heerspink, H.J.; Mayer, G. Multimarker panels in diabetic kidney disease: The way to improved clinical trial design and clinical practice? *Kidney Int. Rep.* **2018**, *4*, 212–221. [CrossRef] [PubMed]
89. Brenner, B.M.; Cooper, M.E.; De Zeeuw, D.; Keane, W.F.; Mitch, W.E.; Parving, H.-H.; Remuzzi, G.; Snapinn, S.M.; Zhang, Z.; Shahinfar, S. Effects of losartan on renal and cardiovascular outcomes in patients with type 2 diabetes and nephropathy. *N. Engl. J. Med.* **2001**, *345*, 861–869. [CrossRef] [PubMed]
90. The GISEN Group (Gruppo Italiano di Studi Epidemiologici in Nefrologia). Randomised placebo-controlled trial of effect of ramipril on decline in glomerular filtration rate and risk of terminal renal failure in proteinuric, non-diabetic nephropathy. *Lancet* **1997**, *349*, 1857–1863. [CrossRef]
91. Heerspink, H.J.L.; Ninomiya, T.; Perkovic, V.; Woodward, M.; Zoungas, S.; Cass, A.; Cooper, M.; Grobbee, D.E.; Mancia, G.; Mogensen, C.E.; et al. Effects of a fixed combination of perindopril and indapamide in patients with type 2 diabetes and chronic kidney disease. *Eur. Hear. J.* **2010**, *31*, 2888–2896. [CrossRef]
92. Perkovic, V.; Jardine, M.J.; Neal, B.; Bompoint, S.; Heerspink, H.J.; Charytan, D.M.; Edwards, R.; Agarwal, R.; Bakris, G.; Bull, S.; et al. Canagliflozin and renal outcomes in type 2 diabetes and nephropathy. *N. Engl. J. Med.* **2019**, *380*, 2295–2306. [CrossRef]
93. Wanner, C.; E Inzucchi, S.; Lachin, J.M.; Fitchett, D.; Von Eynatten, M.; Mattheus, M.; Johansen, O.E.; Woerle, H.J.; Broedl, U.C.; Zinman, B. Empagliflozin and progression of kidney disease in type 2 diabetes. *N. Engl. J. Med.* **2016**, *375*, 323–334. [CrossRef]
94. Heerspink, H.J.L.; Parving, H.H.; Andress, D.L. SONAR Committees and Investigators. Atrasentan and renal events in patients with type 2 diabetes and chronic kidney disease (SONAR): A double-blind, randomised, placebo-controlled trial. *Lancet* **2019**, *393*, 1937–1947. [CrossRef]
95. Perkovic, V.; Ninomiya, T.; Arima, H.; Gallagher, M.; Jardine, M.; Cass, A.; Neal, B.; MacMahon, S.; Chalmers, J.P. Chronic kidney disease, cardiovascular events, and the effects of perindopril-based blood pressure lowering: Data from the PROGRESS study. *J. Am. Soc. Nephrol.* **2007**, *18*, 2766–2772. [CrossRef] [PubMed]
96. De Zeeuw, D.; Remuzzi, G.; Parving, H.-H.; Keane, W.F.; Zhang, Z.; Shahinfar, S.; Snapinn, S.; Cooper, M.E.; Mitch, W.E.; Brenner, B.M. Albuminuria, a therapeutic target for cardiovascular protection in type 2 diabetic patients with nephropathy. *Circulation* **2004**, *110*, 921–927. [CrossRef]
97. Heerspink, H.J.L.; Ninomiya, T.; Persson, F.; Brenner, B.M.; Brunel, P.; Chaturvedi, N.; Desai, A.S.; Haffner, S.M.; McMurray, J.J.; Solomon, S.D.; et al. Is a reduction in albuminuria associated with renal and cardiovascular protection? A post hoc analysis of the ALTITUDE trial. *Diabetes Obes. Metab.* **2016**, *18*, 169–177. [CrossRef] [PubMed]
98. Heerspink, H.J.L.; Gansevoort, R.T. Albuminuria is an appropriate therapeutic target in patients with CKD: The pro view. *Clin. J. Am. Soc. Nephrol.* **2015**, *10*, 1079–1088. [CrossRef]

99. Levey, A.S.; Inker, L.A.; Matsushita, K.; Greene, T.; Willis, K.; Lewis, E.; De Zeeuw, D.; Cheung, A.K.; Coresh, J. GFR decline as an end point for clinical trials in CKD: A scientific workshop sponsored by the National Kidney Foundation and the US Food and Drug Administration. *Am. J. Kidney Dis.* **2014**, *64*, 821–835. [CrossRef]

100. Heerspink, H.J.L.; Tighiouart, H.; Sang, Y.; Ballew, S.H.; Mondal, H.; Matsushita, K.; Coresh, J.; Levey, A.S.; Inker, L.A. GFR decline and subsequent risk of established kidney outcomes: A Meta-analysis of 37 Randomized Controlled Trials. *Am. J. Kidney Dis.* **2014**, *64*, 860–866. [CrossRef]

101. Heerspink, H.J.L.; Weldegiorgis, M.; Inker, L.A.; Gansevoort, R.; Parving, H.-H.; Dwyer, J.P.; Mondal, H.; Coresh, J.; Greene, T.; Levey, A.S.; et al. Estimated GFR decline as a surrogate end point for kidney failure: A post hoc analysis from the reduction of end points in non–insulin-dependent diabetes with the Angiotensin II Antagonist Losartan (RENAAL) Study and Irbesartan Diabetic Nephropathy Trial (IDNT). *Am. J. Kidney Dis.* **2014**, *63*, 244–250. [CrossRef]

102. Steinmann-Niggli, K.; Ziswiler, R.; Küng, M.; Marti, H.P. Inhibition of matrix metalloproteinases attenuates anti-Thy1.1 nephritis. *J. Am. Soc. Nephrol.* **1998**, *9*, 397–407.

103. Aggarwal, H.K.; Jain, D.; Talapatra, P.; Yadav, R.K.; Gupta, T.; Kathuria, K.L. Evaluation of role of doxycycline (a matrix metalloproteinase inhibitor) on renal functions in patients of diabetic nephropathy. *Ren. Fail.* **2010**, *32*, 941–946. [CrossRef]

104. Das, N.A.; Carpenter, A.J.; Belenchia, A.; Aroor, A.R.; Noda, M.; Siebenlist, U.; Chandrasekar, B.; Demarco, V.G. Empagliflozin reduces high glucose-induced oxidative stress and miR-21-dependent TRAF3IP2 induction and RECK suppression, and inhibits human renal proximal tubular epithelial cell migration and epithelial-to-mesenchymal transition. *Cell. Signal.* **2020**, *68*, 109506. [CrossRef] [PubMed]

105. Provenzano, M.; Rivoli, L.; Garofalo, C.; Faga, T.; Pelagi, E.; Perticone, M.; Serra, R.; Michael, A.; Comi, N.; Andreucci, M. Renal resistive index in chronic kidney disease patients: Possible determinants and risk profile. *PLoS ONE* **2020**, *15*, e0230020. [CrossRef] [PubMed]

106. Doi, Y.; Iwashima, Y.; Yoshihara, F.; Kamide, K.; Hayashi, S.-I.; Kubota, Y.; Nakamura, S.; Horio, T.; Kawano, Y. Response to renal resistive index and cardiovascular and renal outcomes in essential hypertension. *Hypertension* **2013**, *61*, e23. [CrossRef] [PubMed]

107. Sugiura, T.; Wada, A. Resistive index predicts renal prognosis in chronic kidney disease. *Nephrol. Dial. Transplant.* **2009**, *24*, 2780–2785. [CrossRef]

108. Solini, A.; Giannini, L.; Seghieri, M.; Vitolo, E.; Taddei, S.; Ghiadoni, L.; Bruno, R.M. Dapagliflozin acutely improves endothelial dysfunction, reduces aortic stiffness and renal resistive index in type 2 diabetic patients: A pilot study. *Cardiovasc. Diabetol.* **2017**, *16*, 138. [CrossRef]

109. Leoncini, G.; Martinoli, C.; Viazzi, F.; Ravera, M.; Parodi, D.; Ratto, E.; Vettoretti, S.; Tomolillo, C.; Derchi, L.E.; Deferrari, G.; et al. Changes in renal resistive index and urinary albumin excretion in hypertensive patients under long-term treatment with lisinopril or nifedipine GITS. *Nephron* **2002**, *90*, 169–173. [CrossRef]

110. Parving, H.-H.; Mauer, M.; Ritz, E. Diabetic nephropathy. In *Brenner and Rector's the Kidney*, 7th ed.; Brenner, B.M., Ed.; Boston Saunders: Cambridge, UK, 2004; pp. 1777–1818.

111. Parving, H.-H.; De Zeeuw, D.; Cooper, M.E.; Remuzzi, G.; Liu, N.; Lunceford, J.; Shahinfar, S.; Wong, P.H.; Lyle, P.A.; Rossing, P.; et al. ACE gene polymorphism and losartan treatment in type 2 diabetic patients with nephropathy. *J. Am. Soc. Nephrol.* **2008**, *19*, 771–779. [CrossRef]

112. Pena, M.J.; Heinzel, A.; Rossing, P.; Parving, H.-H.; Dallmann, G.; Rossing, K.; Andersen, S.; Mayer, B.; Heerspink, H.J.L. Serum metabolites predict response to angiotensin II receptor blockers in patients with diabetes mellitus. *J. Transl. Med.* **2016**, *14*, 203. [CrossRef]

113. Pena, M.J.; Jankowski, J.; Heinze, G.; Kohl, M.; Heinzel, A.; Bakker, S.J.; Gansevoort, R.T.; Rossing, P.; De Zeeuw, D.; Heerspink, H.J.L.; et al. Plasma proteomics classifiers improve risk prediction for renal disease in patients with hypertension or type 2 diabetes. *J. Hypertens.* **2015**, *33*, 2123–2132. [CrossRef]

114. Pencina, M.J.; Parikh, C.R.; Kimmel, P.L.; Cook, N.R.; Coresh, J.; Feldman, H.I.; Foulkes, A.S.; Gimotty, P.A.; Hsu, C.-Y.; Lemley, K.; et al. Statistical methods for building better biomarkers of chronic kidney disease. *Stat. Med.* **2019**, *38*, 1903–1917. [CrossRef]

115. McShane, L.M. Biomarker validation: Context and complexities. *J. Law Med. Ethics* **2019**, *47*, 388–392. [CrossRef]

116. Soveri, I.; Helmersson-Karlqvist, J.; Fellström, B.; Larsson, A. Day-to-day variation of the kidney proximal tubular injury markers urinary cystatin C, KIM1, and NGAL in patients with chronic kidney disease. *Ren. Fail.* **2020**, *42*, 400–404. [CrossRef] [PubMed]
117. LeDue, T.B.; Rifai, N. Preanalytic and analytic sources of variations in C-reactive protein measurement: Implications for cardiovascular disease risk assessment. *Clin. Chem.* **2003**, *49*, 1258–1271. [CrossRef] [PubMed]
118. Schinstock, C.A.; Semret, M.H.; Wagner, S.J.; Borland, T.M.; Bryant, S.C.; Kashani, K.B.; Larson, T.S.; Lieske, J.C. Urinalysis is more specific and urinary neutrophil gelatinase-associated lipocalin is more sensitive for early detection of acute kidney injury. *Nephrol. Dial. Transplant.* **2012**, *28*, 1175–1185. [CrossRef] [PubMed]
119. Jones, G.R.; Albarede, S.; Kesseler, D.; MacKenzie, F.; Mammen, J.; Pedersen, M.; Stavelin, A.; Thelen, M.; Thomas, A.; Twomey, P.J.; et al. Analytical performance specifications for external quality assessment —Definitions and descriptions. *Clin. Chem. Lab. Med.* **2017**, *55*. [CrossRef] [PubMed]
120. Jennings, L.; Van Deerlin, V.M.; Gulley, M.L. Recommended principles and practices for validating clinical molecular pathology tests. *Arch. Pathol. Lab. Med.* **2009**, *133*, 743–755. [PubMed]
121. Tripepi, G.; D'Arrigo, G.; Jager, K.J.; Stel, V.S.; Dekker, F.J.; Zoccali, C. Do we still need cross-sectional studies in Nephrology? Yes we do! *Nephrol. Dial. Transplant.* **2017**, *32*. [CrossRef]
122. Harrell, F.E., Jr.; Lee, K.L.; Mark, D.B. Multivariable prognostic models: Issues in developing models, evaluating assumptions and adequacy, and measuring and reducing errors. *Stat. Med.* **1996**, *15*, 361–387. [CrossRef]
123. Roy, J.; Shou, H.; Xie, D.; Hsu, J.Y.; Yang, W.; Anderson, A.H.; Landis, J.R.; Jepson, C.; He, J.; Liu, K.D.; et al. Statistical methods for cohort studies of CKD: Prediction modeling. *Clin. J. Am. Soc. Nephrol.* **2016**, *12*, 1010–1017. [CrossRef]
124. Tibshirani, R. Regression shrinkage and selection via the lasso. *J. R. Stat. Soc. Ser. B Stat. Methodol.* **1996**, *58*, 267–288. [CrossRef]
125. Pencina, M.J.; D'Agostino, R.B.; Vasan, R.S. Statistical methods for assessment of added usefulness of new biomarkers. *Clin. Chem. Lab. Med.* **2010**, *48*, 1703–1711. [CrossRef] [PubMed]
126. Pepe, M.S.; Kerr, K.F.; Longton, G.; Wang, Z. Testing for improvement in prediction model performance. *Stat. Med.* **2013**, *32*, 1467–1482. [CrossRef] [PubMed]
127. Pencina, M.J.; D'Agostino, R.B., Sr.; Steyerberg, E.W. Extensions of net reclassification improvement calculations to measure usefulness of new biomarkers. *Stat. Med.* **2011**, *30*, 11–21. [CrossRef]
128. Steyerberg, E.W.; Vickers, A.J.; Cook, N.R.; Gerds, T.; Gonen, M.; Obuchowski, N.; Pencina, M.J.; Kattan, M.W. Assessing the performance of prediction models. *Epidemiology* **2010**, *21*, 128–138. [CrossRef] [PubMed]
129. Tangri, N.; Kitsios, G.D.; Inker, L.A.; Griffith, J.; Naimark, D.M.; Walker, S.; Rigatto, C.; Uhlig, K.; Kent, D.M.; Levey, A.S. Risk prediction models for patients with chronic kidney disease. *Ann. Intern. Med.* **2013**, *158*, 596–603. [CrossRef]
130. Andreucci, M.; Faga, T.; Pisani, A.; Perticone, M.; Michael, A. The ischemic/nephrotoxic acute kidney injury and the use of renal biomarkers in clinical practice. *Eur. J. Intern. Med.* **2017**, *39*, 1–8. [CrossRef]
131. Lewis, E.J.; Hunsicker, L.G.; Bain, R.P.; Rohde, R.D. The Effect of angiotensin-converting-enzyme inhibition on diabetic nephropathy. *N. Engl. J. Med.* **1993**, *329*, 1456–1462. [CrossRef]
132. Lewis, E.J.; Hunsicker, L.G.; Clarke, W.R.; Berl, T.; Pohl, M.A.; Lewis, J.B.; Ritz, E.; Atkins, R.C.; Rohde, R.; Raz, I. Renoprotective effect of the angiotensin-receptor antagonist irbesartan in patients with nephropathy due to type 2 diabetes. *N. Engl. J. Med.* **2001**, *345*, 851–860. [CrossRef]
133. De Zeeuw, D.; Heerspink, H.J.L. Time for clinical decision support systems tailoring individual patient therapy to improve renal and cardiovascular outcomes in diabetes and nephropathy. *Nephrol. Dial. Transplant.* **2020**, *35*, ii38–ii42. [CrossRef]
134. Parving, H.-H.; Brenner, B.M.; McMurray, J.J.; De Zeeuw, D.; Haffner, S.M.; Solomon, S.D.; Chaturvedi, N.; Persson, F.; Desai, A.S.; Nicolaides, M.; et al. Cardiorenal end points in a trial of aliskiren for type 2 diabetes. *N. Engl. J. Med.* **2012**, *367*, 2204–2213. [CrossRef]
135. Fried, L.F.; Emanuele, N.; Zhang, J.H.; Brophy, M.; Conner, T.A.; Duckworth, W.C.; Leehey, D.J.; McCullough, P.A.; O'Connor, T.; Palevsky, P.M.; et al. Combined angiotensin inhibition for the treatment of diabetic nephropathy. *N. Engl. J. Med.* **2013**, *369*, 1892–1903. [CrossRef] [PubMed]
136. Heerspink, H.J.; List, J.; Perkovic, V. New clinical trial designs for establishing drug efficacy and safety in a precision medicine era. *Diabetes Obes. Metab.* **2018**, *20*, 14–18. [CrossRef] [PubMed]

137. Lindhardt, M.; Persson, F.; Currie, G.; Pontillo, C.; Beige, J.; Delles, C.; Von Der Leyen, H.; Mischak, H.; Navis, G.; Noutsou, M.; et al. Proteomic prediction and renin angiotensin aldosterone system inhibition prevention of early diabetic nephropathy in type 2 diabetic patients with normoalbuminuria (PRIORITY): Essential study design and rationale of a randomised clinical multicentre trial. *BMJ Open* **2016**, *6*, e010310. [CrossRef] [PubMed]
138. Baigent, C.; Landray, M.; Reith, C.; Emberson, J.R.; Wheeler, D.C.; Tomson, C.; Wanner, C.; Krane, V.; Cass, A.; Craig, J.C.; et al. The effects of lowering LDL cholesterol with simvastatin plus ezetimibe in patients with chronic kidney disease (Study of Heart and Renal Protection): A randomised placebo-controlled trial. *Lancet* **2011**, *377*, 2181–2192. [CrossRef]
139. Woodcock, J.; LaVange, L.M. Master protocols to study multiple therapies, multiple diseases, or both. *N. Engl. J. Med.* **2017**, *377*, 62–70. [CrossRef] [PubMed]
140. Berry, S.M.; Connor, J.T.; Lewis, R.J. The platform trial. *JAMA* **2015**, *313*, 1619–1620. [CrossRef]

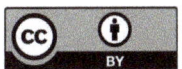

© 2020 by the authors. Licensee MDPI, Basel, Switzerland. This article is an open access article distributed under the terms and conditions of the Creative Commons Attribution (CC BY) license (http://creativecommons.org/licenses/by/4.0/).

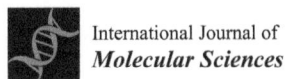

Review

Acute Kidney Injury in Septic Patients Treated by Selected Nephrotoxic Antibiotic Agents—Pathophysiology and Biomarkers—A Review

Nadezda Petejova [1,2,3,*], Arnost Martinek [1,2], Josef Zadrazil [3], Marcela Kanova [4], Viktor Klementa [3], Radka Sigutova [5,6], Ivana Kacirova [5,7], Vladimir Hrabovsky [1,2], Zdenek Svagera [5,6] and David Stejskal [5,6]

1. Department of Internal Medicine, University Hospital Ostrava, 70852 Ostrava, Czech Republic; arnost.martinek@osu.cz (A.M.); vladimir.hrabovsky@fno.cz (V.H.)
2. Department of Clinical Studies Faculty of Medicine, University of Ostrava, 70300 Ostrava, Czech Republic
3. Department of Internal Medicine III—Nephrology, Rheumatology and Endocrinology, University Hospital and Faculty of Medicine and Dentistry, Palacky University Olomouc, 77900 Olomouc, Czech Republic; josef.zadrazil@fnol.cz (J.Z.); viktor.klementa@fnol.cz (V.K.)
4. Department of Anesthesiology and Resuscitation, University Hospital Ostrava, 70852 Ostrava, Czech Republic; marcela.kanova@fno.cz
5. Department of Laboratory Diagnostics Institute of Clinical Biochemistry and Clinical Pharmacology, University Hospital Ostrava, 70852 Ostrava, Czech Republic; radka.sigutova@fno.cz (R.S.); ivana.kacirova@fno.cz (I.K.); zdenek.svagera@fno.cz (Z.S.); david.stejskal@fno.cz (D.S.)
6. Department of Biomedical Sciences Faculty of Medicine, University of Ostrava, 70300 Ostrava, Czech Republic
7. Institute of Clinical Pharmacology Faculty of Medicine, University of Ostrava, 70300 Ostrava, Czech Republic
* Correspondence: petejova@seznam.cz

Received: 23 August 2020; Accepted: 25 September 2020; Published: 26 September 2020

Abstract: Acute kidney injury is a common complication in critically ill patients with sepsis and/or septic shock. Further, some essential antimicrobial treatment drugs are themselves nephrotoxic. For this reason, timely diagnosis and adequate therapeutic management are paramount. Of potential acute kidney injury (AKI) biomarkers, non-protein-coding RNAs are a subject of ongoing research. This review covers the pathophysiology of vancomycin and gentamicin nephrotoxicity in particular, septic AKI and the microRNAs involved in the pathophysiology of both syndromes. PubMED, UptoDate, MEDLINE and Cochrane databases were searched, using the terms: biomarkers, acute kidney injury, antibiotic nephrotoxicity, sepsis, miRNA and nephrotoxicity. A comprehensive review describing pathophysiology and potential biomarkers of septic and toxic acute kidney injury in septic patients was conducted. In addition, five miRNAs: *miR-15a-5p*, *miR-192-5p*, *miR-155-5p*, *miR-486-5p* and *miR-423-5p* specific to septic and toxic acute kidney injury in septic patients, treated by nephrotoxic antibiotic agents (vancomycin and gentamicin) were identified. However, while these are at the stage of clinical testing, preclinical and clinical trials are needed before they can be considered useful biomarkers or therapeutic targets of AKI in the context of antibiotic nephrotoxicity or septic injury.

Keywords: acute kidney injury; gentamicin; sepsis; miRNA; nephrotoxicity; vancomycin

1. Introduction

Acute kidney injury (AKI) is a common and mostly severe clinical syndrome complicating a number of critical illnesses. It has a highly negative impact on patient morbidity, mortality and clinical outcome. The diagnosis is generally based on evaluation of: (1) increase in serum creatinine and/or (2)

decrease in urinary output. According to the KDIGO (Kidney Disease Improving Global Outcomes) classification of 2012, the severity of urinary output deterioration to terminal stages and presentation of an anuria and serum creatinine increase to 353.6 µmol/L is the most serious stage 3 [1]. Further, in 2017, new forms of acute renal impairment were described with AKI lasting at least 7 days after insult and acute kidney disease (AKD) lasting up to 90 days. Renal impairment and serum creatinine levels that had not returned to baseline levels by 90 days resulted in the need for renal replacement therapy (RRT) and/or progression to chronic kidney disease (CKD) [2]. Timely AKI diagnosis, especially in critically ill patients, would enable clinicians to better initiate preventive measures to avoid the need for RRT and obviate the risk of CKD. A number of promising new biomarkers may be able to predict the development or worsening of AKI in intensive care. The most highlighted of these in recent years are noncoding microRNAs in these circumstances. This review focuses on the pathophysiology and potential biomarkers in the detection of AKI after nephrotoxic drugs and/or septic insults with emphasis on specific microRNAs.

2. Epidemiology of Acute Kidney Injury

Acute kidney injury is a relatively frequent complication in critically ill patients in ICUs, especially in those with sepsis. The incidence of AKI in these circumstances, predominantly in situations with presentation of septic shock, may be as high as 47.5% and the overall mortality in critically ill patients with AKI may be more than 60% [3]. According to recent results of a multicenter Chinese study of patients hospitalized in ICUs, the incidence of AKI was 51%, with the majority occurring on the 4th day after admission [4]. A number of factors can contribute to AKI and progression to renal failure, including cardiovascular and hepatic disorders, malignancies, hypovolemia, intoxication, drug nephrotoxicity, anemia and surgical and vascular interventions. Further, many such patients need nephrotoxic iodine contrast drugs for CT scans and other radiological examinations. Therefore, the AKI is often a consequence of multiple factors.

3. Pathophysiology of Sepsis-Induced Acute Kidney Injury

Sepsis is generally characterized as a life-threatening condition induced by any type of infection (e.g., bacterial, viral, mycotic) and the dysregulated response of the host organism, with subsequent organ and tissue dysfunction or failure. The diagnosis has recently been redefined according to the SEPSIS-3 consensus (The Third International Consensus Definitions for Sepsis and Septic Shock) as an increase in the SOFA (Sequential Organ Failure Assessment) score of 2 points or more. For earlier clinical decision-making, the Quick SOFA (qSOFA) criteria can be used as evaluation of: altered mental status, a respiratory rate of 22/min or greater and a systolic blood pressure of 100 mmHg or less [5]. The pathophysiology of sepsis-induced AKI appears to be multifactorial, including, among others, deleterious inflammatory cascade [6]. Underlying explanations of septic AKI development include: (1) alteration of the renal macro- and microcirculation, with subsequent endothelial dysfunction, (2) damage of renal tubular epithelial cells, (3) a change in cellular metabolic pathways and energy consumption, (4) mitochondrial injury, (5) reactive oxygen species (ROS) production and (6) cycle cell arrest [7]. However, the exact mechanism of septic AKI is still unclear. Increase in inflammatory cytokine production and activation of leukocyte activity in the context of a dysregulated immunological and inflammatory response can lead to production of intravascular microthrombi and also reduce intrarenal blood flow and oxygen delivery [8]. Regulation of the immune and adaptive immunity response in renal tubular cells occurs due to activation of the Toll-like receptor (TLRs) family in the cell membrane. There are more than 13 members of this family and they are usually activated by endotoxins. They recognize pathogen-activated molecular patterns (PAMPs) and damage-associated pathogens (DAMPs) with the promotion of leukocyte and intrinsic renal cell activation. Renal tubular cells express TLR-1, -2, -3, -4 and -6, which can be substantially involved in the pathophysiology of tubular cell damage [9,10]. The most important receptor in septic AKI pathophysiology appears to be TLR-4, that can bind the endotoxin lipopolysaccharide (LPS), leading to activation of a number of intracellular signaling pathways via the nuclear-κB (NF-κB) transcription factor. NF-κB response to endotoxin stress leads to activation and release of the inflammatory cytokines TNFα, IL-1, IL-6 and IL-8 [11]. The activation of NF-κB depends on the phosphorylation and degradation of inhibitory κB proteins, triggered by specific kinases [9]. The basic explanation of the pathophysiological pathway in septic AKI development via activation of TLR-4 receptors in proximal tubular cells very likely lies in dysregulation of tubular integrity, with induction of tight junction disruption. This process may contribute to subsequent oliguria and decrease in renal function [12]. A recent animal study (Nakano et al., 2020), where conditional knockout of TLR-4 in proximal tubular cells reduced LPS-induced paracellular leakage of filtrate into the interstitium via TLR-4 showed that the interstitial leakage and accumulation of extracellular fluids lead to anuria and diminished the efficacy of volume resuscitation, which is frequently used in septic AKI to restore renal function [13].

4. Biomarkers of Sepsis-Induced Acute Kidney Injury

Many potential biomarkers have been studied in recent years in the context of sepsis and septic AKI. These can be divided into: (1) standard biomarkers, (2) additional urinary and/or serum biomarkers, (3) metabolomics, (4) other experimental proteomics and (5) microRNAs (miRNAs). Generally, AKI is diagnosed by the standard use of serum creatinine concentration and urinary output, as mentioned, with additional evaluation of serum concentration of urea. In addition, we can include Neutrophile gelatinase-associated lipocalin (NGAL), Cystatin C, Kidney Injury Molecule -1 (KIM-1), Interleukin 18 (IL-18), urinary Insulin-like growth factor-binding protein-7 (IGFBP-7), urinary tissue inhibitor of metalloproteinase 2 (TIMP-2), calprotectin, urine angiotensinogen and liver fatty acid binding protein [14]. In clinical practice, especially in patients with AKI in ICUs, it is very useful to have a biomarker capable of predicting the need for RRT initiation, renal recovery or transition to chronic nephropathy. According to a meta-analysis of 63 studies comprising 15,928 critically ill patients, the best evidence was for blood NGAL and Cystatin C followed by urinary TIMP-2 and IGFBP-7 [15]. However, decision-making in the case of RRT initiation is based on a number of clinical and laboratory findings, not only biomarkers, and none of these is specific to any particular type of AKI [16]. The major limitation of biomarkers in the AKI condition lies in comparing biomarkers to serum creatinine and diuresis, the basic diagnostic tools for AKI [17].

In recent experimental animal models of septic AKI, some potential novel metabolomic biomarkers have been identified using nuclear magnetic resonance spectroscopy on urine, renal tissue and in serum. Alterations in the concentration of several metabolites have been found e.g., lactate, N-acetylglutamine, alanine, pyruvate, myoinositol, glutamine, valine, glucose, ascorbic acid, aminoadipic acid, N-acetylaspartate and betaine and these correlate with serum creatinine and NGAL [18]. Further, many heat shock proteins (HSP) families and their bioactivity are described in various kidney diseases. In ischemic, toxic or other forms of AKI, the following have been found expressed in several renal cell types (podocytes, mesangial cells, tubular cells, fibroblasts, endothelial cells, macrophages): HSP27, HSP70, HSP60, HSP47, HSP90 and HSP32 [19]. Their main role in renal cytoprotection is still under investigation. However, many of them can block the apoptotic death pathway, oxidative stress, cell proliferation and differentiation, mediation of the inflammatory response and inhibit fibrogenesis [19]. A study of 56 critically ill patients, where 17 of them suffered from AKI, revealed that urinary HSP72 levels significantly increased in the period of three days before AKI and remained elevated during AKI diagnosis [20].

5. MiRNAs as Biomarkers of Septic Acute Kidney Injury

Research is currently focused on miRNAs as new potential biomarkers and/or therapeutic tools for many conditions including AKI. MiRNAs are small molecules (18–31 nucleotides) of noncoding RNAs, representing a large part of genetic information not translated from the DNA matrix into final protein production. The evidence of their abundance, developmentally regulated fashion and often subcellular localization points to their important biological role in many biochemical and pathophysiological processes and pathways on the cellular and molecular level [21]. Influence on post-transcriptional gene regulation, cell metabolism, cytokine production, cell differentiation and programmed cell death are only a small percentage of miRNAs' effects and their target genes. In the AKI condition, some act protectively and can become potential therapeutic targets but others can increase the toxic activity and renal damage. Anti-inflammatory and/or anti-apoptotic activity in AKI has been described for the following miRNAs: *miR-10a, miR-21, miR-26a, miR-122, miR-126, miR-146a, miR-199a, miR-296* and *miR-494* [22]. Some miRNAs involved in the pathophysiological inflammatory process of sepsis based on endotoxin (LPS) activation of TLR4 in the signaling pathway of NF-κB activation, pro-inflammatory cytokine production (IL-6, IL-1β, TNFα) and subsequent neutrophil activation, damage of endothelial permeability and tissue injury are: *miR-146 a/b, miR-223, miR-155, miR-203, miR-15a, miR-16, miR-126, miR-199a* and *miR-9*. Each regulates positively or negatively a different part of the biochemical cascade to final cytokine production and tissue damage according to their target genes [23,24]. In the development of septic AKI, severe metabolic alterations of tubular epithelial cells may play a crucial role via *miR-21-3p* influence on the *AKT/CDK2-FOXO1* pathway, with induction of cycle cell arrest and apoptosis [25]. According to one human study (Ge et al., 2017), many other signaling pathways are involved in septic AKI development, including oxidative stress and mitochondrial dysfunction pathways (*HIF-1, PI3K-Akt, mTOR* and *TGFβ*). In septic, critically ill patients, significantly overexpressed *miR-4321* was observed, with the predicted oxidative-stress-associated target genes: *AKT1, MTOR, NOX5, IL17RA* and *IL26* [26]. The mitochondrion is assumed to be a key organelle in the development of septic acute kidney injury, and has major pathophysiological significance in ROS production and apoptosis [27]. In one hybrid human and experimental study including 50 patients with sepsis, an effect was found of *miR-106a* on caspase-3 activity, *Bcl-2* expression and proinflammatory cytokine production after LPS stimulation [28]. The authors found an association between *miR-106a* and an aggravation of LPS-induced inflammation, and apoptosis in sepsis-induced AKI. A target gene for *miR-106a* was established as thrombospondin *THBS2*, which takes part in a number of processes such as regulation of cell motility, death and cytoskeleton formation [28].

6. Medication-Induced AKI in Septic Patients

Drug-induced nephrotoxicity varies from a relatively mild form of acute tubulointerstitial nephritis (ATIN), several types of glomerulonephritis, crystal nephropathy and osmotic nephrosis to acute tubular necrosis represented mostly by severe renal impairment with the need for RRT. The last-mentioned may be associated with development of chronic nephropathy and the need for chronic hemodialysis treatment. The incidence of medication-associated nephrotoxicity accounts for approximately 18–27% of all AKI patients in US hospitals—the main causative drugs are NSAIDs, aminoglycosides, amphotericin B and calcineurin inhibitors [29].

Potentially nephrotoxic medications, which are considered essential and commonly used in sepsis and critically ill patients, are antimicrobial agents (antibiotics, antiviral and antifungal treatment), human albumin in septic shock or proton pump inhibitors to prevent stress ulcers [30] (Table 1). Iodine contrast agents are used for radiocontrast imaging examinations in septic, critically ill patients when there is need for sepsis source finding or surgical interventions [31].

The nephrotoxicity of some antimicrobial drugs is a common problem. Of these, the most nephrotoxic are: vancomycin, aminoglycosides and polymyxins, which cause acute tubular necrosis and apoptosis depending on dose, among other factors. Many antimicrobials and other drugs frequently used in critically ill patients can also cause ATIN, accounting for 60–70% of all ATIN cases [32].

Table 1. Nephrotoxicity of commonly used medications in critically ill patients [30–36].

Medications (Agents)	Clinical and Histological Presentation of Renal Toxicity
Antimicrobials Aminoglycosides Glycopeptides (vancomycin) Polymyxins	acute tubular necrosis, apoptosis, necroptosis, acute oxidative stress, cycle cell arrest
Antimicrobials β-lactams Sulphonamides Macrolides Antiretrovirals (Acyclovir) Rifampin Fluoroquinolones Chloramphenicol **Other medications** Diuretics NSAIDs Proton pump inhibitors	acute tubulointerstitial nephritis
Sulphonamides Antiretrovirals	acute crystalline nephropathy
High-osmolar iodine radiocontrast agents Hydroxyethyl starches and gelatine solutions	increase in ROS production, vasoconstriction, osmotic nephrosis
NSAIDs	altered renal hemodynamics

NSAIDs—nonsteroidal anti-inflammatory drugs, ROS—reactive oxygen species.

7. Vancomycin-Induced Nephrotoxicity Pathophysiology and Biomarkers

Vancomycin is a glycopeptidic antimicrobial agent with substantial bactericidal effect on Gram-positive bacterial infections and is frequently used in the treatment of Methicillin-resistant *Staphylococcus aureus* (MRSA). It also acts against *Streptococcus* sp., *Enterococcus* sp., *Actinomyces* sp., *Clostridium* sp. and *Eubacterium* sp. Its pharmacokinetics and pharmacodynamics are time-dependent, but according to recommendations for vancomycin treatment, the best parameter for evaluating its efficacy is the ratio of the 24 h area under the curve (AUC) to the minimum inhibitory concentration of AUC/MIC ≥400 mg.h/L with an MIC of pathogen <2 mg/L [37,38]. Vancomycin is not metabolized in the human body and is eliminated renally by glomerular filtration. Its binding to plasma proteins is less than 50%, the elimination half-life ranges from 6 to 12 h and volume of distribution is 0.4–1.0 L/kg [37]. The recently revised consensus guidelines of the American Society of Health-System Pharmacists for vancomycin therapy and monitoring for serious MRSA infections (2020) recommends, in adults and pediatric patients, a daily AUC/MIC ratio between 400 to 600 mg.h/L. A higher loading dose (20–25 mg/kg based on actual body weight) should be considered in critically ill patients treated by any type of RRT or in need of continuous vancomycin infusion. In obese patients with serious infections, the maximum loading dose is 3000 mg intravenously [39]. However, vancomycin nephrotoxicity with risk of AKI development is usually associated with higher vancomycin exposure, as measured by AUC_{0-24}. Additionally, a significantly increased risk for nephrotoxicity has been observed in patients with AUC_{0-24} of 563 mg.h/L [40]. However, higher trough vancomycin serum concentrations >16.5 mg/L are also at greatest risk for new onset of AKI in critically ill patients [41]. In these cases, it is very difficult, in clinical practice, to maximize antibiotic efficacy, and, at the same time, to minimize its nephrotoxicity. The pathophysiology of vancomycin nephrotoxicity has been intensively investigated mostly in experimental research. Sakamoto et al. (2017) uncovered the possible nephrotoxic effect based on peroxidation of the mitochondrial membrane cardiolipin by vancomycin-induced production of intracellular ROS and activation of apoptosis in proximal tubular cells [42]. Apoptotic cell death induced by vancomycin may be associated with activation of specific caspases: caspase 9 and caspase 3/7 and extensive ROS production [34]. In the prospective multicenter Sapphire study (NCT01209169 ClinicalTrials.gov) including 723 critically ill adult patients, the pharmacokinetics of two urinary biomarkers TIMP-2 and IGFBP7 were evaluated in patients receiving vancomycin, piperacilin-tazobactam, or their combination. The concentration of biomarkers and the risk of death or need for dialysis treatment within 9 months, were the highest in the combination group. However, the AKI progression to an aggravated stage 2/3 was comparable in vancomycin monotherapy and in the combination treatment [43]. Selected urinary AKI biomarkers—clusterin, cystatin C, NGAL/lipocalin-2, osteopontin and KIM-1—were investigated in animals receiving vancomycin. A higher vancomycin exposure presented by an AUC_{0-24} and maximum serum concentration significantly correlated with increase in urinary AKI biomarkers but did not correlate with histopathological score [44]. Serum creatinine, urinary NGAL and KIM-1 were measured in 87 patients without chronic kidney disease (12.6% developed AKI) before and during the vancomycin therapy. According to the results, both urinary biomarkers NGAL and KIM-1 successfully discriminated patients with and without vancomycin-induced AKI earlier than serum creatinine [45]. However, in one animal study (Pais et al., 2019) KIM-1 and clusterin were more sensitive to vancomycin-induced AKI than NGAL [46].

One possible explanation for vancomycin-induced AKI and tubular cell apoptosis is based on DNA methylation by activation of Methyl-CpG binding domain protein 2 (*MBD2*). Experimental inhibition of *MBD2* can downregulate *miR-301-5p* with subsequent restoration of anti-apoptosis gene expression e.g., hepatoma-derived growth factor (*HDGF*) and microphthalmia-associated transcription factor (*MITF*) and can increase MDM-4 expression for reduction of p53 [47].

8. Gentamicin-Induced Nephrotoxicity Pathophysiology and Biomarkers

Gentamicin is an aminoglycoside concentration-dependent antibiotic agent with bactericidal effects against Gram-negative bacterial pathogens e.g., *Escherichia coli*, *Pseudomonas aeruginosa*, *Proteus* and *Klebsiella*. Renal elimination by glomerular filtration is the predominant type of removal of unchanged gentamicin from the human organism. Gentamicin enters to some extent the proximal tubular cells, where it is accumulated in the lysosomes with alteration of their enzymes [48]. The gentamicin volume of distribution is, approximately, an equivalent to the extracellular body weight, and it generally decreases with age. The gentamicin elimination half-life in adults with physiological renal function is very short and ranges between 2 and 3 h [49]. The incidence of acute renal failure during gentamicin treatment can account for approximately 10–20% of all cases [50]. The nephrotoxicity of gentamicin is a very complex pathophysiological process with both tubular and glomerular involvement (Figure 1). Besides the cellular uptake in proximal convoluted cells and acute tubular necrosis, it can induce mesangial cell contraction and proliferation mediated by platelet-activating factor and also an increase in free intracellular calcium concentration. Moreover, it can induce activation of the phospholipase A2 enzyme and increased production of eicosanoids in mesangial cells, production of ROS and mesangial cell apoptosis [51]. For early detection of progression from minimal to moderate kidney injury in animals treated by gentamicin, the urinary biomarkers clusterin, KIM-1, Cystatin C and NGAL were compared to serum BUN and creatinine. As predictable, all of these biomarkers showed earlier onset changes than the generally used serum BUN and creatinine in AKI diagnosis [52]. Another explanation of gentamicin nephrotoxicity is experimental evaluation of toxicity biomarkers through specific gene expression associated with apoptosis or cell necrosis. Of 10 analyzed genes associated with apoptosis, in four, *TP53*, *CASP3*, *CASP8* and *CASP9*, an increase in expression was found. In addition, the regulation of these genes produced proteins capable of cleaving specific substrates leading to cell death. Moreover, a decrease in antiapoptotic genes e.g., *BCL2L1* has been found [53]. In an experimental study carried out on drug-induced, predominantly tubular (gentamicin and cisplatine) and glomerular (puromycin and doxorubicin) kidney injury, among several commonly downregulated miRNAs, *miR-143-3p* and *miR-122-5p* were proposed as potential tubular and *miR-3473* as glomerular biomarker candidates [54].

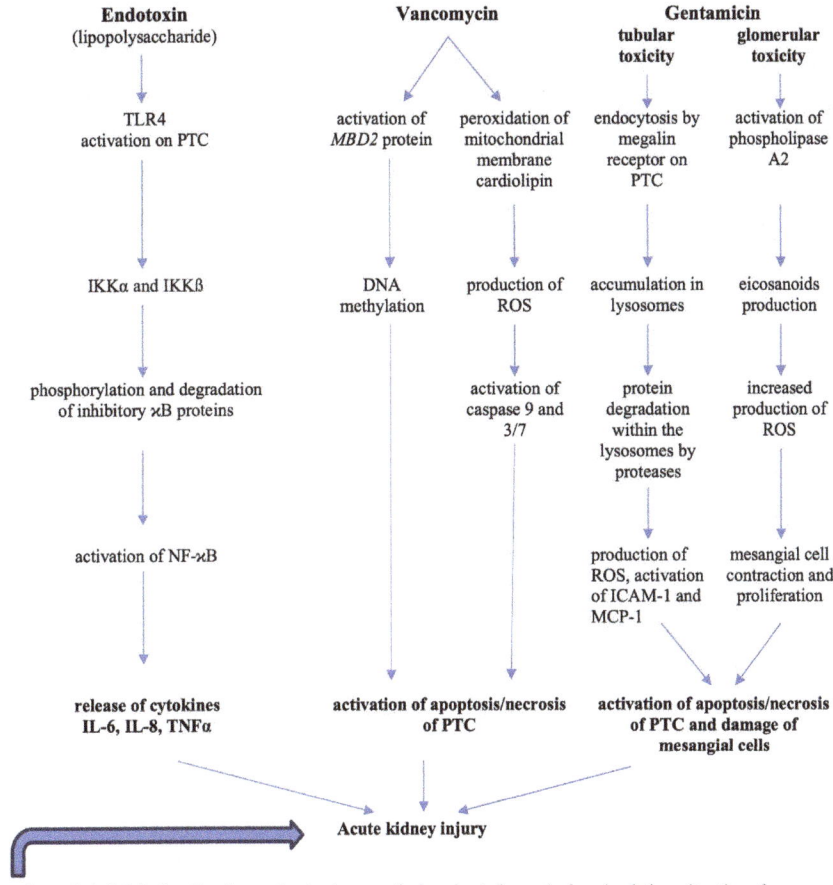

Figure 1. Simplified pathophysiology of acute kidney injury development in sepsis and selected antibiotic treatment [6,10,42,47,48,51,55,56]. DNA—deoxyribonucleic acid, ICAM-1—intercellular adhesion molecule-1, IKK—I-kinase, IL-6—interleukin 6, IL-8—interleukin 8, *MBD2*—Methyl-CpG Binding Domain Protein 2, MCP-1—monocyte chemoattractant protein 1, NF-κB—nuclear factor—kappa B, PTC—proximal tubular cells, ROS—reactive oxygen species, TLR4—Toll-like receptor 4, TNFα—tumor necrosis factor alpha

9. MicroRNAs Associated with AKI Induced by Sepsis or Nephrotoxic Antibiotic Therapy

9.1. miR-15a-5p

The pathogenesis of sepsis AKI development is challenging, and many miRNAs likely participate in the pathophysiological and biochemical pathways involved. *MiR-15a-5p* in a regulatory axis with *XIST* (X inactive specific transcript)/*CUL3* (cullin 3 gene) in septic AKI was investigated in a combined human and animal study from China with LPS as the endotoxin. The lipopolysaccharide inhibited the growth of animal podocytes besides the upregulation of *XIST* and *CUL3* and downregulated *miR-15a-5p*. The inhibition of *XIST* and *miR-15a-5p* enhanced and preserved LPS-induced apoptosis significantly, while the *miR-15a-5p* inhibitor reversed the renal cell apoptosis. Furthermore, overexpression of the *CUL3* gene considerably reduced the LPS and *miR-l5a-5p*-induced apoptosis [57]. Another explanation of sepsis pathophysiology is based on regulation of the crucial inflammatory response of damaged organs with the participation of *miR-15a-5p*. In one animal study (Lou et al., 2020), after the LPS stimulation of macrophages there was an increased expression of *miR-15a-5p* and a release of inflammatory cytokines IL-6, IL-1ß and TNFα in comparison to a control group. Moreover, it has been demonstrated that inhibition of *miR-15a-5p* can decrease the secretion of proinflammatory cytokines by blocking its targeting gene, TNFα induced protein 3-interacting protein 2 (*TNIP2*), and the NF-κB signaling pathway [58]. *MiR-15a-5p* regulates many genes affecting angiogenesis, hematopoietic cells and carcinogenesis and has the effect of suppressing inflammation and fibrosis of peritoneal mesothelial cells induced by peritoneal dialysis [59–61].

9.2. miR-192-5p

In a human study of critically ill patients with sepsis or the nonseptic systemic inflammatory response syndrome, *miR-192-5p* was one of six of the most important circulating RNAs that differentiated sepsis from the nonseptic inflammatory response. *MiR-192-5p* negatively correlated with concentrations of pro-inflammatory cytokines (IL-6, IL-1 and IL-8) and sepsis markers (e.g., CRP). However, no correlation between the *miR-192-5p* concentration and the generally used SOFA score was found [62]. In a proceeding human study, a positive correlation was revealed between *miR-192-5p* and the redox biomarker, peroxiredoxin-1, which is released by immune cells during inflammation [63]. Urinary *miR-192-5p* was studied in animals with ischemia-reperfusion-induced AKI, where its expression in urine was significantly elevated after the ischemic intervention. The results were validated with urine samples from 71 patients who underwent cardiac surgery. The elevation of *miR-192-5p* was detected earlier than KIM-1, that was previously established as a renal injury biomarker [64]. Some other experimental studies on *miR-192-5p* and renal diseases in association with diabetes, hypertension and drug nephrotoxicity, can be added to the complex clinical and pathophysiological review. For example, circulating RNA HIPK3 (homeodomain-interacting protein kinase 3) can bind *miR-192-5p* with upregulation of transcription factor *FOXO1* (forkhead box protein O1) leading to hyperglycemia and insulin resistance [65]. In the kidney, *miRNA-192-5p* contributes to protection against hypertension through the target gene *ATP1B1* (β1 subunit of Na^+/K^+-ATPase), and *miR-192-5p* levels are significantly decreased in humans with hypertension or hypertensive nephrosclerosis [66]. Conversely, there is contrasting data on the kidney-protective role of *miR-192-5p* in association with vancomycin-induced AKI. The antagonism of vancomycin-induced *miR-192-5p* by the miRNA inhibitor led to a decrease of apoptosis in HK2 cells. Moreover, inhibition of p53 can attenuate apoptosis by suppressing *miR-192-5p* in vancomycin-induced AKI [67].

9.3. miR-155-5p

According to the literature, *miR-155* plays a critical role in various pathological and physiological processes, including immunity, inflammation, infection, cancers, hematopoietic cell differentiation, cardiovascular diseases and some genetic malformations [68].

The effects of activation and suppression of *miR-155-5p* in relation to various renal diseases and in sepsis have been investigated in a number of experimental studies [69,70]. Its role in the inflammatory process has been recently studied in an in vitro model of sepsis where inhibition of *miR-155-5p* reduced the expression of IL-6 and IL-8 as pro-inflammatory cytokines by 31% and 14%, respectively. Moreover, its inhibition can reduce the release of heat shock proteins, such as HSP10, by 69%. The latter is released from damaged cells as a stress signal [69]. The HSP10 inhibits lipopolysaccharide-induced inflammatory mediator production and NF-κB activation by inhibiting Toll-like receptor signaling in cell membranes [71]. Endogenous *miR-155* participates on regulation of inflammation and is released from dendritic cells within exosomes. It is subsequently taken up by recipient dendritic cells. Exosomal *miR-155* promoted endotoxin-induced (LPS) inflammation in one study (Alexander et al., 2015) by an increase in TNFα and subsequent increase in IL-6 serum concentration [70]. Gentamicin-induced nephrotoxicity and ischemia-reperfusion injury resulted in increased *miR-155* and *miR-18* in one rodent study [72]. With a higher dose of gentamicin, more significant injury and necrosis of renal epithelial cells were observed. However, contrary to ischemic injury, with the higher dose of gentamicin (300 mg/kg), both miRNAs decreased in the urine and increased in the renal cortex and medulla. The range of *miR-155* target genes is very high, and includes genes for the regulation of e.g., mitochondrial processes, lipid metabolism, kinase-apoptotic pathways and cell proliferation [72].

Experimental modulation of gene expression in salt-sensitive hypertensive animals showed the important role of circular RNAs in the development of hypertensive kidney injury. The authors of one study (Lu et al., 2020) characterized a circular RNA called circNr1h4 derived from the *Nr1h4* (nuclear receptor subfamily 1, group H, member 4) gene that binds to *miR-155-5p* and regulates expression of its target gene—fatty acid reductase 1 (*Far1*). The reaction between *miR-155-5p* and circNr1h4 is basically competitive, where the silencing of circNr1h4 or overexpression of *miR-155-5p* considerably decreased *Far1* levels and increased ROS production. Therefore, *miR-155-5p* may be involved in the pathology of hypertensive kidney injury [73]. The involvement of *miR-155-5p* in the pathophysiological pathway to the development of diabetic kidney disease is probably explained by the signaling axis of *p53* and *sirt1* genes with regulation of autophagic and fibrotic processes in renal tubular injury. MiR-155-5p may be involved in the promotion of renal fibrosis under hypoxia and also in high blood glucose concentration, and is transcriptionally regulated by p53. This allows participation in the regulation of cell growth, the cell cycle, differentiation and apoptosis [74].

9.4. miR-486-5p

One of the most serious causes of acute kidney injury is ischemia-reperfusion injury, often resulting in tubular cell necrosis or apoptosis. In one experimental study (Viñas et al., 2016), the effect of exosomes with *miR-486-5p* derived from endothelial colony-forming cells (ECFCs) on protection against kidney injury was investigated in mice with induced renal ischemia. Infusion of ECFC exosomes into ischemic endothelial kidney cells had a strong functional and histological protective effect, associated with increased kidney *miR-486-5p* levels, decreased phosphatase and tensin homolog (*PTEN*) and activation of the *Akt* pathway [75]. In chronic kidney disease, *miR-486-5p* inhibits the forkhead transcription factor *FOXO1* by downregulation of *PTEN* phosphatase, a negative regulator of *Akt*. *FOXO1* appears to be the predominant mediator of muscle wasting in chronic nephropathy, accelerated by stimulating the ubiquitin proteasome system through activation, e.g., E3 ligases [76]. In one human study (Regmi et al., 2019) involving patients with diabetic nephropathy, decreased serum concentrations of *miR-486-5p* were found and, this negatively correlated with albuminuria, levels of fasting blood glucose and glycated hemoglobin [77].

The association between LPS-induced inflammation and *miR-486-5p* with target *FOXO1* has been studied in vitro in nucleus pulposus cells and intervertebral disc degeneration. Experimentally, it was shown that *miR-486-5p* overexpression led to a decrease of LPS-induced production of inflammatory cytokines IL-1ß, IL-6 and TNFα and protected the nucleus pulposus cells against apoptosis [78].

9.5. miR-423-5p

Ischemia-reperfusion-induced AKI is one possible pathophysiological process, in which *miR-423-5p* may be substantially involved, along with other circulating miRNAs. Experimentally, it has been shown that *miR-423-5p* induces endoplasmic reticulum stress and reactive oxidative stress by inhibiting the *GSTM1* (Glutathione-S-Transferase Mu 1) gene which encodes the glutathione-S-transferase M1 enzyme in ischemia-reperfusion injury [79]. Glutathione-S-transferase is a very potent detoxification enzyme that protects the renal tubular cells against oxidative stress and ROS. The considerable involvement of *miR-423-5p* in the regulation and activation of NF-κB signaling by the *TNIP2* gene has been demonstrated in patients with lupus nephritis [80]. The *TNIP2* gene increases IKKα kinase activity and phosphorylation and induces NF-κB target genes [80]. The exact pathogenesis and factors contributing to renal cell injury here are still under investigation. MiR-423-5p is postulated to suppress podocyte injury in conditions of high blood glucose levels. Overexpression of *miR-423-5p* by negatively regulated Nicotinamide adenine dinucleotide phosphate oxidase-4 (*NOX4*) gene can antagonize high glucose-induced podocyte injury. Moreover, it inhibits ROS production, cell apoptosis, inflammation and subsequent damage of renal cells [81].

The schematic pathophysiology of acute kidney injury in a critically ill patient with sepsis and nephrotoxic antibiotic treatment with selected miRNAs is presented in Figure 2.

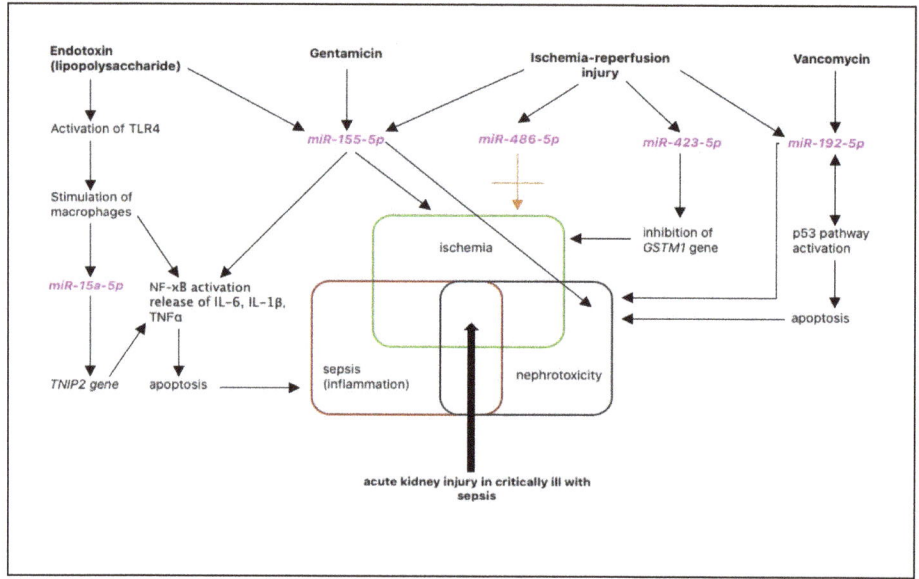

Figure 2. Schematic pathophysiology of acute kidney injury in a critically ill patient with sepsis and nephrotoxic antibiotic treatment with selected miRNAs. AKI—acute kidney injury, *GSTM1*—glutathione-S-transferase Mu 1 gene, IL-6—interleukin 6, IL-1ß—interleukin 1ß, NF-κB—nuclear factor—kappa B, TNFα—tumor necrosis factor alpha, *TNIP2*—tumor necrosis factor alpha induced protein 3-interacting protein 2, TLR4—Toll-like receptor 4.

10. Therapeutic Approaches in Septic Patients with AKI

In the therapeutic approach to AKI in septic critically ill patients, it is essential for clinicians to decide between conservative or invasive measures. The first step is generally the treatment of sepsis by wide-spectrum antimicrobial agents, according to the epidemiologically assumed microbial [30]. Accordingly, there is a need to consider surgical or other intervention to eliminate the potential source of the sepsis. AKI severity, clinical and hemodynamic status as well as metabolic alterations are the basics for RRT or conservative therapy. Many experimental AKI biomarkers including miRNAs have an ancillary role in AKI diagnosis to assist clinicians in decision-making, in primarily preventive approaches. Usually this means dose adjustment of the nephrotoxic agents, stabilization of hemodynamics with controlled volume expansion if needed, preservation of urine output, adequate nutrition and treatment of any metabolic disorder. The crucial use of additive AKI biomarkers besides serum creatinine and urea, are the subject of ongoing research. During the first phase of septic AKI, of clinical importance is optimization of fluid management with adequate fluid resuscitation and avoidance of fluid overload. Physicians have to take into account patient's volume status, urinary output, the type of intravenous fluids and infusion rates [82]. However, fluid overload due to loss of plasmatic proteins and increase in capillary permeability, can lead to fluid accumulation with a worsening of patient clinical status. In the renal parenchyma this increases the renal venous pressure, reduces the renal perfusion pressure and glomerular filtration rate with consequent retention of salt and water [83]. Fluid resuscitation with hemodynamic stabilization and choice of fluids play an important role in the therapeutic approach to both syndromes—sepsis and AKI. The preferred solutions are saline and balanced crystalloids, whereas hydroxyethyl starches and gelatin solutions can be associated with increased risk of AKI in septic patients. In the presence of septic shock, despite adequate volume resuscitation, there is a need for vasoactive drugs to restore renal parenchymal perfusion. In the case of sepsis, for this reason, commonly used drugs are norepinephrine, dopamine, vasopressin and phenylephrine [84].

With severe AKI, metabolic alterations and worsening hemodynamic instability, there is usually an increased need for RRT initiation in intermittent (IRRT) or continuous (CRRT) form. In physical principle and type of RRT or blood purification techniques, there are dialysis, hemofiltration, hemodiafiltration, hemoadsorption by CytoSorb (for severe sepsis) or plasmapheresis. Some RRT methods can be also combined according to clinical or laboratory findings. Close patient status monitoring and adequate supportive measures in cases with absence for urgent RRT initiation are the basic steps in conservative approaches. Thus, the timing for RRT initiation does not play a substantial role in survival in critically ill patients with AKI, especially in cases where conservative approaches can be successfully used [85]. A more comprehensive view was achieved after termination of the French AKIKI (Artificial Kidney Initiation in Kidney Injury) study (ClinicalTrials.gov NCT 01932190) performed in 620 critically ill patients with acute kidney injury. No significant difference in mortality between early and delayed strategies of RRT initiation with a decrease in need for RRT in the delayed approach was found [86]. Hemoadsorption with CytoSorb can be used predominantly in patients suffering from septic shock with careful decision-making, according to the APACHE II score. The basic principle of these blood purification devices, using more effective membranes or columns incorporated in CRRT, is removal of pro-inflammatory cytokines (e.g., IL-6, IL-8, TNFα) and endotoxins to stabilize the patient's hemodynamics and decrease the need for vasopressor therapy [87]. Preserving adequate fluid balance, net ultrafiltration, treatment dose, nutritional support and antibiotic treatment are a vital component of the therapeutic approach in critically ill septic patients [88].

In patients with septic AKI on any type of RRT treatment, what is crucial is the antimicrobial treatment and therapeutic drug monitoring where possible. Many renally eliminated antimicrobial agents in these circumstances undergo changes in pharmacokinetics/pharmacodynamics parameters, including clearance, volume of distribution, binding to plasma proteins and elimination half-life. The dose adjustment has to be individualized according to serum concentration, to achieve the required pharmacodynamics parameters, drug efficacy and decrease the risk of toxicity [89,90]. Other preventive measures such as antioxidants in the case of antibiotic nephrotoxicity are still under investigation.

11. Conclusions

The early diagnosis of AKI, adequate preventive and therapeutic approaches in critically ill septic patients, are still a challenge for clinicians. Some experimental AKI biomarkers are undergoing research to help clinicians with essential, timely detection of renal injury. However, to date, there is no specific biomarker for particular toxic, septic or ischemic renal damage. None of them is able to distinguish between specific insult causing the AKI. For this reason, there is considerable current attention on miRNAs and their pathophysiological role in the human organism.

Author Contributions: N.P. wrote the main text of the manuscript, conceived and designed the underlying scientific project, A.M., J.Z. and D.S. reviewed the manuscript, I.K. contributed with pharmacological consultations, Z.S. and R.S. contributed with biochemical consultations. V.K. collected the scientific research data, M.K. and V.H. contributed with intensive care consultations. All authors have read and agreed to the published version of the manuscript.

Funding: The project is supported by the Ministry of Health Czech Republic—conceptual development of research organization (01-RVO-FNOs/2019).

Conflicts of Interest: The authors declare no conflict of interest related to this manuscript or project.

References

1. Kidney Disease: Improving Global Outcomes (KDIGO) Acute Kidney Injury Work Group. KDIGO Clinical Practice Guideline for Acute Kidney Injury. *Kidney Int. Suppl.* **2012**, *2*, 1–138.
2. Chawla, L.S.; Bellomo, R.; Bihorac, A.; Goldstein, S.L.; Siew, E.D.; Bagshaw, S.M.; Bittleman, D.; Cruz, D.; Endre, Z.; Fitzgerald, R.L.; et al. Acute kidney disease and renal recovery: Consensus report of the Acute Disease Quality Initiative (ADQI) 16 Workgroup. *Nat. Rev. Nephrol.* **2017**, *13*, 241–257. [CrossRef] [PubMed]
3. Uchino, S.; Kellum, J.A.; Bellomo, R.; Doig, G.S.; Morimatsu, H.; Morgera, S.; Schetz, M.; Tan, I.; Bouman, C.; Macedo, E.; et al. Beginning and Ending Supportive Therapy for the Kidney (BEST Kidney) Investigators. Acute renal failure in critically ill patients: A multinational, multicenter study. *JAMA* **2005**, *294*, 813–818.
4. Jiang, L.; Zhu, Y.; Luo, X.; Wen, Y.; Du, B.; Wang, M.; Zhao, Z.; Yin, Y.; Zhu, B.; Xi, X. Epidemiology of acute kidney injury in intensive care units in Beijing: The multi-center BAKIT study. *BMC Nephrol.* **2019**, *20*, 468. [CrossRef] [PubMed]
5. Singer, M.; Deutschman, C.S.; Seymour, C.W.; Shankar-Hari, M.; Annane, D.; Bauer, M.; Bellomo, R.; Bernard, G.R.; Chiche, J.D.; Coopersmith, C.M.; et al. The Third International Consensus Definitions for Sepsis and Septic Shock (Sepsis-3). *JAMA* **2016**, *315*, 801–810. [CrossRef] [PubMed]
6. Poston, J.T.; Koyner, J.L. Sepsis associated acute kidney injury. *BMJ* **2019**, *364*, k4891. [CrossRef]
7. Gómez, H.; Kellum, J.A. Sepsis-induced acute kidney injury. *Curr. Opin. Crit. Care* **2016**, *22*, 546–553. [CrossRef]
8. Ronco, C.; Bellomo, R.; Kellum, J.A. Acute kidney injury. *Lancet* **2019**, *394*, 1949–1964.
9. Anders, H.J.; Banas, B.; Schlöndorff, D. Signaling danger: Toll-like receptors and their potential roles in kidney disease. *J. Am. Soc. Nephrol.* **2004**, *15*, 854–867. [CrossRef]
10. Kawai, T.; Akira, S. Signaling to NF-kappaB by Toll-like receptors. *Trends Mol. Med.* **2007**, *13*, 460–469.
11. Morrell, E.D.; Kellum, J.A.; Pastor-Soler, N.M.; Hallows, K.R. Septic acute kidney injury: Molecular mechanisms and the importance of stratification and targeting therapy. *Crit. Care* **2014**, *18*, 501. [CrossRef] [PubMed]
12. Wei, Q. Novel strategy for septic acute kidney injury rescue: Maintenance of the tubular integrity. *Kidney Int.* **2020**, *97*, 847–849. [PubMed]
13. Nakano, D.; Kitada, K.; Wan, N.; Zhang, Y.; Wiig, H.; Wararat, K.; Yanagita, M.; Lee, S.; Jia, L.; Titze, J.M.; et al. Lipopolysaccharide induces filtrate leakage from renal tubular lumina into the interstitial space via a proximal tubular Toll-like receptor 4-dependent pathway and limits sensitivity to fluid therapy in mice. *Kidney Int.* **2020**, *97*, 904–912. [CrossRef] [PubMed]
14. Kashani, K.; Cheungpasitporn, W.; Ronco, C. Biomarkers of acute kidney injury: The pathway from discovery to clinical adoption. *Clin. Chem. Lab. Med.* **2017**, *55*, 1074–1089. [CrossRef]
15. Klein, S.J.; Brandtner, A.K.; Lehner, G.F.; Ulmer, H.; Bagshaw, S.M.; Wiedermann, C.J.; Joannidis, M. Biomarkers for prediction of renal replacement therapy in acute kidney injury: A systematic review and meta-analysis. *Intensive Care Med.* **2018**, *44*, 323–336. [CrossRef]
16. Schrezenmeier, E.V.; Barasch, J.; Budde, K.; Westhoff, T.; Schmidt-Ott, K.M. Biomarkers in acute kidney injury-pathophysiological basis and clinical performance. *Acta Physiol.* **2017**, *219*, 554–572. [CrossRef]
17. Teo, S.H.; Endre, Z.H. Biomarkers in acute kidney injury (AKI). *Best Pract. Res. Clin. Anaesthesiol.* **2017**, *31*, 331–344. [CrossRef]
18. Izquierdo-Garcia, J.L.; Nin, N.; Cardinal-Fernandez, P.; Rojas, Y.; de Paula, M.; Granados, R.; Martínez-Caro, L.; Ruíz-Cabello, J.; Lorente, J.A. Identification of novel metabolomic biomarkers in an experimental model of septic acute kidney injury. *Am. J. Physiol. Renal Physiol.* **2019**, *316*, F54–F62. [CrossRef]
19. Chebotareva, N.; Bobkova, I.; Shilov, E. Heat shock proteins and kidney disease: Perspectives of HSP therapy. *Cell Stress Chaperones* **2017**, *22*, 319–343. [CrossRef]
20. Morales-Buenrostro, L.E.; Salas-Nolasco, O.I.; Barrera-Chimal, J.; Casas-Aparicio, G.; Irizar-Santana, S.; Pérez-Villalva, R.; Bobadilla, N.A. Hsp72 is a novel biomarker to predict acute kidney injury in critically ill patients. *PLoS ONE* **2014**, *9*, e109407. [CrossRef]
21. Dozmorov, M.G.; Giles, C.B.; Koelsch, K.A.; Wren, J.D. Systematic classification of non-coding RNAs by epigenomic similarity. *BMC Bioinform.* **2013**, *14*, S2. [CrossRef] [PubMed]
22. Fan, P.C.; Chen, C.C.; Chen, Y.C.; Chang, Y.S.; Chu, P.H. MicroRNAs in acute kidney injury. *Hum. Genom.* **2016**, *10*, 29. [CrossRef]

23. Giza, D.E.; Fuentes-Mattei, E.; Bullock, M.D.; Tudor, S.; Goblirsch, M.J.; Fabbri, M.; Lupu, F.; Yeung, S.J.; Vasilescu, C.; Calin, G.A. Cellular and viral microRNAs in sepsis: Mechanisms of action and clinical applications. *Cell Death Differ.* **2016**, *23*, 1906–1918. [CrossRef]
24. Benz, F.; Roy, S.; Trautwein, C.; Roderburg, C.; Luedde, T. Circulating MicroRNAs as Biomarkers for Sepsis. *Int. J. Mol. Sci.* **2016**, *17*, 78. [CrossRef] [PubMed]
25. Lin, Z.; Liu, Z.; Wang, X.; Qiu, C.; Zheng, S. MiR-21-3p Plays a Crucial Role in Metabolism Alteration of Renal Tubular Epithelial Cells during Sepsis Associated Acute Kidney Injury via AKT/CDK2-FOXO1 Pathway. *Biomed. Res. Int.* **2019**, *2019*, 2821731. [CrossRef]
26. Ge, Q.M.; Huang, C.M.; Zhu, X.Y.; Bian, F.; Pan, S.M. Differentially expressed miRNAs in sepsis-induced acute kidney injury target oxidative stress and mitochondrial dysfunction pathways. *PLoS ONE* **2017**, *12*, e0173292. [CrossRef] [PubMed]
27. Ishimoto, Y.; Inagi, R. Mitochondria: A therapeutic target in acute kidney injury. *Nephrol. Dial. Transplant.* **2016**, *31*, 1062–1069. [CrossRef]
28. Shen, Y.; Yu, J.; Jing, Y.; Zhang, J. MiR-106a aggravates sepsis-induced acute kidney injury by targeting THBS2 in mice model. *Acta Cir. Bras.* **2019**, *34*, e201900602. [CrossRef]
29. Taber, S.S.; Pasko, D.A. The epidemiology of drug-induced disorders: The kidney. *Expert Opin. Drug Saf.* **2008**, *7*, 679–690. [CrossRef]
30. Rhodes, A.; Evans, L.E.; Alhazzani, W.; Levy, M.M.; Antonelli, M.; Ferrer, R.; Kumar, A.; Sevransky, J.E.; Sprung, C.L.; Nunnally, M.E.; et al. Surviving Sepsis Campaign: International Guidelines for Management of Sepsis and Septic Shock: 2016. *Intensive Care Med.* **2017**, *43*, 304–377. [CrossRef]
31. Wilhelm-Leen, E.; Montez-Rath, M.E.; Chertow, G. Estimating the Risk of Radiocontrast-Associated Nephropathy. *J. Am. Soc. Nephrol.* **2017**, *28*, 653–659. [CrossRef] [PubMed]
32. Perazella, M.A.; Markowitz, G.S. Drug-induced acute interstitial nephritis. *Nat. Rev. Nephrol.* **2010**, *6*, 461–470. [CrossRef] [PubMed]
33. Petejova, N.; Martinek, A.; Zadrazil, J.; Teplan, V. Acute toxic kidney injury. *Ren. Fail.* **2019**, *41*, 576–594. [CrossRef] [PubMed]
34. Arimura, Y.; Yano, T.; Hirano, M.; Sakamoto, Y.; Egashira, N.; Oishi, R. Mitochondrial superoxide production contributes to vancomycin-induced renal tubular cell apoptosis. *Free Radic. Biol. Med.* **2012**, *52*, 1865–1873. [CrossRef] [PubMed]
35. Moledina, D.G.; Perazella, M.A. PPIs and kidney disease: From AIN to CKD. *J. Nephrol.* **2016**, *29*, 611–616. [CrossRef]
36. Ong, L.Z.; Tambyah, P.A.; Lum, L.H.; Low, Z.J.; Cheng, I.; Murali, T.M.; Wan, M.Q.; Chua, H.R. Aminoglycoside-associated acute kidney injury in elderly patients with and without shock. *J. Antimicrob. Chemother.* **2016**, *71*, 3250–3257. [CrossRef]
37. Rybak, M.J.; Lomaestro, B.M.; Rotschafer, J.C.; Moellering, R.C., Jr.; Craig, W.A.; Billeter, M.; Dalovisio, J.R.; Levine, D.P. Therapeutic monitoring of vancomycin in adults summary of consensus recommendations from the American Society of Health-System Pharmacists, the Infectious Diseases Society of America, and the Society of Infectious Diseases Pharmacists. *Pharmacotherapy* **2009**, *29*, 1275–1279. [CrossRef]
38. Zamoner, W.; Prado, I.R.S.; Balbi, A.L.; Ponce, D. Vancomycin dosing, monitoring and toxicity: Critical review of the clinical practice. *Clin. Exp. Pharmacol. Physiol.* **2019**. [CrossRef]
39. Rybak, M.J.; Le, J.; Lodise, T.P.; Levine, D.P.; Bradley, J.S.; Liu, C.; Mueller, B.A.; Pai, M.P.; Wong-Beringer, A.; Rotschafer, J.C.; et al. Executive Summary: Therapeutic Monitoring of Vancomycin for Serious Methicillin-Resistant Staphylococcus aureus Infections: A Revised Consensus Guideline and Review of the American Society of Health-System Pharmacists, the Infectious Diseases Society of America, the Pediatric Infectious Diseases Society, and the Society of Infectious Diseases Pharmacists. *Pharmacotherapy* **2020**, *40*, 363–367.
40. Chavada, R.; Ghosh, N.; Sandaradura, I.; Maley, M.; Van Hal, S.J. Establishment of an AUC_{0-24} Threshold for Nephrotoxicity Is a Step towards Individualized Vancomycin Dosing for Methicillin-Resistant Staphylococcus aureus Bacteremia. *Antimicrob. Agents Chemother.* **2017**, *61*. [CrossRef]
41. Hanrahan, T.P.; Kotapati, C.; Roberts, M.J.; Rowland, J.; Lipman, J.; Roberts, J.A.; Udy, A. Factors associated with vancomycin nephrotoxicity in the critically ill. *Anaesth. Intensive Care* **2015**, *43*, 594–599. [CrossRef] [PubMed]

42. Sakamoto, Y.; Yano, T.; Hanada, Y.; Takeshita, A.; Inagaki, F.; Masuda, S.; Matsunaga, N.; Koyanagi, S.; Ohdo, S. Vancomycin induces reactive oxygen species-dependent apoptosis via mitochondrial cardiolipin peroxidation in renal tubular epithelial cells. *Eur. J. Pharmacol.* **2017**, *800*, 48–56. [CrossRef] [PubMed]
43. Kane-Gill, S.L.; Ostermann, M.; Shi, J.; Joyce, E.L.; Kellum, J.A. Evaluating Renal Stress Using Pharmacokinetic Urinary Biomarker Data in Critically Ill Patients Receiving Vancomycin and/or Piperacillin-Tazobactam: A Secondary Analysis of the Multicenter Sapphire Study. *Drug Saf.* **2019**, *42*, 1149–1155. [CrossRef] [PubMed]
44. Rhodes, N.J.; Prozialeck, W.C.; Lodise, T.P.; Venkatesan, N.; O'Donnell, J.N.; Pais, G.; Cluff, C.; Lamar, P.C.; Neely, M.N.; Gulati, A.; et al. Evaluation of Vancomycin Exposures Associated with Elevations in Novel Urinary Biomarkers of Acute Kidney Injury in Vancomycin-Treated Rats. *Antimicrob. Agents Chemother.* **2016**, *60*, 5742–5751. [CrossRef] [PubMed]
45. Pang, H.M.; Qin, X.L.; Liu, T.T.; Wei, W.X.; Cheng, D.H.; Lu, H.; Guo, Q.; Jing, L. Urinary kidney injury molecule-1 and neutrophil gelatinase-associated lipocalin as early biomarkers for predicting vancomycin-associated acute kidney injury: A prospective study. *Eur. Rev. Med. Pharmacol. Sci.* **2017**, *21*, 4203–4213. [PubMed]
46. Pais, G.M.; Avedissian, S.N.; O'Donnell, J.N.; Rhodes, N.J.; Lodise, T.P.; Prozialeck, W.C.; Lamar, P.C.; Cluff, C.; Gulati, A.; Fitzgerald, J.C.; et al. Comparative Performance of Urinary Biomarkers for Vancomycin-Induced Kidney Injury According to Timeline of Injury. *Antimicrob. Agents Chemother.* **2019**, *63*. [CrossRef]
47. Wang, J.; Li, H.; Qiu, S.; Dong, Z.; Xiang, X.; Zhang, D. MBD2 upregulates miR-301a-5p to induce kidney cell apoptosis during vancomycin-induced AKI. *Cell Death Dis.* **2017**, *8*, e3120. [CrossRef]
48. Olbricht, C.J.; Fink, M.; Gutjahr, E. Alterations in lysosomal enzymes of the proximal tubule in gentamicin nephrotoxicity. *Kidney Int.* **1991**, *39*, 639–646. [CrossRef]
49. Gentamicin 40 mg/mL Injection. Available online: https://www.medicines.org.uk/emc/product/6531/smpc (accessed on 7 July 2020).
50. Romero, F.; Pérez, M.; Chávez, M.; Parra, G.; Durante, P. Effect of uric acid on gentamicin-induced nephrotoxicity in rats-role of matrix metalloproteinases 2 and 9. *Basic Clin. Pharmacol. Toxicol.* **2009**, *105*, 416–424. [CrossRef]
51. Martínez-Salgado, C.; López-Hernández, F.J.; López-Novoa, J.M. Glomerular nephrotoxicity of aminoglycosides. *Toxicol. Appl. Pharmacol.* **2007**, *223*, 86–98. [CrossRef]
52. Udupa, V.; Prakash, V. Gentamicin induced acute renal damage and its evaluation using urinary biomarkers in rats. *Toxicol. Rep.* **2018**, *6*, 91–99. [CrossRef] [PubMed]
53. Campos, M.A.A.; de Almeida, L.A.; Grossi, M.F.; Tagliati, C.A. In vitro evaluation of biomarkers of nephrotoxicity through gene expression using gentamicin. *J. Biochem. Mol. Toxicol.* **2018**, *32*, e22189. [CrossRef] [PubMed]
54. Kagawa, T.; Zarybnicky, T.; Omi, T.; Shirai, Y.; Toyokuni, S.; Oda, S.; Yokoi, T. A scrutiny of circulating microRNA biomarkers for drug-induced tubular and glomerular injury in rats. *Toxicology* **2019**, *415*, 26–36. [CrossRef] [PubMed]
55. Hori, Y.; Aoki, N.; Kuwahara, S.; Hosojima, M.; Kaseda, R.; Goto, S.; Iida, T.; De, S.; Kabasawa, H.; Kaneko, R.; et al. Megalin Blockade with Cilastatin Suppresses Drug-Induced Nephrotoxicity. *J. Am. Soc. Nephrol.* **2017**, *28*, 1783–1791. [CrossRef]
56. Balakumar, P.; Rohilla, A.; Thangathirupathi, A. Gentamicin-induced nephrotoxicity: Do we have a promising therapeutic approach to blunt it? *Pharmacol. Res.* **2010**, *62*, 179–186. [CrossRef]
57. Xu, G.; Mo, L.; Wu, C.; Shen, X.; Dong, H.; Yu, L.; Pan, P.; Pan, K. The *miR-15a-5p-XIST-CUL3* regulatory axis is important for sepsis-induced acute kidney injury. *Ren. Fail.* **2019**, *41*, 955–966. [CrossRef]
58. Lou, Y.; Huang, Z. microRNA-15a-5p participates in sepsis by regulating the inflammatory response of macrophages and targeting TNIP2. *Exp. Ther. Med.* **2020**, *19*, 3060–3068. [CrossRef]
59. Wang, Z.M.; Wan, X.H.; Sang, G.Y.; Zhao, J.D.; Zhu, Q.Y.; Wang, D.M. miR-15a-5p suppresses endometrial cancer cell growth via Wnt/β-catenin signaling pathway by inhibiting WNT3A. *Eur. Rev. Med. Pharmacol. Sci.* **2017**, *21*, 4810–4818.
60. Chen, D.; Wu, D.; Shao, K.; Ye, B.; Huang, J.; Gao, Y. MiR-15a-5p negatively regulates cell survival and metastasis by targeting CXCL10 in chronic myeloid leukemia. *Am. J. Transl. Res.* **2017**, *9*, 4308–4316.
61. Shang, J.; He, Q.; Chen, Y.; Yu, D.; Sun, L.; Cheng, G.; Liu, D.; Xiao, J.; Zhao, Z. miR-15a-5p suppresses inflammation and fibrosis of peritoneal mesothelial cells induced by peritoneal dialysis via targeting VEGFA. *J. Cell. Physiol.* **2019**, *234*, 9746–9755. [CrossRef]

62. Caserta, S.; Kern, F.; Cohen, J.; Drage, S.; Newbury, S.F.; Llewelyn, M.J. Circulating Plasma microRNAs can differentiate Human Sepsis and Systemic Inflammatory Response Syndrome (SIRS). *Sci. Rep.* **2016**, *6*, 28006. [CrossRef] [PubMed]
63. Caserta, S.; Mengozzi, M.; Kern, F.; Newbury, S.F.; Ghezzi, P.; Llewelyn, M.J. Severity of Systemic Inflammatory Response Syndrome Affects the Blood Levels of Circulating Inflammatory-Relevant MicroRNAs. *Front. Immunol.* **2018**, *8*, 1977. [CrossRef] [PubMed]
64. Zou, Y.F.; Wen, D.; Zhao, Q.; Shen, P.Y.; Shi, H.; Zhao, Q.; Chen, Y.X.; Zhang, W. Urinary MicroRNA-30c-5p and MicroRNA-192-5p as potential biomarkers of ischemia-reperfusion-induced kidney injury. *Exp. Biol. Med.* **2017**, *242*, 657–667. [CrossRef] [PubMed]
65. Cai, H.; Jiang, Z.; Yang, X.; Lin, J.; Cai, Q.; Li, X. Circular RNA HIPK3 contributes to hyperglycemia and insulin homeostasis by sponging miR-192-5p and upregulating transcription factor forkhead box O1. *Endocr. J.* **2020**, *67*, 397–408. [CrossRef] [PubMed]
66. Baker, M.A.; Wang, F.; Liu, Y.; Kriegel, A.J.; Geurts, A.M.; Usa, K.; Xue, H.; Wang, D.; Kong, Y.; Liang, M. MiR-192-5p in the Kidney Protects Against the Development of Hypertension. *Hypertension* **2019**, *73*, 399–406. [CrossRef] [PubMed]
67. Chen, J.; Wang, J.; Li, H.; Wang, S.; Xiang, X.; Zhang, D. p53 activates miR-192-5p to mediate vancomycin induced AKI. *Sci. Rep.* **2016**, *6*, 38868. [CrossRef]
68. Elton, T.S.; Selemon, H.; Elton, S.M.; Parinandi, N.L. Regulation of the MIR155 host gene in physiological and pathological processes. *Gene* **2013**, *532*, 1–12. [CrossRef]
69. Pfeiffer, D.; Roßmanith, E.; Lang, I.; Falkenhagen, D. miR-146a, miR-146b, and miR-155 increase expression of IL-6 and IL-8 and support HSP10 in an In vitro sepsis model. *PLoS ONE* **2017**, *12*, e0179850. [CrossRef]
70. Alexander, M.; Hu, R.; Runtsch, M.C.; Kagele, D.A.; Mosbruger, T.L.; Tolmachova, T.; Seabra, M.C.; Round, J.L.; Ward, D.M.; O'Connell, R.M. Exosome-delivered microRNAs modulate the inflammatory response to endotoxin. *Nat. Commun.* **2015**, *6*, 7321. [CrossRef] [PubMed]
71. Johnson, B.J.; Le, T.T.; Dobbin, C.A.; Banovic, T.; Howard, C.B.; Flores, F.D.M.L.; Vanags, D.; Naylor, D.J.; Hill, G.R.; Suhrbier, A. Heat shock protein 10 inhibits lipopolysaccharide-induced inflammatory mediator production. *J. Biol. Chem.* **2005**, *280*, 4037–4047. [CrossRef] [PubMed]
72. Saikumar, J.; Hoffmann, D.; Kim, T.M.; Gonzalez, V.R.; Zhang, Q.; Goering, P.L.; Brown, R.P.; Bijol, V.; Park, P.J.; Waikar, S.S.; et al. Expression, circulation, and excretion profile of microRNA-21, -155, and -18a following acute kidney injury. *Toxicol. Sci.* **2012**, *129*, 256–267. [CrossRef] [PubMed]
73. Lu, C.; Chen, B.; Chen, C.; Li, H.; Wang, D.; Tan, Y.; Weng, H. CircNr1h4 regulates the pathological process of renal injury in salt-sensitive hypertensive mice by targeting miR-155-5p. *J. Cell. Mol. Med.* **2020**, *24*, 1700–1712. [CrossRef] [PubMed]
74. Wang, Y.; Zheng, Z.J.; Jia, Y.J.; Yang, Y.L.; Xue, Y.M. Role of p53/miR-155-5p/sirt1 loop in renal tubular injury of diabetic kidney disease. *J. Transl. Med.* **2018**, *16*, 146. [CrossRef] [PubMed]
75. Viñas, J.L.; Burger, D.; Zimpelmann, J.; Haneef, R.; Knoll, W.; Campbell, P.; Gutsol, A.; Carter, A.; Allan, D.S.; Burns, K.D. Transfer of microRNA-486-5p from human endothelial colony forming cell-derived exosomes reduces ischemic kidney injury. *Kidney Int.* **2016**, *90*, 1238–1250. [CrossRef]
76. Xu, J.; Li, R.; Workeneh, B.; Dong, Y.; Wang, X.; Hu, Z. Transcription factor FoxO1, the dominant mediator of muscle wasting in chronic kidney disease, is inhibited by microRNA-486. *Kidney Int.* **2012**, *82*, 401–411. [CrossRef]
77. Regmi, A.; Liu, G.; Zhong, X.; Hu, S.; Ma, R.; Gou, L.; Zafar, M.I.; Chen, L. Evaluation of Serum microRNAs in Patients with Diabetic Kidney Disease: A Nested Case-Controlled Study and Bioinformatics Analysis. *Med. Sci. Monit.* **2019**, *25*, 1699–1708. [CrossRef]
78. Chai, X.; Si, H.; Song, J.; Chong, Y.; Wang, J.; Zhao, G. miR-486-5p Inhibits Inflammatory Response, Matrix Degradation and Apoptosis of Nucleus Pulposus Cells through Directly Targeting FOXO1 in Intervertebral Disc Degeneration. *Cell. Physiol. Biochem.* **2019**, *52*, 109–118.
79. Yuan, X.P.; Liu, L.S.; Chen, C.B.; Zhou, J.; Zheng, Y.T.; Wang, X.P.; Han, M.; Wang, C.X. MicroRNA-423-5p facilitates hypoxia/reoxygenation-induced apoptosis in renal proximal tubular epithelial cells by targeting GSTM1 via endoplasmic reticulum stress. *Oncotarget* **2017**, *8*, 82064–82077. [CrossRef]
80. Wang, W.; Gao, J.; Wang, F. MiR-663a/MiR-423-5p are involved in the pathogenesis of lupus nephritis via modulating the activation of NF-κB by targeting TNIP2. *Am. J. Transl. Res.* **2017**, *9*, 3796–3803.

81. Xu, Y.; Zhang, J.; Fan, L.; He, X. miR-423-5p suppresses high-glucose-induced podocyte injury by targeting Nox4. *Biochem. Biophys. Res. Commun.* **2018**, *505*, 339–345. [CrossRef]
82. Montomoli, J.; Donati, A.; Ince, C. Acute Kidney Injury and Fluid Resuscitation in Septic Patients: Are We Protecting the Kidney? *Nephron* **2019**, *143*, 170–173. [CrossRef] [PubMed]
83. O'Connor, M.E.; Prowle, J.R. Fluid Overload. *Crit. Care Clin.* **2015**, *31*, 803–821. [CrossRef] [PubMed]
84. Bellomo, R.; Kellum, J.A.; Ronco, C.; Wald, R.; Martensson, J.; Maiden, M.; Bagshaw, S.M.; Glassford, N.J.; Lankadeva, Y.; Vaara, S.T.; et al. Acute kidney injury in sepsis. *Intensive Care Med.* **2017**, *43*, 816–828. [CrossRef] [PubMed]
85. Gaudry, S.; Hajage, D.; Benichou, N.; Chaïbi, K.; Barbar, S.; Zarbock, A.; Lumlertgul, N.; Wald, R.; Bagshaw, S.M.; Srisawat, N.; et al. Delayed versus early initiation of renal replacement therapy for severe acute kidney injury: A systematic review and individual patient data meta-analysis of randomised clinical trials. *Lancet* **2020**, *395*, 1506–1515. [CrossRef]
86. Gaudry, S.; Hajage, D.; Schortgen, F.; Martin-Lefevre, L.; Pons, B.; Boulet, E.; Boyer, A.; Chevrel, G.; Lerolle, N.; Carpentier, D.; et al. Initiation Strategies for Renal-Replacement Therapy in the Intensive Care Unit. *N. Engl. J. Med.* **2016**, *375*, 122–133. [CrossRef]
87. Karkar, A.; Ronco, C. Prescription of CRRT: A pathway to optimize therapy. *Ann. Intensive Care* **2020**, *10*, 32. [CrossRef]
88. Romagnoli, S.; Ricci, Z.; Ronco, C. CRRT for sepsis-induced acute kidney injury. *Curr. Opin. Crit. Care* **2018**, *24*, 483–492. [CrossRef]
89. Petejova, N.; Martinek, A.; Zahalkova, J.; Duricova, J.; Brozmannova, H.; Urbanek, K.; Grundmann, M.; Plasek, J.; Kacirova, I. Vancomycin pharmacokinetics during high-volume continuous venovenous hemofiltration in critically ill septic patients. *Biomed. Pap. Med. Faculty Univ. Palacky Olomouc Czech Repub.* **2014**, *158*, 65–72. [CrossRef]
90. Petejova, N.; Zahalkova, J.; Duricova, J.; Kacirova, I.; Brozmanova, H.; Urbanek, K.; Grundmann, M.; Martinek, A. Gentamicin pharmacokinetics during continuous venovenous hemofiltration in critically ill septic patients. *J. Chemother.* **2012**, *24*, 107–112. [CrossRef]

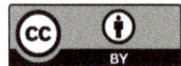

© 2020 by the authors. Licensee MDPI, Basel, Switzerland. This article is an open access article distributed under the terms and conditions of the Creative Commons Attribution (CC BY) license (http://creativecommons.org/licenses/by/4.0/).

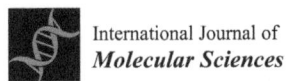

International Journal of
Molecular Sciences

Review

Roles Played by Biomarkers of Kidney Injury in Patients with Upper Urinary Tract Obstruction

Satoshi Washino [1,*], Keiko Hosohata [2] and Tomoaki Miyagawa [1]

[1] Department of Urology, Jichi Medical University Saitama Medical Center, 1-847, Amanuma-cho, Omiya-ku, Saitama 330-8503, Japan; sh2-miya@jichi.ac.jp
[2] Education and Research Center for Clinical Pharmacy, Osaka University of Pharmaceutical Sciences, 4-20-1 Nasahara, Takatsuki 569-1094, Japan; hosohata@gly.oups.ac.jp
* Correspondence: suwajiisan@yahoo.co.jp

Received: 28 June 2020; Accepted: 29 July 2020; Published: 31 July 2020

Abstract: Partial or complete obstruction of the urinary tract is a common and challenging urological condition caused by a variety of conditions, including ureteral calculi, ureteral pelvic junction obstruction, ureteral stricture, and malignant ureteral obstruction. The condition, which may develop in patients of any age, induces tubular and interstitial injury followed by inflammatory cell infiltration and interstitial fibrosis, eventually impairing renal function. The serum creatinine level is commonly used to evaluate global renal function but is not sensitive to early changes in the glomerular filtration rate and unilateral renal damage. Biomarkers of acute kidney injury are useful for the early detection and monitoring of kidney injury induced by upper urinary tract obstruction. These markers include levels of neutrophil gelatinase-associated lipocalin (NGAL), monocyte chemotactic protein-1, kidney injury molecule 1, N-acetyl-b-D-glucosaminidase, and vanin-1 in the urine and serum NGAL and cystatin C concentrations. This review summarizes the pathophysiology of kidney injury caused by upper urinary tract obstruction, the roles played by emerging biomarkers of obstructive nephropathy, the mechanisms involved, and the clinical utility and limitations of the biomarkers.

Keywords: upper urinary tract obstruction; kidney injury; biomarkers; neutrophil gelatinase-associated lipocalin; monocyte chemotactic protein-1; kidney injury molecule 1; cystatin C; vanin-1

1. Introduction

Upper urinary tract obstruction (UUTO) is a common and challenging urological condition caused by a variety of diseases, such as ureteropelvic junction obstruction (UPJO), ureteral calculi, ureteral strictures, and malignant ureteral obstruction. The condition may occur in patients of any age. Surgical intervention is necessary for moderate to severe cases, depending on the cause of the obstruction.

Hydronephrosis, or swelling in one or both kidneys due to incomplete emptying, is often observed in UUTO patients. However, the extent of hydronephrosis does not necessarily reflect the severity of UUTO. Obstruction may be minimal despite moderate to severe hydronephrosis, or it may be severe without obvious hydronephrosis. Renal scans together with determination of the glomerular filtration rate constitute the standard method of evaluating the presence and severity of UUTO. These examinations can be time-consuming and distressing especially to the child, and are not sensitive or specific enough to identify those kidneys that require treatment in all cases. Additionally, renal scans are expensive and not always available. Therefore, there is a great need for the development of new methods to stratify and monitor patients, and the biomarker research field is a promising approach for this purpose. Urinary as well as serum proteins provide information of the physiological condition in the kidney and have the potential to be used as prognostic tools for early disease detection and the choice of the optimal treatment and monitoring [1]. The present review summarizes the pathophysiology of kidney injury caused by UUTO, the roles played by emerging biomarkers of obstructive nephropathy, the mechanisms involved, and the clinical utility and limitations of the biomarkers.

2. Upper Urinary Tract Obstruction

2.1. UPJO

Congenital obstructive nephropathy reflects maldevelopment of the urinary tract in utero. Most commonly, lesions lie in the ureteropelvic junction (UPJ), causing chronic renal failure. Rapid diagnosis and treatment are essential to preserving function and slowing renal damage. The prevalence is one in 1500 live births [2]. Although UPJO is less common in adults, the condition is not rare [3]. In addition to having a congenital cause, acquired stenosis of the UPJ may follow an upper urinary tract infection, the development of stones, trauma, or ischemia. Vessels that compress or distort the UPJ when crossing the urinary tract may obstruct ureteral outflow in adults.

2.2. Ureteral Calculi

Urinary tract stones are very common. The prevalence is 1–19.1% in Asia, 5–9% in Europe, and 7–13% in North America [4,5]. Although most small stones pass spontaneously, some do not, causing UUTO with or without infection. Surgical intervention (shock wave or ureteroscopic lithotripsy) is required to prevent the impairment of renal function [6]. Even after stones are removed, some patients develop ureteral strictures that may continue to impair renal function.

2.3. Ureteral Strictures

A ureteral stricture is a narrowing of the ureter that causes an obstruction. Strictures cause significant morbidity and mortality from renal failure. Benign strictures are typically caused by ischemia or inflammation. Causes include radiation, trauma associated with calculus impaction, pelvic surgery, and ureteroscopy [7]. Moderate to severe strictures require surgical intervention, such as balloon dilation, endoureterotomy, or stricture resection.

2.4. Malignant Ureteral Obstruction

A malignant ureteral obstruction develops secondary to a malignant tumor. A primary tumor may infiltrate the ureteral wall and compress the ureter, swollen lymph nodes may wrap around the ureter, edema and retroperitoneal fibrosis that develop after radiotherapy may distort the ureter or cause luminal stenosis, or ureter elasticity may be weakened [8]. The condition may be unilateral or bilateral. Clinical removal of the obstruction and rapid improvement in renal function are the aims of treatment. Although ureteral stenting or nephrostomy is performed in severe cases, these procedures reduce the quality of life. Markers of severity are required.

3. The Pathophysiology of Kidney Injury Caused by UUTO (Figure 1)

Urinary tract obstruction affects renal function in many ways. The increase in intratubular hydrostatic pressure [9] triggers renopathogenic effects via three proposed mechanisms: tubular ischemia caused by hypoperfusion, pressure-induced mechanical stretching or compression of tubular cells, and altered urinary shear stress. The latter two mechanisms are likely the primary causes of obstructive renal injury [10], being associated with the dysregulation of many cytokines, growth factors, enzymes, and cytoskeletal proteins. Changes in early renal hemodynamics are followed by structural and functional changes in the entire nephron. The earliest stage of UUTO is associated with an increase in renal blood flow 1–2 h in duration [10]. The intrarenal renin–angiotensin–aldosterone system is then activated, which causes pre- and post-glomerular vasoconstriction and resultant drops in renal blood flow, medullary oxygen tension, and the glomerular filtration rate [11,12]. The increased intra-renal angiotensin II activates nuclear factor kappa B, triggering cytokine release and reactive oxygen species (ROS) production [2,10,13,14]. Adhesion molecules such as selectins attract infiltrating macrophages, monocyte chemotactic protein-1 (MCP-1) is upregulated, and tumor necrosis factor-α (TNF-α) is released. Monocytes and macrophages are attracted to the tubular interstitium of the UUTO kidney [2,14,15]. Activated macrophages infiltrate the interstitium, sustaining the inflammatory response by releasing cytokines such as transforming growth factor-β1 (TGF-β1) and TNF-α and ROS [16]. ROS mediate the profibrotic action of TGF-β1, and renal fibrosis proceeds via the epithelial–mesenchymal transition (EMT) of renal tubular epithelial cells. The outcome is interstitial fibrosis caused by increased deposition of the extracellular matrix, cellular infiltration, tubular apoptosis, and the EMT [17]. The mechanical stretching of tubular cells, ischemia, and oxidative stress that follow ureteral obstruction cause tubular cell death [18,19]. Mild injury triggers apoptosis, while tubulointerstitial atrophy after obstruction causes cell deletion. The apoptotic bodies are phagocytosed by neighboring tubular cells or directly shed into the tubular lumen, reestablishing homeostasis. When the injury is severe, necrosis is likely to be the predominant cause of cell loss [19,20]. Increased apoptosis and/or necrosis activates cell infiltration, interstitial cell proliferation, and interstitial fibrosis (Figure 1).

Hydrostatic pressure stretches tubular cells and creates urinary shear stress, inducing intrarenal angiotensin II activation followed by the release of cytokines and adhesion molecules, in turn triggering macrophage infiltration, the production of reactive oxygen species (ROS), and decreased renal blood flow (RBF). The drop in RBF triggers renal ischemia, and the increase of hydrostatic pressure and ROS causes tubular cell death. Monocyte chemotactic protein-1 (MCP-1), tumor necrosis factor-α (TNF-α) and transforming growth factor-β1 (TGF-β1) released from activated macrophages, ROS, and/or tubular cell death induce the epithelial–mesenchymal transition (EMT) and fibroblast proliferation. Eventually the renal parenchyma is transformed into fibrotic tissue.

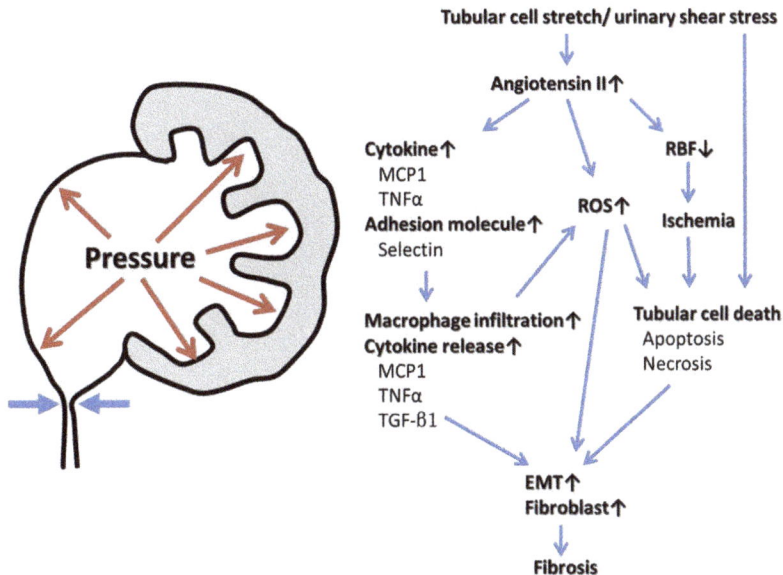

Figure 1. Mechanisms of UUTO causing kidney injury and fibrosis.

4. Imaging Studies and Their Limitations

Technetium 99m (^{99m}Tc) mertiatide, ^{99m}Tc diethylene triamine penta-acetic acid, or ^{99m}Tc dimercaptosuccinic acid renal scans (with or without diuresis) are commonly used to evaluate the presence and severity of UUTO in patients with hydronephrosis. Patients are divided into those with no, partial, or complete obstruction and with or without renal function [21–23]. Urgent surgical relief of complete obstruction is essential, otherwise the kidney will rapidly become nonfunctional. A partial obstruction is a resistance to outflow that, if left untreated, will lead to a loss of kidney function. If renal function is lost, surgery is not considered unless the kidney may be infected. Although renal scans are the standard method of evaluating the presence and severity of UUTO, they are expensive and expose patients to radiation, and repeat scans should be avoided. Furthermore, they do not reveal kidney damage per se, and the equipment is not widely available.

5. Biomarkers of UUTO

Urinary and serum biomarkers facilitate the evaluation of renal damage in UUTO patients. An ideal biomarker is assessed noninvasively in a simple manner, is highly sensitive and specific in terms of early detection, and exhibits a wide dynamic range and cutoff values, allowing for risk stratification. Diagnostic utility improves when pelvic urine samples (compared to bladder urine) are used [23,24]. However, the collection of renal pelvic urine is invasive, requiring the placement of an indwelling ureteral catheter via cystoscopy under X-ray guidance, and thus it is difficult to repeatedly collect renal pelvic urine. Biomarkers of kidney injury evaluate glomerular function and renal tubular damage. Serum creatinine (SCr) and cystatin C are representative glomerular function biomarkers. Levels of neutrophil gelatinase-associated lipocalin (NGAL), MCP-1, kidney injury molecule 1 (KIM-1), N-acetyl-b-D-glucosaminidase (NAG), and liver type fatty acid-binding protein (L-FABP) are used to evaluate proximal tubule damage.

5.1. Biomarkers of Glomerular Function

5.1.1. SCr

SCr concentrations are widely used to assess kidney function. However, accumulating evidence indicates that measurements of SCr levels do not always detect kidney disease early, and individual variability in SCr generation rates limits the utility of these tests in terms of identifying and assessing the severity of kidney injury [25]. Furthermore, UUTO often affects the unilateral upper urinary tract. The contralateral kidney can compensate for the loss of renal function.

5.1.2. Cystatin C

Cystatin C is an endogenous cysteine protease inhibitor of molecular weight 13.3 kDa secreted by most nucleated cells [26]. It is an ideal filtration marker, being produced at a stable rate, freely filtered without tubular secretion, and completely catabolized in the proximal tubule [27]. Cystatin C is distributed only in the extracellular space and thus reflects changes in the glomerular filtration rate more precisely than creatinine, which is distributed in all body water [28]. In one study, the serum cystatin C level strongly predicted all-cause acute kidney injury (AKI). The area under the curve (AUC; the receiver operating characteristic curve [ROC]) was 0.89 [29]. Use of the urine cystatin C level for early detection of AKI after cardiac surgery allows for the diagnosis of tubular damage and dysfunction [30]. Serum cystatin C is a useful biomarker for AKI in patients in the intensive care unit (ICU) [31,32] with contrast-induced AKI [29,33]. In one study, preoperative serum cystatin C levels were significantly higher in children with UPJO compared to controls and decreased after surgery (Table 1) [26], and the AUC-ROC value of serum cystatin C indicating UPJO was 0.72 (Table 1) [26,34]. In another study, serum cystatin C levels increased in adults with ureteral calculi as hydronephrosis increased and differed significantly between patients with no and mild hydronephrosis, while SCr levels did not [35]. Multivariate logistic regression showed that only the serum cystatin C level was an independent risk factor for hydronephrosis. By contrast, the urine cystatin C level is less useful as a UUTO biomarker. In two independent studies of children with UUTO, urine cystatin C levels did not differ between patients and controls (Table 1) [24,36].

Table 1. Urinary and serum biomarkers for pediatric and adults UUTO.

Biomarkers		Author, Ref.	Publish Year	Disease	Pts Number	Mean or Median Age of Pts	Laterality of Affected Kidneys	Source of Samples	Comparison of Values, p-Value	AUC-ROC	Comparison of Group
Urinary NGAL	Ped	Pavlaki A, 26	2020	UPJO	22 Obst, 19 Non-obst, 17Cts	3.0 months	Uni	Bl	0.01, Obst vs. Cts	0.61	Obst + Non-obst vs. Cts
		Kostic D, 34	2019	HN	37 Obst, 45 Cts	5.0 months	Uni + Bi	Bl	NA	0.80	Obst vs. Cts
		Yu L, 46	2019	UPJO	17 Pts, 17 Cts	NA	Uni + Bi	Bl	0.0004, Pts vs. Cts	0.90	Pts vs. Cts
		Bienias B, 45	2018	UPJO	28 Obst, 17 Non-obst, 21 Cts	11 years	Uni	Bl	<0.05, Obst vs. Cts	0.66	Obst vs. Cts
		Gupta S, 47	2018	UPJO	30 Pts, 15 Cts	4.7 years	Uni	Bl	0.0009, Pts vs. Cts	0.80	Pts vs. Cts
		Karakus S, 36	2016	UPJO	13 Obst, 14 Non-obst, 9 Cts	3.9 years	Uni	Bl	0.032, Obst vs. Cts	0.85	Obst vs. Cts
		Noyan A, 48	2015	UPJO	26 Pts, 36 Non-obst, 20 Cts	21 months	NA	Bl	<0.05, Obst vs. Cts	0.68	Obst vs. Cts
		Madsen MG, 24	2013	UPJO	24 Pts, 13 Cts	6.5 years	Uni	Rp	NS, Pts vs. Cts	NA	NA
								Bl	<0.05, Pts vs. Cts	NA	NA
		Wasilewska A, 49	2011	UPJO	20 Obst, 20 Non-obst, 25 Cts	2.2 years	Uni	Bl	<0.01, Obst vs. Cts	0.81	Obst vs. Cts
								Rp	<0.01, Obst vs. Cts	NA	NA
	Adul	Washino S, 23	2019	UUTO	28 Pts, 21 Cts	54 years	Uni	Bl	<0.05, Pts vs. Cts	0.70	Pts vs. Cts
		Olvera-Posada D, 51	2017	HN	24 Obst 20 Non-obst, 11Cts	58.5 years	Uni	Rp	<0.01, Pts vs. Cts	0.76	Pts vs. Cts
		Urbschat A, 50	2014	Ureteral calculi	53 Pts, 52 Cts	44 years	Uni	Bl	0.009, Obst vs. Cts	NA	NA
								Bl	<0.05, Obst vs. Cts	NA	NA
Urinary MCP-1	Ped	Yu L, 46	2019	UPJO	17 Pts, 17 Cts	NA	Uni + Bi	Bl	0.0005, Pts vs. Cts	0.89	Pts vs. Cts
		Karakus S, 36	2016	UPJO	13 Obst, 14 Non-obst, 9 Cts	3.9 years	Uni	Bl	0.002, Obst vs. Cts	0.93	Obst + Non-obst vs. Ct
		Mohammadjafari H, 68	2014	HN	24 Obst, 18 Non-obst	6.5 years	Uni + Bi	Bl	0.012, Obst vs. Cts	0.73	Obst vs. Non obst
		Madsen MG, 24	2013	UPJO	28 Pts, 13 Cts	6.5 Years	Uni	Bl	<0.05, Pts vs. Cts	0.78	Pts vs. Cts
								Rp	<0.05, Pts vs. Cts	0.89	Pts vs. Cts
		Taranta-Janusz K, 69	2012	HN	15 Obst, 21 Non-obst, 19 Cts	0.25 years	Uni	Bl	<0.05, Obst vs. Cts	0.70	Pts vs. Cts
		Bartoli F, 70	2011	UPJO	12 Obst, 36 Non-obst, 30 Cts	NA	NA	Rp	<0.01, Obst vs. Cts	NA	NA
		Grandaliano G, 59	2000	UPJO	24 Pts, 15 Cts	NA	NA	Bl	<0.001, Obst vs. Cts	NA	NA
								Bl	<0.01, Pts vs. Cts	NA	NA
Urinary KIM-1	Ped	Kostic D, 34	2019	HN	37 Obst vs. 45 Cts	5.0 months	Uni + Bi	Bl	NA	0.70	Obst vs. Cts
		Bienias B, 45	2018	UPJO	28 Obst, 17 Non-obst, 21 Cts	11 years	Uni	Bl	<0.05, Obst vs. Cts	0.65	Obst vs. Cts
		Karakus S, 36	2016	UPJO	13 Obstr, 14 Non-obst, 9 Cts	3.9 years	Uni	Bl	0.001, Obst vs. Cts	0.89	Obst + Non-obst vs. Ct
		Noyan A, 48	2015	UPJO	26 Pts, 36 Non-obst, 20 Cts	21 months	NA	Bl	NS, Obst vs. Cts	NA	Obst vs. Cts
		Wasilewska A, 49	2011	UPJO	20 Obst, 20 Non-obst, 25 Cts	2.2 years	Uni	Bl	<0.01, Obst vs. Cts	0.80	Obst + Non-obst vs. Ct
								Rp	<0.01, Obst vs. Cts	NA	NA
	Adul	Washino S, 23	2019	HN	28 Pts, 21 Cts	54 years	Uni	Bl	NS, Pts vs. Cts	0.57	NA
								Rp	<0.01, Pts vs. Cts	0.88	NA
		Olvera-Posada D, 51	2017	HN	24 Obst 20 Non-obst, 11Cts	58.5 years	Uni	Bl	0.02, Obst vs. Cts	0.73	Obst vs. Cts
		Urbschat A, 50	2014	Ureteral calculi	53 Pts, 52 Cts	44 years	Uni	Bl	NS, Pts vs. Cts	NA	NA

Table 1. Cont.

Biomarkers		Author, Ref.	Publish Year	Disease	Pts Number	Mean or Median Age of Pts	Laterality of Affected Kidneys	Source of Samples	Comparison of Values, p-Value	AUC-ROC	Comparison of Group
Urinary NAG	Ped	Skalova S, 84	2007	HN	31 Pts, 262 reference Cts	2.3 years	Uni + Bi	Bl	0.002, Pts vs. Cts	NA	NA
		Mohammadjafari H, 68	2014	HN	24 Obst, 18 Non-obst	6.5 years	Uni + Bi	Bl	NS, Obst vs. Non-obst	0.67	Obst vs. Non-obst
	Adul	Washino S, 23	2019	HN	28 Pts, 21 Cts	54 years	Uni	Bl	<0.01, Pts vs. Cts	0.74	Pts vs. Cts
								Rp	<0.001 Pts vs. Cts	0.91	Pts vs. Cts
Urinary L-FABP	Ped	Noyan A, 48	2015	UPJO	26 Pts, 36 Non-obst, 20 Cts	21 months	NA	Bl	NS, Obst vs. Cts	NA	NA
Urinary Vanin-1	Adul	Washino S, 23	2019	HN	28 Pts, 21 Cts	54 years	Uni	Bl	<0.05, Pts vs. Cts	0.63	Pts vs. Cts
								Rp	<0.0001, Pts vs. Cts	0.98	Pts vs. Cts
Urinary α-GST	Ped	Bienias B, 45	2018	UPJO	28 Obst, 17 Non-obst, 21 Cts	11 years	Uni	Bl	<0.05, Obst vs. Cts	0.90	Obst vs. Cts
Urinary CyC	Ped	Kostic D, 34	2019	HN	37 Obst vs. 45 Cts	5.0 months	Uni + Bi	Bl	NA	0.71	Obst vs. Cts
		Karakus S, 36	2016	UPJO	13 Obst, 14 Non-obst, 9 Cts	3.9 years	Uni	Bl	NS, Obst vs. Cts	NA	NA
		Madsen MG, 24	2012	UPJO	24 Pts, 13 Cts	8.0 years	Uni	Bl	NS, Pts vs. Cts	NA	NA
								Rp	NS, Pts vs. Cts	NA	NA
Serum NGAL	Ped	Bienias B, 45	2018	UPJO	28 Obst, 17 Non-obst, 21 Cts	11 years	Uni	S	<0.05, Obst vs. Cts	1.00	Obst vs. Cts
	Adul	Urbschat A, 50	2014	Ureteral calculi	53 Pts, 52 Cts	44 years	Uni	S	<0.01, Pts vs. Cts	NA	NA
Serum CyC	Ped	Pavlaki A, 26	2020	UPJO	22 Obst, 19 Non-obst, 17Cts	3 months	Uni	S	0.01, Obst vs. Cts	0.72	Obst + Non-obst vs. Cts
		Kostic D, 34	2019	HN	37 Obst vs. 45 Cts	5.0 months	Uni + Bi	S	NA	0.72	Obst vs. Cts
	Adul	Mao W, 35	2020	Ureteral calculi	160 HN, 40 Non-HN	52 years	Uni	S	<0.001, HN vs. Non-HN	0.66	HN vs. Non-HN

Abbreviation: NGAL: neutrophil gelatinase-associated lipocalin; MCP-1: monocyte chemotactic protein-1; KIM-1: kidney injury molecule 1; NAG: N-acetyl-b-D-glucosaminidase; L-FABP: liver type fatty acid-binding protein; α-GST: α-glutathione S-transferases; CyC: Cystatin C. Ped: pediatrics; Adul: adults; UPJO: ureteropelvic junction obstruction; HN: hydronpehrosis; Pts: patients; Obst: patients with obstructive hydronephrosis; Non-obst: patients with non-obstructive hydronephrosis; Cts: controls; NA: not assessed; Uni: unilateral; Bi: bilateral; Bl: bladder; Rp: renal pelvis; S: serum; NS: not significant; AUC-ROC: area under curve in receiver operating characteristics.

5.2. Biomarkers of Renal Tubular Damage

5.2.1. NGAL

Human NGAL, a ubiquitous 25 kDa protein, was initially isolated from human neutrophils [37]. NGAL is expressed in small amounts in cells other than neutrophils, including lung, spleen, and kidney cells, and is thought to inhibit bacterial growth, scavenge iron, and induce epithelial growth [38]. NGAL can be secreted by epithelial cells, and it is markedly elevated in patients exhibiting an inflammatory immune response and defects in lipid metabolism, intracellular iron transport, renal tubular repair, or differentiation of kidney progenitor cells into tubular epithelial cells [39]. In the kidney, NGAL is secreted into the urine from the ascending limb of the loop of Henle to the collecting ducts, being synthesized in the distal nephron [40]. NGAL is small, freely filtered, and easily assayed in urine. The urine NGAL level is an early and sensitive biomarker of kidney injury [41]. The serum or urine NGAL level is a clinically useful biomarker of various types of AKI, including AKI after kidney transplantation [42], contrast medium-induced AKI [43], and AKI in critical care settings [44]. In children with UUTO, urine NGAL levels are significantly higher in bladder urine and/or renal pelvic urine compared to controls, correlate inversely with worsening obstruction, and decrease after surgery (Table 1) [26,36,45–49]. The AUC-ROC value for UUTO in children is 0.61–0.90 for bladder urine NGAL [26,36,45–48]. In adults with UUTO, the urine NGAL level increases in those with obstructive nephropathy (AUC-ROCs of 0.70 for bladder urine and 0.76 for renal pelvic urine) and decreases after relief of the obstruction [23,50,51]. Serum NGAL levels are significantly higher than in controls [45,50]. However, the use of NGAL as a biomarker of kidney injury induced by UUTO has several limitations. Age affects the predictive performance: NGAL better predicts AKI in children than in adults [52]. Serum and urine NGAL levels may be influenced by conditions other than UUTO, including chronic hypertension, systemic infection, inflammation, anemia, hypoxia, or malignancy [53–55]. The many sources of NGAL can render it difficult to identify the underlying pathology [40].

5.2.2. MCP-1

MCP-1, a 13 kDa protein, is a potent attractant of monocytes and a member of the CC subfamily [56]. It is produced by many types of cells, including epithelial, endothelial, and smooth muscle cells; fibroblasts, astrocytes, and monocytes; and microglial cells. MCP-1 recruits monocytes, memory T-cells, and dendritic cells to sites of tissue injury and infection; monocytes and macrophages are the major sources of MCP-1 [57]. MCP-1 mRNA is undetectable in the normal kidney, but MCP-1 gene expression is markedly increased at the tubulointerstitial level in UPJO biopsy samples and correlates with the extent of monocyte infiltration [58,59]. In one experimental study, mice deficient in MCP-1 exhibited significantly decreased survival and increased renal damage after ischemia/reperfusion-induced renal tubular injury in the absence of macrophage accumulation [60]. Kidneys and primary tubular epithelial cells from such mice exhibited increased apoptosis after ischemia, which indicates that MCP-1 protects the kidney from the acute inflammatory response that develops after kidney injury. MCP-1 is one of the most promising biomarkers of kidney injury [61]. Elevated MCP-1 levels are associated with immune system-mediated kidney injury [62,63], diabetic nephropathy [64], and autosomal-dominant polycystic kidney disease [65]. In a mouse model of UUTO, serum and urine MCP-1 levels increased significantly compared to those of control mice [66]. mRNA expression and urinary excretion of MCP-1 correlate with the extent of the obstruction, subsequent renal damage, and hydronephrosis. Urine levels of MCP-1 decrease after release of the obstruction [67]. Urine MCP-1 levels are significantly increased in UPJO groups compared to controls and fall significantly after surgery [24,36,46,59,68–70]. The AUC-ROC values in terms of the presence of UUTO are 0.70–0.93 for bladder urine MCP-1 and 0.89 for renal pelvic urine MCP-1 (Table 1) [24,36,46,68,69]. An inverse correlation is evident between the level of MCP-1 in renal pelvic urine and mertiatide clearance by the affected kidney [59,69]. Urine MCP-1 levels usefully distinguish between UPJO (which requires pyeloplasty) and the absence of an obstructive dilation of the renal pelvis. They can be used to monitor the resolution of kidney damage after surgery for UUTO [36]. Serum MCP-1 levels increase in patients with AKI after cardiac surgery and in those with chronic kidney damage [60,71,72], but no study has yet evaluated the serum MCP-1 level as a biomarker of UUTO in a clinical setting.

5.2.3. KIM-1

KIM-1 is a type I membrane protein of 104 kDa composed of a 14 kDa membrane-bound fragment and a 90 kDa soluble portion [73]. It was isolated from T-cells, exhibits various functions, and was termed T-cell immunoglobulin-and-mucin-domain-containing molecule-1 (TIM-1) [73]. Normal kidney tissue rarely expresses KIM-1, but kidneys acutely injured by ischemia, hypoxia, toxicity, or renal tubular interstitial/polycystic kidney disease do [74]. The ectodomain of KIM-1 (90 kD) is cleaved by matrix metalloproteinases and is found in urine after injury to the kidney proximal tubules [75]. Acute KIM-1 overexpression in proximal, renal tubular epithelial cells after ischemia, hypoxia, or toxicity promotes the transformation of these cells into semi-professional phagocytic cells. KIM-1 is a phosphatidylserine receptor of the liposome surface and identifies both apoptotic bodies and phosphatidylserine, triggering further phagocytosis [74,76]. The upregulation of KIM-1 by injured tubular epithelial cells facilitates the clearance of apoptotic cells, protecting against AKI. Apart from mediating phagocytosis, KIM-1 assists in repairing injury to cells [77]. It is a valuable biomarker of AKI. Urine and/or serum KIM-1 levels increase after ischemic kidney injury [75] and in patients with diabetic nephropathy [78], IgA nephropathy [79], and kidney injury after renal transplantation [80]. In an animal model, serum and urine KIM-1 levels were useful for the early diagnosis of obstructive nephropathy-induced AKI [81,82]. In a mouse model, serum KIM-1 levels increased after UUTO, peaking on day 3, and remained detectable for 14 days [82]. In a rat model, the urine KIM-1 level began to increase on day 1 after UUTO and remained high until day 7 [81]. In children with UUTO, urine KIM1 levels correlated inversely with worsening obstruction and decreased after surgery [34,36,45,48,49]. The AUC-ROC value for the prediction of childhood UUTO is 0.65–0.89 for the bladder urine KIM-1 level (Table 1) [34,36,45,49]. In adults with UUTO, the urine KIM-1 level is a useful marker of obstructive nephropathy (AUCs of 0.57–0.73 for bladder urine and 0.88 for renal pelvic urine) [23,50,51]. Xie found that the urine KIM-1 level after surgery to treat UUTO predicted renal function deterioration [83].

5.2.4. NAG

NAG, a 130–140 kDa protein, is a lysosomal enzyme distributed in various human tissue [84]. NAG is not filtered through the glomeruli. In the kidney, it is found predominantly in lysosomes of proximal tubular cells. The small amount of NAG normally present in the urine is exocytosed by these cells. Although the function of NAG in the kidney remains unknown, it is a marker of tubular cell function or damage [85]. Increased NAG excretion in urine is caused exclusively by proximal tubular cell injury. Accumulating evidence indicates that urine NAG levels correlate with exposure to nephrotoxic drugs, delayed allograft nephropathy, diabetic nephropathy, and AKI [85]. Urine NAG levels are elevated in patients with upper urinary tract infection, nephrolithiasis, and reflux nephropathy [86,87]. In children with UUTO, urine NAG levels were significantly higher in those with hydronephrosis (with or without a vesicoureteral reflux) than healthy controls or cystitis patients [88,89]. The NAG level in renal pelvic urine is 7-fold higher and that in bladder urine 1.7-fold higher than in normal controls [89]. Mohammad found that the AUC-ROC value for bladder NAG was 0.67 in children with UUTO [68]. Skalova reported that although the urine NAG level was significantly higher in patients with hydronephrosis compared to healthy controls, there were no differences between children with unilateral and bilateral hydronephrosis and no correlation between the urine NAG level and the grade of hydronephrosis [90]. In summary, urine NAG levels usefully detect childhood UUTO but do not reflect its severity. In one study of adults with UUTO, levels of NAG in bladder and renal pelvic urine were 2.5- and five-fold higher than those of normal controls (AUC-ROC values of 0.74 for bladder urine and 0.91 for renal pelvic urine) and decreased after treatment [23].

5.2.5. L-FABP

L-FABP, which is expressed by both the normal and diseased human kidney, has been found in both the convoluted and straight portions of human proximal tubules [91]. Mammalian intracellular FABP is a 14 kDa protein encoded by a member of a large multigene family within a superfamily of lipid-binding proteins [92]. Nine tissue-specific FABPs have been identified: L (liver), I (intestinal), H (muscle and heart), A (adipocyte), E (epidermal), IL (ileal), B (brain), M (myelin), and T (testis). All FABPs primarily regulate fatty acid metabolism and intracellular transport [93]. L-FABP is expressed not only in the liver but also in the intestine, pancreas, stomach, lung, and kidney [94]. Serum and/or urine L-FABP levels are useful biomarkers of kidney injury after renal transplantation [95], in critical care patients with AKI [96], and in those with contrast-induced AKI [97] and diabetic nephropathy [98]. However, the utility of L-FABP for predicting UUTO remains controversial. Xie found that urine L-FABP levels after UUTO surgery predicted the deterioration of renal function [83]. Furthermore, in one study of patients with vesicoureteral refluxes, the urine L-FABP level was significantly higher than in controls [99]. However, Noyan found that urine L-FABP levels did not differ significantly between children with hydronephrosis and controls [48].

5.3. Novel Biomarkers of UUTO

5.3.1. Vanin-1

Vanin-1, a 53 kDa protein, is expressed in the brush borders of the proximal tubule of the kidney [100]. By catabolizing panteheine to cysteamine and pantothenic acid (a precursor of coenzymes), it has roles in metabolism and energy production. The function of kidney vanin-1 remains to be established. However, the fact that vanin-1 is located specifically in the brush borders suggests that the enzyme plays a pivotal role in pantothenic acid salvage and recycling. The proximal tubular cells bear microvilli with large apical surface areas within which many transporters and channels are found [101]. Vanin-1 in cellular membranes is anchored to glycosylphosphatidylinositol. The anchor may be cleaved and soluble vanin-1 then secreted or released into the extracellular matrix in response to various stimuli [102].

Urine vanin-1 levels are increased in patients with drug-induced AKI [103] and UUTO [23], and in rat models with high salt-induced kidney damage [104], diabetic nephropathy [105], and UUTO [102]. UUTO inhibits urine flow and increases intratubular pressure, causing renal tubular damage. Vanin-1 is then secreted into the urine by renal tubular cells. The level of vanin-1 in renal pelvic urine correlates highly with the severity of urinary tract obstruction [23]. The level of vanin-1 in renal pelvic urine is highly predictive (AUC-ROC value 0.98) of adult UUTO, more predictive than NGAL, KIM-1, or NAG levels. Vanin-1 levels decrease following UUTO relief in patients with moderate to severe UUTO [23].

5.3.2. α-Glutathione S-Transferase (GST)

GST, a 28 kDa protein, is a cytosolic enzyme. The isoforms α and π (α-GST, π-GST) are typical of the human kidney [106]. α-GST is expressed in proximal tubular epithelial cells, and π-GST is expressed in distal tubular epithelial cells [45]. Both isoforms of GST are released from injured cells into the urine and were recently suggested to be promising biomarkers of kidney injury [107] in the context of cyclosporine-induced nephrotoxicity, cadmium exposure, administration of nephrotoxic antibiotics, acute transplant rejection [106], and critical illness in the ICU [106,108]. Recently, the utility of the α-GST and π-GST level in terms of predicting UUTO was explored. Children with UPJO exhibited significantly higher urinary α-GST excretion than controls. Urinary AUC-ROC values for UUTO detection were 0.90 for α-GST and 0.3 for π-GST. The predictive performance of α-GST was superior to that of urinary NGAL or KIM-1 [45].

5.3.3. Tissue inhibitor of metalloproteinases-2 (TIMP-2)/ insulin-like growth factor-binding protein 7 (IGFBP7)

TIMP-2 and IGFBP7 are new AKI biomarkers. In 2014, Food and Drug Administration approved TIMP-2/ IGFBP7 to be used in ICU patients to predict the risk of developing moderate to severe AKI [109]. TIMP-2 has a molecular weight of approximately 24 kDa and IGFBP7 has a molecular mass of 29 kDa [110]. Both of them are expressed and secreted by renal tubular cells, and involved in G1 cell cycle arrest during the early phases of cellular stress or injury caused by various insults (e.g., sepsis, ischemia, oxidative stress, and toxins) [111]. TIMP-2/ IGFBP7 shows the best accuracy among AKI biomarkers in patients with various types of AKI condition including AKI after kidney transplantation and AKI in critical care settings, sepsis and platinum-based chemotherapy, and chronic kidney damage induced by diabetes mellitus and congestive heart failure [112,113]. However, no study has yet evaluated the TIMP-2/ IGFBP7 as a biomarker of UUTO in an animal study or a clinical setting, and therefore it is urgently necessary.

5.4. Comparison of Biomarkers

Several studies have compared the utility of NAGL, KIM-1, and/or L-FABP levels as biomarkers of childhood UUTO. In studies, urine and/or serum NAGL levels outperformed urine KIM-1 or L-FABP levels [48,49]. In one study, striking increases in serum and urine NGAL levels were evident in patients with obstructive nephropathy, whereas urine KIM-1 levels did not differ significantly between patients and controls, which suggests that KIM-1 is not sensitive in this setting [50]. In another study, urine NGAL levels were significantly higher in patients with both hydronephrosis and obstruction than in those with hydronephrosis but no obstruction or normal controls. Urine KIM-1 and L-FABP levels did not differ significantly among the groups [48]. Patients with renal colic who also exhibited hydronephrosis had significantly higher urine NAG and NGAL, but not KIM-1, levels than did patients without hydronephrosis [114]. In a mouse model of ischemia/reperfusion kidney injury, serum and urine KIM-1 levels increased during the acute phase and declined gradually in the chronic phase, while serum and urine NGAL levels increased continuously during the transition from AKI to chronic kidney disease, which suggests that NGAL is a valuable biomarker in this setting [41]. This may explain why NGAL is a better biomarker of UUTO than KIM-1. However, one predictive model of worsening kidney function after surgery found that urine KIM-1 and L-FABP levels more reliably predicted kidney deterioration after surgical removal of ureteral stones than did urine NGAL levels [83].

MCP-1 is one of the best biomarkers of childhood UUTO. In one study, urine MCP-1 levels were significantly higher in a pyeloplasty group than a non-obstruction group, while urine NGAL and KIM-1 levels did not differ significantly between the groups [36]. In another study, urine MCP-1 levels were significantly higher in patients with hydronephrosis who required surgery than in those who did not; urine NAG levels did not differ significantly between the groups [68]. In one study, the AUC-ROC values of bladder urine MCP-1 and NGAL in children with UPJO were 0.89 and 0.90, respectively, higher than those of bladder urine interleukin-6 (0.78) or TGF-β1 (0.67) [46].

5.5. Panel Assessment of Biomarkers

No single biomarker is specific for UUTO, and given the multifactorial nature of obstruction, not all obstructions can be identified using a single biomarker [24]. In children with UPJO, combined NGAL/MCP-1 assessment improved diagnostic performance compared to assessment of either biomarker alone [46]. In another study on such children, the AUC-ROC values were 0.63 for SCr, 0.72 for serum cystatin C, 0.80 for urinary NGAL, 0.70 for urinary KIM-1, and 0.70 for urinary cystatin C. The AUC-ROCs of combinations of these biomarkers were higher than those of the single biomarkers, being highest (0.88) for urinary NGAL + urinary cystatin C + serum cystatin C [34]. In critically ill patients with AKI, a combination of urine NGAL and L-FABP levels, sepsis status, blood lactate level, and stratification using the Acute Physiology and Chronic Health Evaluation score improved AKI predictive performance (AUC-ROC 0.94) compared to NGAL alone (AUC-ROC 0.86) or

L-FABP alone (AUC-ROC 0.84) [43]. In a model predicting worsening kidney function after surgery in UUTO patients, the AUC-ROC of the preoperative combination of urinary biomarkers L-FABP, KIM-1, and NGAL was 0.97, higher than the highest AUC of a single biomarker (0.91 for L-FABP) [83].

6. Current Limitations and Future Directions

Most obstructions of the upper urinary tract are unilateral. Reduced glomerular filtration in the affected kidney and the obstruction per se decreases the amount of any biomarker that reaches the bladder, which explains why the biomarker AUC-ROCs of bladder urine are generally lower than those of renal pelvic urine [23,24]. Combinations of serum and bladder biomarker levels may thus be optimal. However, serum values of biomarkers have been less studied than urine values in UUTO patients. Only serum cystatin C and NGAL levels are clinically useful. Serum markers that are highly predictive of UUTO should be sought. Combinations of serum and urinary biomarkers facilitate the diagnosis of UUTO, risk stratification, clinical decision making, and monitoring.

Age affects the predictive performance of biomarkers [52]. Acute and/or chronic kidney injury is a condition frequently found in elderly population with comorbidities, which may alter the value of biomarkers. This would be the reason why NGAL better predicts AKI in children than in adults [52].

Both urinary and serum UUTO biomarkers lack specificity. Increases may be associated with conditions other than UUTO or even non-kidney conditions. Increases in MCP-1 are associated with liver cirrhosis [115] and sleep apnea syndrome [116], increases in NGAL are associated with cardiovascular ischemia, heart failure, atherosclerosis, and pneumonia [117,118], and increases in L-FABP are associated with various liver diseases [119,120]. However, panel assessment may compensate for the lack of specificity.

7. Conclusions

Renal scans are standard in evaluations of the presence and severity of UUTO, but they are expensive, are not always available, and expose patients to radiation. Many urinary and serum biomarkers have been studied in children and adults with UUTO. MCP-1 and NGAL, the most extensively studied, are the most likely to be optimal. Recently, novel biomarkers (vanin-1 and α-GST) have outperformed traditional biomarkers in terms of evaluating UUTO, but further work must explore whether this is the case in all UUTO settings. No single biomarker is adequately sensitive or specific. Panel assessment affords mutual biomarker compensation and improves predictive performance. The obstruction per se and reduced glomerular filtration in the affected kidney decrease the amount of any biomarker reaching the bladder, limiting the performance of bladder urine biomarkers. However, combinations of serum and bladder urinary biomarkers improve performance. Panel assessment of urinary and serum biomarkers facilitates the diagnosis of UUTO, risk stratification, clinical decision making, and monitoring.

Author Contributions: Development of the idea: S.W. Review and Editing: S.W. and K.H. Supervision: T.M. All authors have read and agreed to the published version of the manuscript.

Funding: This research received no external funding.

Conflicts of Interest: The authors declare no conflict of interest.

Abbreviations

AKI	Acute kidney injury
AUC	Area under curve
GST	Glutathione S-transferases
IGFBP7	Insulin-like growth factor-binding protein 7
KIM-1	Kidney injury molecule 1
L-FABP	Liver type fatty acid-binding protein
MCP-1	Monocyte chemotactic protein-1
NAG	N-acetyl-b-D-glucosaminidase

NGAL	Neutrophil gelatinase-associated lipocalin
ROC	Receiver operating characteristic
ROS	Reactive oxygen species
SCr	Serum creatinine
TNF-α	Tumor necrosis factor-α
TIMP-2	Tissue inhibitor of metalloproteinases-2
TGF-β1	Transforming growth factor-β1
UPJ	Ureteropelvic junction
UPJO	Ureteropelvic junction obstruction
UUTO	Upper urinary tract obstruction

References

1. Mesrobian, H.-G.O.; Mitchell, M.E.; See, W.A.; Halligan, B.D.; Carlson, B.E.; Greene, A.S.; Wakim, B.T. Candidate Urinary Biomarker Discovery in Ureteropelvic Junction Obstruction: A Proteomic Approach. *J. Urol.* **2010**, *184*, 709–714. [CrossRef] [PubMed]
2. Chevalier, R.L.; Thornhill, B.A.; Forbes, M.S.; Kiley, S.C. Mechanisms of renal injury and progression of renal disease in congenital obstructive nephropathy. *Pediatr. Nephrol.* **2009**, *25*, 687–697. [CrossRef] [PubMed]
3. Grasso, M.; Caruso, R.P.; Phillips, C.K. UPJ Obstruction in the Adult Population: Are Crossing Vessels Significant? *Rev. Urol.* **2001**, *3*, 42–51. [PubMed]
4. Liu, Y.; Chen, Y.; Liao, B.; Luo, D.; Wang, K.-J.; Li, H.; Zeng, G. Epidemiology of urolithiasis in Asia. *Asian J. Urol.* **2018**, *5*, 205–214. [CrossRef]
5. Sorokin, I.; Mamoulakis, C.; Miyazawa, K.; Rodgers, A.; Talati, J.; Lotan, Y. Epidemiology of stone disease across the world. *World J. Urol.* **2017**, *35*, 1301–1320. [CrossRef]
6. Türk, C.; Neisius, A.; Petrik, A.; Seitz, C.; Skolarikos, A.; Thomas, K. EAU Guideline for Urolithiasis 2020. Available online: https://uroweb.org/guideline/urolithiasis/ (accessed on 15 June 2020).
7. Tran, H.; Arsovska, O.; Paterson, R.F.; Chew, B.H. Evaluation of risk factors and treatment options in patients with ureteral stricture disease at a single institution. *Can. Urol. Assoc. J.* **2015**, *9*, 921–924. [CrossRef]
8. Chen, Y.; Liu, C.-Y.; Zhang, Z.-H.; Xu, P.-C.; Chen, D.-G.; Fan, X.-H.; Ma, J.-C.; Xu, Y.-P. Malignant ureteral obstruction: Experience and comparative analysis of metallic versus ordinary polymer ureteral stents. *World J. Surg. Oncol.* **2019**, *17*, 74. [CrossRef]
9. Chevalier, R.L. Chronic Partial Ureteral Obstruction in the Neonatal Guinea Pig. II. Pressure Gradients Affecting Glomerular Filtration Rate. *Pediatr. Res.* **1984**, *18*, 1271–1277. [CrossRef]
10. Klein, J.; Gonzalez, J.; Miravete, M.; Caubet, C.; Chaaya, R.; Decramer, S.; Bandin, F.; Bascands, J.L.; Buffin-Meyer, B.; Schanstra, J.P. Congenital ureteropelvic junction obstruction: Human disease and animal models. *Int. J. Exp. Pathol.* **2010**, *92*, 168–192. [CrossRef]
11. Cachat, F.; Lange-Sperandio, B.; Chang, A.Y.; Kiley, S.C.; Thornhill, B.A.; Forbes, M.S.; Chevalier, R.L. Ureteral obstruction in neonatal mice elicits segment-specific tubular cell responses leading to nephron loss11See Editorial by Woolf, p. 761. *Kidney Int.* **2003**, *63*, 564–575. [CrossRef]
12. Klimova, E.M.; Aparicio-Trejo, O.E.; Tapia, E.; Pedraza-Chaverri, J. Unilateral Ureteral Obstruction as a Model to Investigate Fibrosis-Attenuating Treatments. *Biomolecules* **2019**, *9*, 141. [CrossRef] [PubMed]
13. Ratliff, R.B.; Abdulmahdi, W.; Pawar, R.; Wolin, M.S. Oxidant Mechanisms in Renal Injury and Disease. *Antioxid Redox Signal.* **2016**, *25*, 119–146. [CrossRef] [PubMed]
14. Jackson, L.; Woodward, M.; Coward, R.J. The molecular biology of pelvi-ureteric junction obstruction. *Pediatr. Nephrol.* **2017**, *33*, 553–571. [CrossRef] [PubMed]
15. Lee, W.-C.; Jao, H.-Y.; Hsu, J.-D.; Lee, Y.-R.; Wu, M.-J.; Kao, Y.-L.; Lee, H.-J. Apple polyphenols reduce inflammation response of the kidneys in unilateral ureteral obstruction rats. *J. Funct. Foods* **2014**, *11*, 1–11. [CrossRef]
16. Madsen, M.G. Urinary biomarkers in hydronephrosis. *Dan. Med. J.* **2013**, *60*, B4582. [PubMed]
17. Xia, Z.-E.; Xi, J.-L.; Shi, L. 3,3′-Diindolylmethane ameliorates renal fibrosis through the inhibition of renal fibroblast activation in vivo and in vitro. *Ren. Fail.* **2018**, *40*, 447–454. [CrossRef]

18. Nilsson, L.; Madsen, K.; Krag, S.; Frøkiær, J.; Jensen, B.L.; Nørregaard, R. Disruption of cyclooxygenase type 2 exacerbates apoptosis and renal damage during obstructive nephropathy. *Am. J. Physiol. Physiol.* **2015**, *309*, F1035–F1048. [CrossRef]
19. Mei, W.; Peng, Z.; Tang, D.; Yang, H.; Tao, L.; Lu, M.; Liu, C.; Deng, Z.; Xiao, Y.; Liu, J.; et al. Peroxiredoxin 1 inhibits the oxidative stress induced apoptosis in renal tubulointerstitial fibrosis. *Nephrology* **2015**, *20*, 832–842. [CrossRef]
20. Xu, Y.; Ruan, S.; Wu, X.; Chen, H.; Zheng, K.; Fu, B. Autophagy and apoptosis in tubular cells following unilateral ureteral obstruction are associated with mitochondrial oxidative stress. *Int. J. Mol. Med.* **2013**, *31*, 628–636. [CrossRef]
21. Taylor, A.T. Radionuclides in nephrourology, Part 2: Pitfalls and diagnostic applications. *J. Nucl. Med.* **2014**, *55*, 786–798. [CrossRef]
22. Akbal, C.; Şahan, A.; Garayev, A.; Şekerci, Ç.A.; Sulukaya, M.; Alpay, H.; Tarcan, T.; Şimşek, F. Assessment of Differential Renal Function in Children with Hydronephrosis: Comparison of DMSA and MAG-3. *J. Urol. Surg.* **2015**, *2*, 129–134. [CrossRef]
23. Washino, S.; Hosohata, K.; Oshima, M.; Okochi, T.; Konishi, T.; Nakamura, Y.; Saito, K.; Miyagawa, T. A Novel Biomarker for Acute Kidney Injury, Vanin-1, for Obstructive Nephropathy: A Prospective Cohort Pilot Study. *Int. J. Mol. Sci.* **2019**, *20*, 899. [CrossRef] [PubMed]
24. Madsen, M.G.; Nørregaard, R.; Palmfeldt, J.; Olsen, L.H.; Frøkiær, J.; Jørgensen, T.M. Epidermal growth factor and monocyte chemotactic peptide-1: Potential biomarkers of urinary tract obstruction in children with hydronephrosis. *J. Pediatr. Urol.* **2013**, *9*, 838–845. [CrossRef] [PubMed]
25. Lopez-Giacoman, S.; Madero, M. Biomarkers in chronic kidney disease, from kidney function to kidney damage. *World J. Nephrol.* **2015**, *4*, 57–73. [CrossRef] [PubMed]
26. Pavlaki, A.; Printza, N.; Farmaki, E.; Stabouli, S.; Taparkou, A.; Sterpi, M.; Dotis, J.; Papachristou, F. The role of urinary NGAL and serum cystatin C in assessing the severity of ureteropelvic junction obstruction in infants. *Pediatr. Nephrol.* **2019**, *35*, 163–170. [CrossRef]
27. Inker, L.A.; Okparavero, A. Cystatin C as a marker of glomerular filtration rate. *Curr. Opin. Nephrol. Hypertens.* **2011**, *20*, 631–639. [CrossRef]
28. Slort, P.R.; Ozden, N.; Pape, L.; Offner, G.; Tromp, W.F.; Wilhelm, A.J.; Bokenkamp, A. Comparing cystatin C and creatinine in the diagnosis of pediatric acute renal allograft dysfunction. *Pediatr. Nephrol.* **2011**, *27*, 843–849. [CrossRef]
29. Yong, Z.; Pei, X.; Zhu, B.; Yuan, H.; Zhao, W. Predictive value of serum cystatin C for acute kidney injury in adults: A meta-analysis of prospective cohort trials. *Sci. Rep.* **2017**, *7*, 41012. [CrossRef]
30. Koyner, J.L.; Vaidya, V.S.; Bennett, M.R.; Ma, Q.; Worcester, E.; Akhter, S.A.; Raman, J.; Jeevanandam, V.; O'Connor, M.F.; Devarajan, P.; et al. Urinary Biomarkers in the Clinical Prognosis and Early Detection of Acute Kidney Injury. *Clin. J. Am. Soc. Nephrol.* **2010**, *5*, 2154–2165. [CrossRef]
31. Chen, S.; Shi, J.-S.; Yibulayin, X.; Wu, T.-S.; Yang, X.-W.; Zhang, J.; Baiheti, P. Cystatin C is a moderate predictor of acute kidney injury in the early stage of traumatic hemorrhagic shock. *Exp. Ther. Med.* **2015**, *10*, 237–240. [CrossRef]
32. Haase-Fielitz, A.; Bellomo, R.; Devarajan, P.; Story, D.F.; Matalanis, G.; Dragun, D.; Haase, M. Novel and conventional serum biomarkers predicting acute kidney injury in adult cardiac surgery—A prospective cohort study. *Crit. Care Med.* **2009**, *37*, 553–560. [CrossRef] [PubMed]
33. Shukla, A.N.; Juneja, M.; Patel, H.; Shah, K.H.; Konat, A.; Thakkar, B.M.; Madan, T.; Prajapati, J. Diagnostic accuracy of serum cystatin C for early recognition of contrast induced nephropathy in Western Indians undergoing cardiac catheterization. *Indian Hear. J.* **2016**, *69*, 311–315. [CrossRef] [PubMed]
34. Kostic, D.; Beozzo, G.; Couto, S.B.D.; Kato, A.; Lima, L.; Palmeira, P.; Krebs, V.; Bunduki, V.; Francisco, R.P.; Zugaib, M.; et al. The role of renal biomarkers to predict the need of surgery in congenital urinary tract obstruction in infants. *J. Pediatr. Urol.* **2019**, *15*, 242.e1–242.e9. [CrossRef]
35. Mao, W.; Liu, S.; Wang, K.; Wang, M.; Shi, H.; Liu, Q.; Bao, M.; Peng, B.; Geng, J. Cystatin C in Evaluating Renal Function in Ureteral Calculi Hydronephrosis in Adults. *Kidney Blood Press. Res.* **2019**, *45*, 109–121. [CrossRef] [PubMed]
36. Karakus, S.; Oktar, T.; Kucukgergin, C.; Kalelioğlu, I.; Seckin, S.; Atar, A.; Ander, H.; Ziylan, O. Urinary IP-10, MCP-1, NGAL, Cystatin-C, and KIM-1 Levels in Prenatally Diagnosed Unilateral Hydronephrosis: The Search for an Ideal Biomarker. *Urology* **2016**, *87*, 185–192. [CrossRef] [PubMed]

37. Guo, L.; Zhu, B.; Yuan, H.; Zhao, W. Evaluation of serum neutrophil gelatinase-associated lipocalin in older patients with chronic kidney disease. *Aging Med.* **2020**, *3*, 35–42. [CrossRef] [PubMed]
38. Zwiers, A.J.M.; De Wildt, S.N.; Van Rosmalen, J.; De Rijke, Y.B.; Buijs, E.A.B.; Tibboel, D.; Cransberg, K. Urinary neutrophil gelatinase-associated lipocalin identifies critically ill young children with acute kidney injury following intensive care admission: A prospective cohort study. *Crit. Care* **2015**, *19*, 1–14. [CrossRef]
39. Liu, X.; Guan, Y.; Xu, S.; Li, Q.; Sun, Y.; Han, R.; Jiang, C. Early Predictors of Acute Kidney Injury: A Narrative Review. *Kidney Blood Press. Res.* **2016**, *41*, 680–700. [CrossRef]
40. Schmidt-Ott, K.M.; Mori, K.; Li, J.Y.; Kalandadze, A.; Cohen, D.J.; Devarajan, P.; Barasch, J. Dual Action of Neutrophil Gelatinase–Associated Lipocalin. *J. Am. Soc. Nephrol.* **2007**, *18*, 407–413. [CrossRef]
41. Dong, Y.; Zhang, Q.; Wen, J.; Chen, T.; He, L.; Wang, Y.; Yin, J.; Wu, R.; Xue, R.; Li, S.; et al. Ischemic Duration and Frequency Determines AKI-to-CKD Progression Monitored by Dynamic Changes of Tubular Biomarkers in IRI Mice. *Front. Physiol.* **2019**, *10*, 153. [CrossRef]
42. Cappuccilli, M.; Capelli, I.; Comai, G.; Cianciolo, G.; La Manna, G. Neutrophil Gelatinase-Associated Lipocalin as a Biomarker of Allograft Function After Renal Transplantation: Evaluation of the Current Status and Future Insights. *Artif. Organs* **2017**, *42*, 8–14. [CrossRef] [PubMed]
43. Nusca, A.; Miglionico, M.; Proscia, C.; Ragni, L.; Carassiti, M.; Pepe, F.L.; Di Sciascio, G. Early prediction of contrast-induced acute kidney injury by a "bedside" assessment of Neutrophil Gelatinase-Associated Lipocalin during elective percutaneous coronary interventions. *PLoS ONE* **2018**, *13*, e0197833. [CrossRef] [PubMed]
44. Asada, T.; Isshiki, R.; Hayase, N.; Sumida, M.; Inokuchi, R.; Noiri, E.; Nangaku, M.; Yahagi, N.; Doi, K. Impact of clinical context on acute kidney injury biomarker performances: Differences between neutrophil gelatinase-associated lipocalin and L-type fatty acid-binding protein. *Sci. Rep.* **2016**, *6*, 33077. [CrossRef] [PubMed]
45. Bieniaś, B.; Sikora, P. Potential Novel Biomarkers of Obstructive Nephropathy in Children with Hydronephrosis. *Dis. Markers* **2018**, *2018*, 1–9. [CrossRef]
46. Yu, L.; Zhou, L.; Li, Q.; Li, S.; Luo, X.; Zhang, C.; Wu, B.; Brooks, J.D.; Sun, H. Elevated urinary lipocalin-2, interleukin-6 and monocyte chemoattractant protein-1 levels in children with congenital ureteropelvic junction obstruction. *J. Pediatr. Urol.* **2019**, *15*, 44.e1–44.e7. [CrossRef]
47. Gupta, S.; Jackson, A.R.; DaJusta, D.; McLeod, D.; Alpert, S.; Jayanthi, V.R.; McHugh, K.; Schwaderer, A.; Becknell, B.; Ching, C. Urinary antimicrobial peptides: Potential novel biomarkers of obstructive uropathy. *J. Pediatr. Urol.* **2018**, *14*, 238.e1–238.e6. [CrossRef]
48. Noyan, A.; Parmaksız, G.; Dursun, H.; Ezer, S.S.; Anarat, R.; Cengiz, N.; Parmaksız, G. Urinary NGAL, KIM-1 and L-FABP concentrations in antenatal hydronephrosis. *J. Pediatr. Urol.* **2015**, *11*, 249.e1–249.e6. [CrossRef]
49. Wasilewska, A.; Taranta-Janusz, K.; Debek, W.; Zoch-Zwierz, W.; Kuroczycka-Saniutycz, E. KIM-1 and NGAL: New markers of obstructive nephropathy. *Pediatr. Nephrol.* **2011**, *26*, 579–586. [CrossRef]
50. Urbschat, A.; Gauer, S.; Paulus, P.; Reissig, M.; Weipert, C.; Ramos-Lopez, E.; Hofmann, R.; Hadji, P.; Geiger, H.; Obermüller, N. Serum and urinary NGAL but not KIM-1 raises in human postrenal AKI. *Eur. J. Clin. Investig.* **2014**, *44*, 652–659. [CrossRef]
51. Olvera-Posada, D.; Dayarathna, T.; Dion, M.; Alenezi, H.; Sener, A.; Denstedt, J.D.; Pautler, S.E.; Razvi, H. KIM-1 Is a Potential Urinary Biomarker of Obstruction: Results from a Prospective Cohort Study. *J. Endourol.* **2017**, *31*, 111–118. [CrossRef]
52. Devarajan, P. Neutrophil gelatinase-associated lipocalin: A promising biomarker for human acute kidney injury. *Biomark. Med.* **2010**, *4*, 265–280. [CrossRef] [PubMed]
53. Devarajan, P. Neutrophil gelatinase-associated lipocalin: New paths for an old shuttle. *Cancer Ther.* **2007**, *5*, 463–470. [PubMed]
54. Choi, J.W.; Fujii, T.; Fujii, N. Elevated Plasma Neutrophil Gelatinase-Associated Lipocalin Level as a Risk Factor for Anemia in Patients with Systemic Inflammation. *BioMed Res. Int.* **2016**, *2016*, 1–8. [CrossRef] [PubMed]
55. Ning, M.; Mao, X.; Niu, Y.; Tang, B.; Shen, H. Usefulness and limitations of neutrophil gelatinase-associated lipocalin in the assessment of kidney diseases. *J. Lab. Precis. Med.* **2018**, *3*, 1. [CrossRef]
56. Gu, L.; Tseng, S.C.; Rollins, B.J. Monocyte chemoattractant protein-1. *Chem. Immunol.* **1999**, *72*, 7–29.
57. Gschwandtner, M.; Derler, R.; Midwood, K.S. More Than Just Attractive: How CCL2 Influences Myeloid Cell Behavior Beyond Chemotaxis. *Front. Immunol.* **2019**, *10*, 2759. [CrossRef]

58. Grandaliano, G.; Gesualdo, L.; Ranieri, E.; Monno, R.; Montinaro, V.; Marra, F.; Schena, F.P. Monocyte chemotactic peptide-1 expression in acute and chronic human nephritides: A pathogenetic role in interstitial monocytes recruitment. *J. Am. Soc. Nephrol.* **1996**, *7*, 906–913.
59. Grandaliano, G.; Gesualdo, L.; Bartoli, F.; Ranieri, E.; Monno, R.; Leggio, A.; Paradies, G.; Caldarulo, E.; Infante, B.; Schena, F.P. MCP-1 and EGF renal expression and urine excretion in human congenital obstructive nephropathy. *Kidney Int.* **2000**, *58*, 182–192. [CrossRef]
60. Stroo, I.; Claessen, N.; Teske, G.J.D.; Butter, L.M.; Florquin, S.; Leemans, J.C. Deficiency for the Chemokine Monocyte Chemoattractant Protein-1 Aggravates Tubular Damage after Renal Ischemia/Reperfusion Injury. *PLoS ONE* **2015**, *10*, e0123203. [CrossRef]
61. Moledina, D.G.; Isguven, S.; McArthur, E.; Thiessen-Philbrook, H.; Garg, A.X.; Shlipak, M.; Whitlock, R.; Kavsak, P.A.; Coca, S.G.; Parikh, C.R.; et al. Plasma Monocyte Chemotactic Protein-1 Is Associated With Acute Kidney Injury and Death After Cardiac Operations. *Ann. Thorac. Surg.* **2017**, *104*, 613–620. [CrossRef]
62. Tam, F.W.K.; Ong, A.C. Renal monocyte chemoattractant protein-1: An emerging universal biomarker and therapeutic target for kidney diseases? *Nephrol. Dial. Transplant.* **2019**, *35*, 198–203. [CrossRef]
63. Kronbichler, A.; Kerschbaum, J.; Gründlinger, G.; Leierer, J.; Mayer, G.; Rudnicki, M.A. Evaluation and validation of biomarkers in granulomatosis with polyangiitis and microscopic polyangiitis. *Nephrol. Dial. Transplant.* **2015**, *31*, 930–936. [CrossRef] [PubMed]
64. Nowak, N.; Skupien, J.; Smiles, A.M.; Yamanouchi, M.; Niewczas, M.; Galecki, A.T.; Duffin, K.L.; Breyer, M.D.; Pullen, N.; Bonventre, J.V.; et al. Markers of early progressive renal decline in type 2 diabetes suggest different implications for etiological studies and prognostic tests development. *Kidney Int.* **2018**, *93*, 1198–1206. [CrossRef] [PubMed]
65. Grantham, J.J.; Chapman, A.B.; Blais, J.; Czerwiec, F.S.; Devuyst, O.; Gansevoort, R.T.; Higashihara, E.; Krasa, H.; Zhou, W.; Ouyang, J.; et al. Tolvaptan suppresses monocyte chemotactic protein-1 excretion in autosomal-dominant polycystic kidney disease. *Nephrol. Dial. Transplant.* **2017**, *32*, 969–975. [CrossRef] [PubMed]
66. Munshi, R.; Johnson, A.; Siew, E.D.; Ikizler, T.A.; Ware, L.B.; Wurfel, M.M.; Himmelfarb, J.; Zager, R.A. MCP-1 Gene Activation Marks Acute Kidney Injury. *J. Am. Soc. Nephrol.* **2010**, *22*, 165–175. [CrossRef]
67. Stephan, M.; Conrad, S.; Eggert, T.; Heuer, R.; Fernandez, S.; Huland, H. Urinary concentration and tissue messenger RNA expression of monocyte chemoattractant protein-1 as an indicator of the degree of hydronephrotic atrophy in partial ureteral obstruction. *J. Urol.* **2002**, *167*, 1497–1502. [CrossRef]
68. Mohammadjafari, H.; Rafiei, A.; Mousavi, S.A.; Alaee, A.; Yeganeh, Y. Role of Urinary Levels of Endothelin-1, Monocyte Chemotactic Peptide-1, andN-Acetyl Glucosaminidase in Predicting the Severity of Obstruction in Hydronephrotic Neonates. *Korean J. Urol.* **2014**, *55*, 670–676. [CrossRef]
69. Taranta-Janusz, K.; Wasilewska, A.; Debek, W.; Waszkiewicz-Stojda, M. Urinary cytokine profiles in unilateral congenital hydronephrosis. *Pediatr. Nephrol.* **2012**, *27*, 2107–2113. [CrossRef]
70. Bartoli, F.; Penza, R.; Aceto, G.; Niglio, F.; D'Addato, O.; Pastore, V.; Campanella, V.; Magaldi, S.; Lasalandra, C.; Di Bitonto, G.; et al. Urinary epidermal growth factor, monocyte chemotactic protein-1, and beta2-microglobulin in children with ureteropelvic junction obstruction. *J. Pediatr. Surg.* **2011**, *46*, 530–536. [CrossRef]
71. Musiał, K.; Bargenda, A.; Drożdż, D.; Zwolińska, D. New Markers of Inflammation and Tubular Damage in Children with Chronic Kidney Disease. *Dis. Markers* **2017**, *2017*, 1–5. [CrossRef]
72. Gregg, L.P.; Tio, M.C.; Li, X.; Adams-Huet, B.; De Lemos, J.A.; Hedayati, S.S. Association of Monocyte Chemoattractant Protein-1 with Death and Atherosclerotic Events in Chronic Kidney Disease. *Am. J. Nephrol.* **2018**, *47*, 395–405. [CrossRef] [PubMed]
73. Ichimura, T.; Bonventre, J.V.; Bailly, V.; Wei, H.; Hession, C.A.; Cate, R.L.; Sanicola, M. Kidney Injury Molecule-1 (KIM-1), a Putative Epithelial Cell Adhesion Molecule Containing a Novel Immunoglobulin Domain, Is Up-regulated in Renal Cells after Injury. *J. Biol. Chem.* **1998**, *273*, 4135–4142. [CrossRef] [PubMed]
74. Song, J.; Yu, J.; Prayogo, G.W.; Cao, W.; Wu, Y.; Jia, Z.; Zhang, A. Understanding kidney injury molecule 1: A novel immune factor in kidney pathophysiology. *Am. J. Transl. Res.* **2019**, *11*, 1219–1229.
75. Han, W.K.; Bailly, V.; Abichandani, R.; Thadhani, R.; Bonventre, J.V. Kidney Injury Molecule-1 (KIM-1): A novel biomarker for human renal proximal tubule injury. *Kidney Int.* **2002**, *62*, 237–244. [CrossRef] [PubMed]

76. Ichimura, T.; Asseldonk, E.J.; Humphreys, B.D.; Gunaratnam, L.; Duffield, J.S.; Bonventre, J.V. Kidney injury molecule–1 is a phosphatidylserine receptor that confers a phagocytic phenotype on epithelial cells. *J. Clin. Investig.* **2008**, *118*, 1657–1668. [CrossRef] [PubMed]
77. Ismail, O.Z.; Zhang, X.; Bonventre, J.V.; Gunaratnam, L. G protein α12 (Gα12) is a negative regulator of kidney injury molecule-1-mediated efferocytosis. *Am. J. Physiol. Physiol.* **2016**, *310*, F607–F620. [CrossRef]
78. Satirapoj, B.; Pooluea, P.; Nata, N.; Supasyndh, O. Urinary biomarkers of tubular injury to predict renal progression and end stage renal disease in type 2 diabetes mellitus with advanced nephropathy: A prospective cohort study. *J. Diabetes Complicat.* **2019**, *33*, 675–681. [CrossRef]
79. Peters, H.P.; Waanders, F.; Meijer, E.; Brand, J.V.D.; Steenbergen, E.J.; Van Goor, H.; Wetzels, J.F. High urinary excretion of kidney injury molecule-1 is an independent predictor of end-stage renal disease in patients with IgA nephropathy. *Nephrol. Dial. Transplant.* **2011**, *26*, 3581–3588. [CrossRef]
80. Zhang, P.; Rothblum, L.; Han, W.; Blasick, T.; Potdar, S.; Bonventre, J.V. Kidney injury molecule-1 expression in transplant biopsies is a sensitive measure of cell injury. *Kidney Int.* **2008**, *73*, 608–614. [CrossRef]
81. Jin, Y.; Shao, X.; Sun, B.; Miao, C.; Li, Z.; Shi, Y. Urinary kidney injury molecule-1 as an early diagnostic biomarker of obstructive acute kidney injury and development of a rapid detection method. *Mol. Med. Rep.* **2017**, *15*, 1229–1235. [CrossRef]
82. Tian, L.; Shao, X.; Xie, Y.; Wang, Q.; Che, X.; Zhang, M.; Xu, W.; Xu, Y.; Mou, S.; Ni, Z. Kidney Injury Molecule-1 is Elevated in Nephropathy and Mediates Macrophage Activation via the Mapk Signalling Pathway. *Cell. Physiol. Biochem.* **2017**, *41*, 769–783. [CrossRef] [PubMed]
83. Xie, Y.; Xue, W.; Shao, X.; Che, X.; Xu, W.; Ni, Z.; Mou, S. Analysis of a Urinary Biomarker Panel for Obstructive Nephropathy and Clinical Outcomes. *PLoS ONE* **2014**, *9*, e112865. [CrossRef] [PubMed]
84. Skálová, S. The diagnostic role of urinary N-acetyl-beta-D-glucosaminidase (NAG) activity in the detection of renal tubular impairment. *Acta Medica* **2005**, *48*, 75–80. [PubMed]
85. Bosomworth, M.P.; Aparicio, S.R.; Hay, A.W. Urine N-acetyl- -D-glucosaminidase—A marker of tubular damage? *Nephrol. Dial. Transplant.* **1999**, *14*, 620–626. [CrossRef] [PubMed]
86. Hong, N.; Lee, M.; Park, S.; Lee, Y.H.; Jin, S.M.; Kim, J.H.; Lee, B.W. Elevated urinary N-acetyl-beta-D-glucosaminidase is associated with high glycoalbumin-to-hemoglobin A1c ratio in type 1 diabetes patients with early diabetic kidney disease. *Sci. Rep.* **2018**, *8*, 6710. [CrossRef]
87. Demir, A.D.; Goknar, N.; Oktem, F.; Ozkaya, E.; Yazici, M.; Torun, E.; Vehapoglu, A.; Kucukkoc, M. Renal tubular function and urinary N-acetyl-beta-d-glucosaminidase and kidney injury molecule-1 levels in asthmatic children. *Int. J. Immunopathol. Pharmacol.* **2016**, *29*, 626–631. [CrossRef]
88. Ali, R.J.; Al-Obaidi, F.H.; Arif, H.S. The Role of Urinary N-acetyl Beta-D-glucosaminidase in Children with Urological Problems. *Oman Med. J.* **2014**, *29*, 285–288. [CrossRef]
89. Carr, M.C.; Peters, C.A.; Retik, A.B.; Mandell, J. Urinary levels of the renal tubular enzyme N-acetyl-beta-D-glucosaminidase in unilateral obstructive uropathy. *J. Urol.* **1994**, *151*, 442–445. [CrossRef]
90. Skálová, S.; Rejtar, P.; Kutilek, S. Increased urinary N-acetyl-beta-D-glucosaminidase activity in children with hydronephrosis. *Int. Braz. Urol.* **2007**, *33*, 80–86. [CrossRef]
91. Kamijo-Ikemori, A.; Sugaya, T.; Matsui, K.; Yokoyama, T.; Kimura, K. Roles of human liver type fatty acid binding protein in kidney disease clarified using hL-FABP chromosomal transgenic mice. *Nephrology* **2011**, *16*, 539–544. [CrossRef]
92. Yamamoto, T.; Noiri, E.; Ono, Y.; Doi, K.; Negishi, K.; Kamijo, A.; Kimura, K.; Fujita, T.; Kinukawa, T.; Taniguchi, H.; et al. Renal L-Type Fatty Acid–Binding Protein in Acute Ischemic Injury. *J. Am. Soc. Nephrol.* **2007**, *18*, 2894–2902. [CrossRef] [PubMed]
93. Furuhashi, M. Fatty Acid-Binding Protein 4 in Cardiovascular and Metabolic Diseases. *J. Atheroscler. Thromb.* **2019**, *26*, 216–232. [CrossRef] [PubMed]
94. Graupera, I.; Coll, M.; Pose, E.; Elia, C.; Piano, S.; Sola, E.; Blaya, D.; Huelin, P.; Solé, C.; Moreira, R.; et al. Adipocyte Fatty-Acid Binding Protein is Overexpressed in Cirrhosis and Correlates with Clinical Outcomes. *Sci. Rep.* **2017**, *7*, 1829. [CrossRef] [PubMed]
95. Kawai, A.; Kusaka, M.; Kitagawa, F.; Ishii, J.; Fukami, N.; Maruyama, T.; Sasaki, H.; Shiroki, R.; Kurahashi, H.; Hoshinaga, K. Serum liver-type fatty acid-binding protein predicts recovery of graft function after kidney transplantation from donors after cardiac death. *Clin. Transplant.* **2014**, *28*, 749–754. [CrossRef]

96. Parr, S.K.; Clark, A.J.; Bian, A.; Shintani, A.K.; Wickersham, N.E.; Ware, L.B.; Ikizler, T.A.; Siew, E.D. Urinary L-FABP predicts poor outcomes in critically ill patients with early acute kidney injury. *Kidney Int.* **2014**, *87*, 640–648. [CrossRef]
97. Connolly, M.; Kinnin, M.; Mc Eneaney, D.; Menown, I.; Kurth, M.J.; Lamont, J.; Morgan, N.; Harbinson, M. Prediction of contrast induced acute kidney injury using novel biomarkers following contrast coronary angiography. *QJM Int. J. Med.* **2017**, *111*, 103–110. [CrossRef]
98. Panduru, N.M.; Forsblom, C.; Saraheimo, M.; Thorn, L.; Bierhaus, A.; Humpert, P.M.; Groop, P.-H. Urinary Liver-Type Fatty Acid–Binding Protein and Progression of Diabetic Nephropathy in Type 1 Diabetes. *Diabetes Care* **2013**, *36*, 2077–2083. [CrossRef]
99. Parmaksız, G.; Noyan, A.; Dursun, H.; Ince, E.; Anarat, R.; Cengiz, N. Role of new biomarkers for predicting renal scarring in vesicoureteral reflux: NGAL, KIM-1, and L-FABP. *Pediatr. Nephrol.* **2015**, *31*, 97–103. [CrossRef]
100. Bartucci, R.; Salvati, A.; Olinga, P.; Boersma, Y.L. Vanin 1: Its Physiological Function and Role in Diseases. *Int. J. Mol. Sci.* **2019**, *20*, 3891. [CrossRef]
101. Wessely, O.; Cerqueira, D.M.; Tran, U.; Kumar, V.; Hassey, J.M.; Romaker, D. The bigger the better: Determining nephron size in kidney. *Pediatr. Nephrol.* **2013**, *29*, 525–530. [CrossRef]
102. Hosohata, K.; Jin, D.; Takai, S.; Iwanaga, K. Vanin-1 in Renal Pelvic Urine Reflects Kidney Injury in a Rat Model of Hydronephrosis. *Int. J. Mol. Sci.* **2018**, *19*, 3186. [CrossRef] [PubMed]
103. Hosohata, K.; Washino, S.; Kubo, T.; Natsui, S.; Fujisaki, A.; Kurokawa, S.; Ando, H.; Fujimura, A.; Morita, T. Early prediction of cisplatin-induced nephrotoxicity by urinary vanin-1 in patients with urothelial carcinoma. *Toxicology* **2016**, *360*, 71–75. [CrossRef] [PubMed]
104. Hosohata, K.; Jin, D.; Takai, S.; Iwanaga, K. Involvement of Vanin-1 in Ameliorating Effect of Oxidative Renal Tubular Injury in Dahl-Salt Sensitive Rats. *Int. J. Mol. Sci.* **2019**, *20*, 4481. [CrossRef] [PubMed]
105. Fugmann, T.; Borgia, B.; Révész, C.; Godó, M.; Forsblom, C.; Hamar, P.; Holthofer, H.; Neri, D.; Roesli, C. Proteomic identification of vanin-1 as a marker of kidney damage in a rat model of type 1 diabetic nephropathy. *Kidney Int.* **2011**, *80*, 272–281. [CrossRef] [PubMed]
106. Sundberg, A.; Appelkvist, E.L.; Dallner, G.; Nilsson, R. Glutathione Transferases in the Urine: Sensitive Methods for Detection of Kidney Damage Induced by Nephrotoxic Agents in Humans. *Environ. Health Perspect.* **1994**, *102*, 293. [CrossRef]
107. Andreucci, M.; Faga, T.; Pisani, A.; Perticone, M.; Michael, A. The ischemic/nephrotoxic acute kidney injury and the use of renal biomarkers in clinical practice. *Eur. J. Intern. Med.* **2017**, *39*, 1–8. [CrossRef]
108. Walshe, C.M.; Odejayi, F.; Ng, S.; Marsh, B. Urinary glutathione S-transferase as an early marker for renal dysfunction in patients admitted to intensive care with sepsis. *Crit. Care Resusc. J. Australas. Acad. Crit. Care Med.* **2009**, *11*, 204–209.
109. Vijayan, A.; Faubel, S.; Askenazi, D.J.; Cerda, J.; Fissell, W.H.; Heung, M.; Humphreys, B.D.; Koyner, J.L.; Liu, K.D.; Mour, G.; et al. Clinical use of the urine biomarker [TIMP-2] × [IGFBP7] for acute kidney injury risk assessment. *Am. J. Kidney Dis.* **2016**, *68*, 19–28. [CrossRef]
110. Emlet, D.R.; Pastor-Soler, N.; Marciszyn, A.; Wen, X.; Gomez, H.; Humphries, W.H.; Morrisroe, S.; Volpe, J.K.; Kellum, J.A. Insulin-like growth factor binding protein 7 and tissue inhibitor of metalloproteinases-2: Differential expression and secretion in human kidney tubule cells. *Am. J. Physiol. Physiol.* **2016**, *312*, F284–F296. [CrossRef]
111. Ortega, L.M.; Heung, M. The use of cell cycle arrest biomarkers in the early detection of acute kidney injury. Is this the new renal troponin? *Nefrologia* **2018**, *38*, 361–367. [CrossRef]
112. Heung, M.; Ortega, L.M.; Chawla, L.S.; Wunderink, R.G.; Self, W.H.; Koyner, J.L.; Shi, J.; Kellum, J.A. Sapphire and Topaz Investigators Common chronic conditions do not affect performance of cell cycle arrest biomarkers for risk stratification of acute kidney injury. *Nephrol. Dial. Transplant.* **2016**, *31*, 1633–1640. [CrossRef] [PubMed]
113. Fan, W.; Ankawi, G.; Zhang, J.; Digvijay, K.; Giavarina, D.; Yin, Y.; Ronco, C. Current understanding and future directions in the application of TIMP-2 and IGFBP7 in AKI clinical practice. *Clin. Chem. Lab. Med.* **2019**, *57*, 567–576. [CrossRef] [PubMed]
114. Tasdemir, M.; Fucucuoglu, D.; Kucuk, S.H.; Erol, M.; Yigit, O.; Bilge, I. Urinary biomarkers in the early detection and follow-up of tubular injury in childhood urolithiasis. *Clin. Exp. Nephrol.* **2018**, *22*, 133–141. [CrossRef] [PubMed]

115. Graupera, I.; Sola, E.; Fabrellas, N.; Moreira, R.; Sole, C.; Huelin, P.; De La Prada, G.; Pose, E.; Ariza, X.; Risso, A.; et al. Urine Monocyte Chemoattractant Protein-1 Is an Independent Predictive Factor of Hospital Readmission and Survival in Cirrhosis. *PLoS ONE* **2016**, *11*, e0157371. [CrossRef]
116. Fanfulla, F.; Rotondi, M.; Morrone, E.; Coperchini, F.; Lodigiani, S.; Trentin, R.; Maccabruni, V.; Chiovato, L. Sleep hypoxia and not obesity is the main determinant of the increasing monocyte chemoattractant protein-1 (MCP-1) in patients with obstructive sleep apnoea. *ERJ Open Res.* **2017**, *3*, P70. [CrossRef]
117. Buonafine, M.; Martinez-Martinez, E.; Jaisser, F. More than a simple biomarker: The role of NGAL in cardiovascular and renal diseases. *Clin. Sci.* **2018**, *132*, 909–923. [CrossRef]
118. Kim, J.W.; Hong, D.Y.; Lee, K.R.; Kim, S.Y.; Baek, K.J.; Park, S.O. Usefulness of plasma neutrophil gelatinase-associated lipocalin concentration for predicting the severity and mortality of patients with community-acquired pneumonia. *Clin. Chim. Acta* **2016**, *462*, 140–145. [CrossRef]
119. Tanoğlu, A.; Beyazit, Y. Liver fatty acid-binding protein may be a useful marker for non-alcoholic fatty liver disease but obesity is a major concern. *Wien. Klin. Wochenschr.* **2016**, *128*, 304. [CrossRef]
120. Eguchi, A.; Hasegawa, H.; Iwasa, M.; Tamai, Y.; Ohata, K.; Oikawa, T.; Sugaya, T.; Takei, Y. Serum Liver-Type Fatty Acid-Binding Protein Is a Possible Prognostic Factor in Human Chronic Liver Diseases From Chronic Hepatitis to Liver Cirrhosis and Hepatocellular Carcinoma. *Hepatol. Commun.* **2019**, *3*, 825–837. [CrossRef]

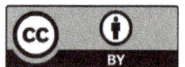

© 2020 by the authors. Licensee MDPI, Basel, Switzerland. This article is an open access article distributed under the terms and conditions of the Creative Commons Attribution (CC BY) license (http://creativecommons.org/licenses/by/4.0/).

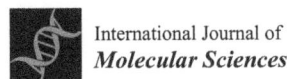

Review

Aminopeptidases in Cardiovascular and Renal Function. Role as Predictive Renal Injury Biomarkers

Félix Vargas [1], Rosemary Wangesteen [2], Isabel Rodríguez-Gómez [1] and Joaquín García-Estañ [3],*

1. Depto. Fisiologia, Fac. Medicina, Universidad de Granada, 18071 Granada, Spain; fvargas@ugr.es (F.V.); isabelrg@ugr.es (I.R.-G.)
2. Depto. Ciencias de la salud, Universidad de Jaén, 23071 Jaén, Spain; rwanges@ujaen.es
3. Depto. Fisiologia, Fac. Medicina, IMIB, Universidad de Murcia, 30120 Murcia, Spain
* Correspondence: jgestan@um.es

Received: 23 June 2020; Accepted: 3 August 2020; Published: 5 August 2020

Abstract: Aminopeptidases (APs) are metalloenzymes that hydrolyze peptides and polypeptides by scission of the N-terminus amino acid and that also participate in the intracellular final digestion of proteins. APs play an important role in protein maturation, signal transduction, and cell-cycle control, among other processes. These enzymes are especially relevant in the control of cardiovascular and renal functions. APs participate in the regulation of the systemic and local renin–angiotensin system and also modulate the activity of neuropeptides, kinins, immunomodulatory peptides, and cytokines, even contributing to cholesterol uptake and angiogenesis. This review focuses on the role of four key APs, aspartyl-, alanyl-, glutamyl-, and leucyl-cystinyl-aminopeptidases, in the control of blood pressure (BP) and renal function and on their association with different cardiovascular and renal diseases. In this context, the effects of AP inhibitors are analyzed as therapeutic tools for BP control and renal diseases. Their role as urinary biomarkers of renal injury is also explored. The enzymatic activities of urinary APs, which act as hydrolyzing peptides on the luminal surface of the renal tubule, have emerged as early predictive renal injury biomarkers in both acute and chronic renal nephropathies, including those induced by nephrotoxic agents, obesity, hypertension, or diabetes. Hence, the analysis of urinary AP appears to be a promising diagnostic and prognostic approach to renal disease in both research and clinical settings.

Keywords: urinary aminopeptidases; biomarkers; arterial hypertension; renal function

---

1. Aminopeptidases in the Renin–Angiotensin System

The renin–angiotensin system (RAS) plays an essential role in blood pressure (BP) control, via vascular, renal, brain, and other mechanisms. Abnormalities in RAS activity may lead to the development of arterial hypertension and other cardiovascular and renal diseases. Blockade of this system is an effective therapeutic measure against numerous diseases, and RAS compounds have been found in the kidney, brain, and other tissues. Over recent years, our knowledge of the components of the RAS has increased, including numerous angiotensin peptides with diverse biological activities mediated by different receptor subtypes [1,2].

The enzymatic cascade of the RAS is depicted in Figure 1. It is initiated by angiotensinogen, an alfa 2 globulin of hepatic origin, which generates angiotensin I (AngI) through the enzymatic action of renin on the extreme amino-terminus. The decapeptide AngI is a substrate for angiotensin-converting enzyme (ACE), which splits the dipeptide His-Leu from the extreme carboxy-terminus to generate the octapeptide AngII [1], the major effector peptide of the RAS, which bind to two major receptors, AT1 and AT2, that generally oppose each other.

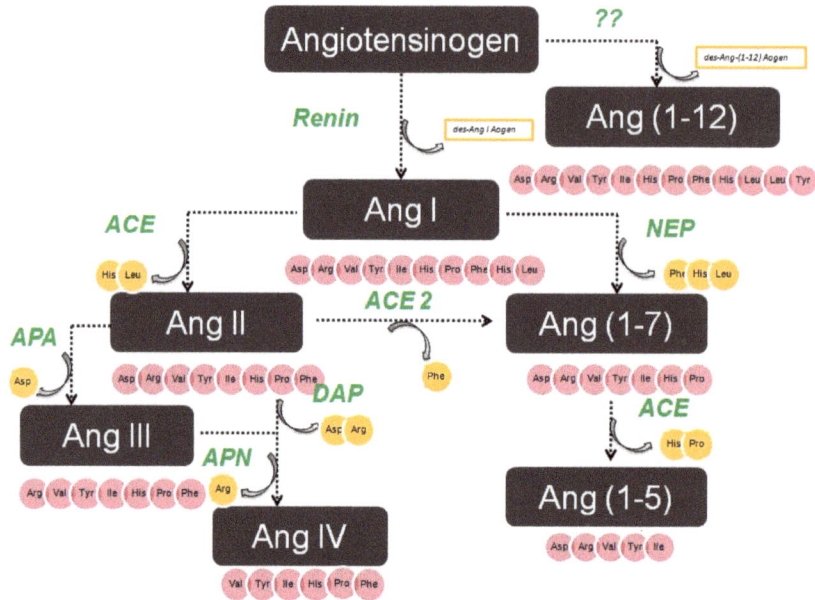

Figure 1. The renin–angiotensin system.

Action of glutamyl aminopeptidase (APA) on AngII removes the Asp residue N-terminus to generate the heptapeptide AngIII. AngIII can also be generated by an AngII-independent pathway via the nonapeptide [des-Asp1]AngI, produced from AngI by AspAP, which is converted to AngIII via ACE. APA also participates in the formation of Ang(1-7), which can also be transformed into Ang(2-7) through cleaving of the Asp-Arg bond.

In the extreme N-terminus, membrane alanyl aminopeptidase N (APN) removes Arg to give hexapeptide angiotensin IV (AngIV). AngIV is also transformed into Ang(3-7) by carboxypeptidase P (Carb-P) and propyl oligopeptidase through scission of the Pro-Phe carboxy-terminus.

ACE2 can also transform AngII into Ang(1-7) through hydrolysis of Phe by Carb-P or through scission of the dipeptide Phe-His from Ang(1-9) [1–4].

Aminopeptidase B (APB), also known as arginine aminopeptidase (Arg-AP), cleaves basic amino acids at the N-terminus. It participates in the conversion of AngIII to AngIV.

Although not part of the RAS, both neuropeptides oxytocin and vasopressin are cleaved at the N-terminus of cysteine next to tyrosine by cystinyl aminopeptidase (CAP), a rat homolog of insulin-regulated AP (IRAP) [5].

All these enzymes are globally called "angiotensinases" because they are responsible for the generation of systemic and local peptides (angiotensins) related to the regulation of BP and the excretion of sodium and water. These enzymes determine the proportions of bioactive compounds.

AngI is biologically inactive, but AngII and AngIII act as agonists for AT1 and AT2 receptors, thereby mediating pressor and dipsogenic effects [6,7]. AngIV has a low affinity for AT1 and AT2 receptors but high affinity and specificity for the AT4 receptor subtype. Interaction with the AT1 receptor subtype reduces the pressor effect of AngIV. A counterregulatory system to the AngII-AngIII/AT1 receptor system is composed of ACE2 and Ang(1-7), which activate the Mas receptor [6–8]. This system induces vasodilatory, antifibrotic, antihypertrophic, and antiproliferative effects.

2. Aminopeptidases in Arterial Hypertension

A list of the most common aminopeptidases with their enzyme commission (EC) numbers and their main abbreviations is shown in Table 1. As was introduced in the previous paragraph, aminopeptidases (Aps) generate the active compounds of the RAS and play an essential role in BP control and sodium handling [9]. APs can also degrade certain peptidergic hormones or neuropeptides such as vasopressin, cholecystokinin, and enkephalins [10]. For this reason, APs have been analyzed in plasma, kidney, and other tissues related to BP control in several rat models of hypertension.

Table 1. Types of aminopeptidases showing their most common abbreviations.

Enzyme	EC Number	Abbreviations
Leucyl AP	3.4.11.1	LAP
Membrane alanyl AP	3.4.11.2	APN, AlaAP
Cystinyl AP	3.4.11.3	CysAP, CAP
Prolyl AP	3.4.11.5	PIP
Aminopeptidase B	3.4.11.6	APB, ArgAP
Glutamyl AP	3.4.11.7	APA, GluAP, EAP
Aminopeptidase P	3.4.11.9	APP
Cytosol alanyl AP	3.4.11.14	AAP, AlaAP
Methionyl AP	3.4.11.18	eMetAP
Aspartyl AP	3.4.11.21	AspAP, DNPEP
Arginyl AP	3.4.22.16	iRAP, APR

Thus, reduced renal membrane-bound APA, iRAP, and APN activities were observed in a reduced renal mass saline model, and reduced APA activity was detected in a two-kidney one-clip Goldblatt hypertension model [11]. In the low renal mass model, a positive correlation was found in both soluble CAP and APN activities between the neurohypophysis and the adrenal gland, but this was not observed in the normotensive rats [12].

The relationship between APs and arterial hypertension has been explored with greater precision. For instance, it has been proposed that endoplasmic reticulum AP 1 (ERAP1) and ERAP2 regulate BP by inactivation of AngII, and these two APs, which also hydrolyze amino acids from the N-terminus of various human antigens and peptide hormones, are widely expressed in human tissues, including heart, endothelial cells, and kidney [13–15]. In vitro, ERAP1 transforms AngII into AngIII and AngIV [14], while ERAP2 converts AngIII to AngIV [15]. ERAP 1 was initially identified as a placental leucine AP that degrades AngII and III and transforms kallidin into bradykinin in vitro, thus has a role in BP regulation [14].

In this sense, several interesting papers have been published. In an in vivo study, an increase in circulating levels of ERAP1 was found to reduce BP and AngII levels [16]. In a genetic study, an association was detected between variants of the gene encoding Arg528 and the development of essential hypertension in a Japanese population [17]. In an investigation of 45 genetic variants of ERAP1 and ERAP2 in 17,255 Caucasian females from the Women's Genome Health Study, ERAP1 was found to be related to increased BP [18]. The ERAP1 genotype also appears to be involved in the reduction of left ventricular mass produced by some antihypertensive treatments [19]. Thus, all these data indicate a possible role for ERAP1 in BP regulation and ventricular remodeling. Finally, other genetic studies have associated variants of ERAP1 and ERAP2 genes with preeclampsia [20], hemolytic uremia [21], and hypertension [17].

Aminopeptidases after Antihypertensive Therapy

Various systemic antihypertensive treatments can alter the activities of brain and systemic APs associated with effects on BP. Thus, in a rat study by Banegas et al. [22], unilateral brain lesions in the nigrostriatal system produced simultaneous and paralleled changes in BP and in brain and plasma AP activities. Later, the same group [23] examined the participation of APs in the metabolism of some angiotensins, vasopressin, cholecystokinin, and enkephalins in the plasma and hypothalamus of spontaneous hypertensive (SHR) rats under normal conditions and after beta-blocker treatment with propranolol. In this rat strain, AP activity in response to propranolol administration differed between plasma and hypothalamus, thus suggesting an interaction between APs and the autonomic nervous system. Moreover, these authors also reported that treatment with ACE inhibitors captopril, propranolol, or the nitric oxide synthesis inhibitor L-NAME, induced a marked modification of brain patterns of neuropeptidase activity in SHR rats [24].

The BP-lowering effect of a diet enriched in extra virgin olive oil in rats was analyzed by Villarejo et al. [25] who observed that rats receiving this diet showed augmented APN and AspAP activity in the renal cortex, suggesting a greater degradation of AngIII and AngIV and an increased generation of the antihypertensive Ang(2-10). Hence, the glomerular formation of Ang(2-10) might compensate the well-known pressor effects of AngII on the glomerular vasculature in this model of hypertension.

Taken together, the data reported in this section indicate that BP changes induced by antihypertensive or prohypertensive drugs are associated with modifications in AP activity. However, no definitive conclusions can be drawn about the functional role of APs in the pathogenesis of hypertension.

3. Brain APA

Aminopeptidase A (APA) is a 109 kDa homodimeric zinc-metallopeptidase that catalyzes the cleavage of glutamatic and aspartatic amino acid residues from the N-terminus of polypeptides. It is encoded by the ENPEP gene and is also known as glutamyl aminopeptidase, gp160, or CD249.

Numerous studies have demonstrated the major role of brain AngIII and both APA and APN in the control of BP and in arterial hypertension [26]. Thus, the intracerebroventricular (icv) injection of APA to induce the transformation of AngII into AngIII was found to elevate BP in normotensive WKY and SHR animals [27]. In contrast, the icv administration of APN, which hydrolyzes AngIII, reduced the BP in WKY rats and to a greater degree in SHR animals [28]. A study of the icv administration of analogs of AngII and AngIII to SHR rats found that a greater BP increase was induced by AngIII than with AngII [29], thus indicating that a major BP reduction is produced by the inhibition of APA activity and consequent interference in the transformation of AngII to AngIII [30], which suggests a greater contribution of brain AngIII than AngII to the BP increase (Figure 2).

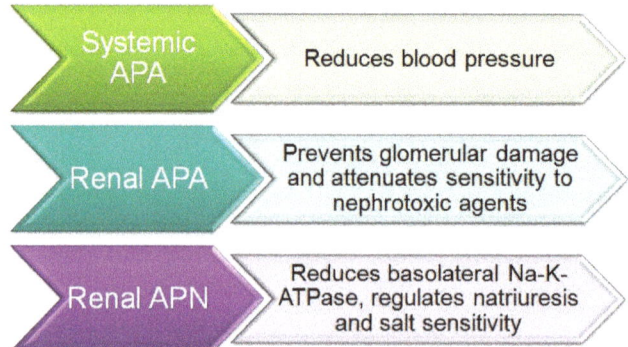

Figure 2. Systemic aminopeptidase A (APA) and aminopeptidase N (APN) in blood pressure control.

Systemic and Renal APA

APA is a membrane-bound enzyme with a major presence in the kidney, in multiple tissues [31], and in a soluble form in the blood, probably due to the cleavage of membrane-bound APA [32]. APA, which thas also been called angiotensinase [33], transforms AngII, the most active systemic peptide, to AngIII, limiting the rate of angiotensin generation [34,35].

The importance of APA in BP control is evidenced by the BP reduction that follows the administration of purified APA [1] and by the BP increase induced by APA inhibitors [36]. In addition, APA-deficient mice are characterized by a high BP and an increased responsiveness to AngII [37]. These data support a role for APA in the regulation of BP under physiological conditions and in hypertensive humans and experimental models.

A study of SHR rats found that a decrease in kidney APA was related to an increase in RAS activity, whereas the administration of APA produced a dose-related reduction in systolic BP [38], showing a 2300-fold increase in activity in comparison to the AT1 blocker candesartan [39]. APA abnormalities have also been observed in the Goldblatt hypertension model [40]. Thus, Prieto et al. [41] reported decreased APA levels in the renal cortex of clipped and non-clipped kidneys in this model, suggesting the involvement of APA in augmenting the AngII-induced reabsorption of sodium and water. Renal RAS is also increased in Dahl salt-sensitive (DSS) rats [42]; in this model, age-related glomerular injury is associated with an increasing elevation of AngII levels because sclerotic glomeruli are less active in synthesizing APA [43]. In human subjects, serum APA activity increases in an age-dependent manner in both men and women [44], and this may be in relation to the metabolic clearance of AngII [45].

At the renal level, Velez et al. [46] observed an increased sensitivity to glomerular damage in APA-deficient BALB/c mice. The authors injected the APA-knockout (KO) mice with a nephrotoxic serum and observed glomerular hyalinosis and albuminuria at 96 h post-administration, whereas no renal injury was observed in the wild-type controls. Likewise, the 4-week infusion of AngII reduced podocyte nephrin levels in APA-KO mice but not in wild-type controls. These data indicate that the degradation of AngII induced by APA plays a protective role in glomerular injury.

Taken together, the above data indicate that an increase in systemic APA protects against hypertension. Conversely, a reduction in the activity of this enzyme maintains high levels of AngII and therefore promotes hypertension (Figure 2). As a conclusion, increased APA activity in the brain raises BP through an increased generation of AngIII, which is the main AT1 receptor agonist in the brain, whereas increased APA activity in the peripheral circulation lowers BP through the degradation of AngII (Figure 2).

4. APN

Aminopeptidase N (APN), also called leucine aminopeptidase and alanyl aminopeptidase, is a homodimeric, membrane-bound, zinc-dependent aminopeptidase [47]. APN cleaves AngIII to AngIV via the scission of arginine at the extreme N-terminus, which indicates its participation in the regulation of tissue and systemic RAS [48]. APN is highly expressed in the central nervous system and kidneys [47,49,50] and may develop multiple actions [47] besides peptide cleavage [51,52]. For this reason, APN is known as a "moonlighting protein" [53].

4.1. Brain APN in BP Regulation

Studies in rodents suggest the participation of brain APN in BP regulation [54]. Thus, icv administration of APN decreased BP in WKY and SHR animals, with more effect in the hypersensitive rats [55]. Conversely, icv administration of bestatin and amistatin, APN inhibitors, raised BP and induced a dipsogenic response in WKY and SHR animals (Figure 3) [55]. The paraventricular nucleus of the hypothalamus appears to be the target for APN in the brain, because its microinfusion at this site reduced BP in both SHR and WKY rats [56,57]. Central APN exerts its effects by transforming the pressor AngIII in the brain into AngIV. In this way, the pressor response induced by icv AngIII is potentiated by the APN antagonists bestatin and amistatin [38,58]. In line with these observations, administration of an angiotensin antagonist was found to inhibit the increase in BP produced by the icv administration of APN inhibitors [30,57].

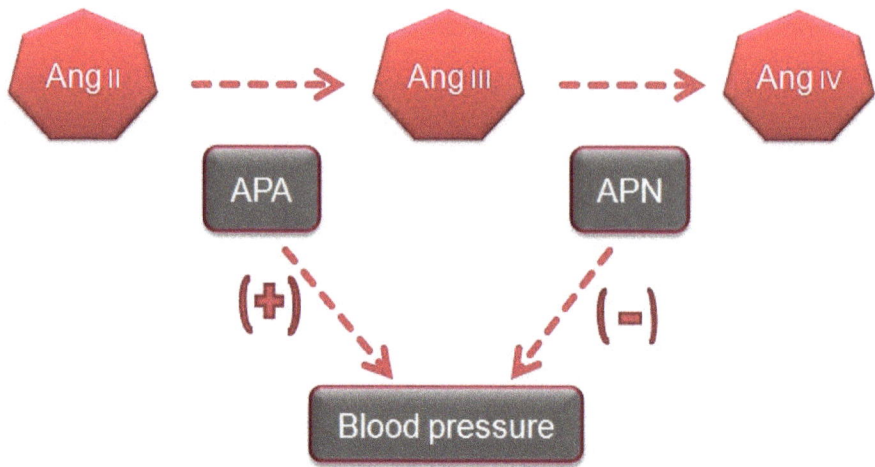

Figure 3. Systemic and renal APA and APN in the control of blood pressure and renal function.

4.2. Renal APN in BP Control

APN is widely distributed in the kidney and has been detected in glomeruli, mesangial cells, and on the luminal surface of tubules [47,58]. Renal APN generates AngIV [59,60], and infusion of AngIV in the renal artery increased sodium excretion [61–63], an effect related to the reduced activity of basolateral tubular Na-K-ATPase [64]. This mechanism may also participate in the adaptive response to increased salt intake, thus protecting against hypertension. Moreover, abnormalities in renal APN have also been observed in several models of experimental hypertension. Thus, the Goldblatt model showed increased APN activity in the renal cortex of the non-clipped kidney [41] and APN protein abundance and activity in the kidney were increased in Dahl salt-resistant versus Dahl salt-sensitive animals (64). APN has also been associated with essential hypertension in humans [65].

APN as a Regulator of Salt Sensitivity

Renal APN regulates mechanisms that facilitate renal sodium excretion after increased saline intake, producing a coordinated decrease in Na-K-ATPase abundance on the basal side of the tubule (by endocytosis) and a reduction in sodium transporters (by internalization) [66–68].

APN abundance is higher in Dahl salt-resistant rats. In these animals, APN may reduce basolateral Na^+-K^+-ATPase as a protective mechanism in response to the increased saline intake [64]. Reduced tissue and plasma APN levels have also been reported in the L-NAME model but not in the controls [68]. In conclusion, renal tubule levels of APN can regulate sodium excretion and, therefore, salt sensitivity and BP.

4.3. Other Actions of APN Related to the Cardiovascular System

APN activation has been reported in diabetic nephropathy, renal damage, connective vascular disease, and cerebral ischemia [69]. In mice, APN is also essential for inflammatory trafficking after coronary artery occlusion and for sustaining the reparative response [70]. Hence, APN blockade of APN is a therapeutic approach to these vascular abnormalities.

Stimulation of AT4 receptors by APN-generated AngIV exerts proangiogenic action. Thus, APN is augmented in pathologic angiogenesis, especially in tumor vasculature [71], and APN blockade reduces angiogenesis in vivo [72]. In APN-null mice, angiogenesis alterations are manifested in pathological situations but not under physiological conditions [73]. According to these observations, APN activity promotes angiogenesis in various conditions and its blockade prevents new blood vessel growth. Indeed, molecular imaging of APN has been used to detect and monitor multiple types of cancer and the surface of vasculature undergoing angiogenesis in cardiac regeneration [74]. Hence, APN is a potential biomarker of angiogenesis and therapeutic tool.

5. Therapeutic Strategies to Treat Arterial Hypertension with Aminopeptidases

The vast majority of studies on the control of BP and treatment of hypertension have addressed the blockade of AngII or its receptors, and there has been less research on the regulation of other angiotensin peptides. Thus, blockade of the brain RAS has been found to simultaneously decrease sympathetic tone, vasopressin release, and baroreflex activity, thereby reducing cardiac output and peripheral resistance [75].

An action on central or peripheral APs represents a new approach to the treatment of hypertension. Thus, new antihypertensive treatments have been developed based on potent orally-active inhibitors of APA or activators of aspartyl-aminopeptidase (DNPEP), since brain aspartyl aminopeptidase exerts BP-lowering effects by transforming AngI into angiotensin 2-10. Currently, the search for new antihypertensive compounds that affect the RAS multi-enzyme cascade is an important line of research.

5.1. Inhibition of APA

The icv administration of EC33, a specific APA inhibitor, prevented the BP increase produced by the icv administration of AngII in SHR animals, indicating that the central response to AngII requires its transformation into AngIII by APA. A marked BP decrease has also been observed in conscious SHR and DOCA-salt hypertensive rats after the icv infusion of EC33 [76,77]. In contrast, the peripheral iv infusion of EC33 did not reduce BP, indicating that EC33 does not cross the blood–brain barrier and/or is inactive in systemic circulation.

The BP of SHR rats increased after the central icv administration of APA [78], probably due to an increased endogenous generation of AngIII, whereas APA blockade with an antiserum attenuated the pressor response to AngII by around 60% [78]. It is interesting to note that a selective APA inhibitor (RB150) with antihypertensive properties can be given either intravenously [77] or orally [79] because it can cross the blood–brain barrier.

The peripheral activity of the AT1 receptor depends on the transformation of AngII into AngIII by APA [80]. Thus, antihypertensive effects were observed in SHR rats after the systemic administration of recombinant APA [81] at a dose that was one-tenth of the usual candesartan dose [82]; the joint i.v. administration of APA and APN attenuated the pressor effect of AngII in normal rats and treatment with APA reduced the BP of SHR rats to normal levels [83].

Considered together, these data clearly demonstrate that APA reduces BP, while abnormalities in APA activity promote hypertension, as supported by the lower renal APA activity in SHR versus WKY rats [84]. The administration of APA has therefore been proposed for the treatment of acute heart failure, acute hypertensive crisis, preeclampsia, and hypertensive encephalopathy, among other hypertensive emergencies [85,86].

5.2. APN Blockade in the Treatment of Hypertension

The administration of PC18, an inhibitor of APN, generates a pressor response through the accumulation of endogenous AngIII, which is mediated via the AT1 receptor. In this way, pretreatment with the AT1 blocker losartan can suppress the pressor response, while the AT2 antagonist PD123319 is unable to prevent the BP increase [87]. The enhanced proximal tubular sodium reabsorption of SHR rats is prevented by the intrarenal infusion of PC18 [88]. This finding indicates that the blockade of

AngIII degradation achieved by APN inhibition improved sodium excretion in the proximal tubule of these rats when it was administered in the renal interstitium [89]. Hence, the transformation of AngII into AngIII is required for this natriuretic response, which is not affected by the AT1 blocker candesartan. Research on the usefulness of APN inhibitors to treat hypertensive patients is at an early stage, and further studies are required.

6. APs as Urinary Biomarkers of Renal Injury

Serum creatinine and blood urea nitrogen (BUN) are widely used markers of renal disease, but their sensitivity and specificity are limited, and they are not useful in distinguishing the stages of acute kidney injury (AKI) [90]. They lack sensitivity because they increase only when the renal lesion is evident. Thus, serum creatinine levels rise gradually, and the kidneys have already lost half of their functionality by the time normal levels are doubled [91,92]. Besides, normal levels of these markers can be affected by protein-rich diets, intestinal bleeding, muscle disease, and dehydration, generating false positives in the diagnosis of renal disease. There is a need for biomarkers to allow an earlier diagnosis of AKI, a better prediction of renal disease severity, and an improved assessment of adverse effects in drug development [90].

Various urinary biomarkers for the early detection of AKI have emerged over recent years [91,92], including tubular enzymes that are increased in urine after damage to the tubular epithelium [92], which can precede or even trigger renal dysfunction. Major advantages of urinary markers include the non-invasiveness of the sampling and their usefulness to elucidate the size and localization of tubular cell lesions and to detect the presence of necrosis or other alterations that evoke renal dysfunction [93]. The measurement of urinary enzymes and other urinary biomarkers may therefore be a valuable tool to obtain an early diagnosis during initial stages of renal disease and to follow its progression or regression, facilitating prediction of the prognosis. Urinary APs are considered promising and useful biomarkers of renal disease of different pathophysiological origin, and an automated photometric assay has been developed for their measurement [94].

APA, APN, and CAP are present in the brush border membrane of renal tubular cells [95], have molecular weights above 140 kDa, and are highly organ-specific. These conditions ensure the tubular origin of these urinary enzymes, which cannot pass easily into the urine through the glomerular barrier (Figure 4).

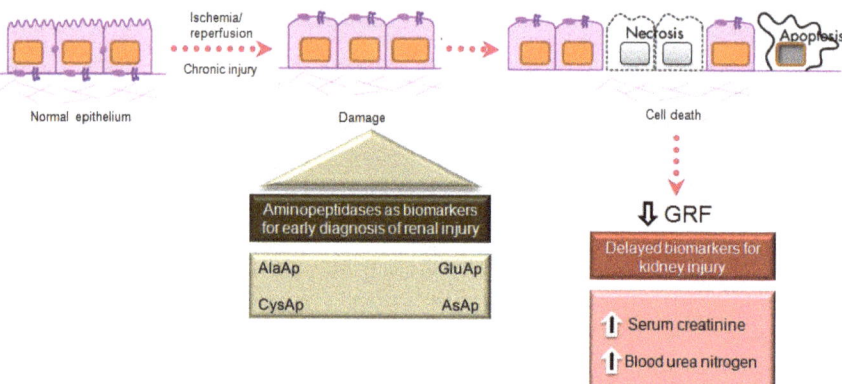

Figure 4. Main aminopeptidases studied as biomarkers of acute and chronic kidney injury.

APs participate in AngII metabolism, forming part of the renal renin–angiotensin–aldosterone system (RAAS) [96], which is elevated in renal diseases. One of these enzymes, alanine aminopeptidase (APN), is a brush border enzyme that was proposed in the early 1970s as a urinary marker of renal disease [97]. Later, Marchewka et al. [98] demonstrated that the measurement of APN and its isoforms was of diagnostic relevance in nephrolithiasis. They also observed significantly higher APN excretion in patients with glomerulonephritis than in controls and a positive correlation between urinary protein concentrations and APN activity [99]. Their findings supported the association between proteinuria and elevated activity of renal tubular brush border enzymes reported in other studies of chronic glomerulonephritis [100]. As an explanation of this association, these authors [99] proposed that the protein present in the ultrafiltrate produces a release of APN from the external membrane of renal tubule microvilli. Because of its external localization, its release into the urine can be caused by a weak destructive action and is not necessarily linked to disruption of the integrity of kidney tubule cells [101].

Jung et al. [102] reported that the urinary excretion of APN, alkaline phosphatase, γ-glutamyltransferase, and N-acetyl-β-D-glucosaminidase is age-dependent in humans. These enzymes were determined in random morning urine samples from 442 individuals aged from 5 days to 58 years, and their creatinine-normalized activity significantly decreased with increasing age. APN activity has also been proposed as a biomarker of the nephrotoxicity induced by vancomycin [101] or amphotericin B [103] in experimental models and in several human diseases, such as glomerulopathy [104], IgA nephropathy [105], and diabetes [106]. However, conflicting results have been published on its usefulness as a biomarker of renal function in kidney transplantation patients [107,108].

Acute Kidney Injury

AKI is defined by an abrupt increase in serum creatinine during the 48 h period after an insult responsible for functional or structural changes in the kidney, and it is mainly caused by the acute apoptosis or necrosis of renal tubular cells [109]. The early detection of AKI is a current preclinical and clinical research priority. The administration of nephrotoxic drugs that alter tubular function is the most common experimental model to relate the excretion of different biomarkers to renal dysfunction. Cisplatin is an antineoplastic drug with a potent nephrotoxic effect, mainly due to its action on the proximal tubule, causing AKI in experimental animal models and patients [110,111]. Its administration induces tubular and glomerular disturbances that lead to the development of interstitial fibrosis [112].

Our group investigated whether urinary activities of APN, APA, and CAP could serve as biomarkers of renal dysfunction by using a rat model of cisplatin-induced nephrotoxicity [113]. Their activity was determined in urine samples collected at 24, 48, and 72 h after cisplatin injection. Their urinary activity at 24 h post-injection was correlated with two renal function indicators (plasma creatinine and creatinine clearance) and their activity at two weeks post-injection was correlated with two indicators of structural damage (renal hypertrophy and interstitial fibrosis). A comparative analysis was also performed with other proposed urinary biomarkers of kidney injury, i.e., albumin, proteinuria, NAG, and NGAL. The area under the curve (AUC) was calculated to quantify the sensitivity and specificity of each marker to distinguish cisplatin-treated from control rats at 24 h post-injection (Figure 5). APN, APA, CAP, and DNPEP had an AUC value greater than 0.5, indicating that these enzymes are early biomarkers of kidney injury in cisplatin-treated rats. The greatest specificity and sensitivity values were observed for APN, which was the best variable to discriminate between treated and untreated animals, whereas an AUC value below 0.5 was observed for NAG and NGAL at this time point. A significant correlation was also found between AP activities at day 1 post-injection and functional and structural variables at day 14. It can therefore be concluded that the urinary activities of these APs may serve as early and predictive biomarkers of cisplatin-induced renal dysfunction. The measurement of urinary AP activities can be useful in preclinical research for the early detection and follow-up of renal damage and for the evaluation of drug nephrotoxicity, and it may offer a useful prognostic and diagnostic tool for renal diseases in the clinical setting.

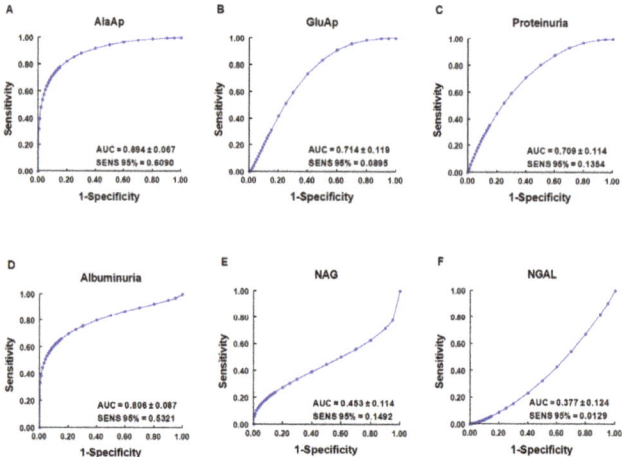

Figure 5. ROC curves showing specificity and sensitivity for APN (AlaAp) (**A**), APA (GluAp) (**B**), proteinuria (**C**), albuminuria (**D**), N-acetyl-β-D-glucosaminidase (NAG) (**E**), and neutrophil gelatinase-associated lipocalin (NGAL) (**F**) to differentiate cisplatin-treated rats from control rats 24 h after injection of saline, 3.5 or 7 mg/kg of cisplatin (n = 8 each group). All cisplatin-treated rats displayed tubular dysplasia and interstitial fibrosis 14 days after injection. Urinary markers were expressed in daily total activity or excretion per 100 g of body weight. AUC = area under the curve. SENS 95 % = calculated sensitivity at 95 % of specificity.

7. Quantification of Urinary APs

APs activities can be readily quantified in biological samples by kinetic methods using photometric [94] or fluorometric [113] assays. Widely applied immunological techniques such as immunoblotting or ELISA can be used to analyze the amount/expression of these proteins in biological samples. Our group used ELISA and Western blot to measure the amount of APN excreted in the urine of cisplatin-treated rats and correlated its excretion 24 h post-injection with increased serum creatinine and decreased body weight at two weeks [114]. In addition, the quantification of APN by ELISA showed a very high correlation with urinary APA activity. The above findings confirm that the immunological determination of this enzyme can also serve as an early marker of renal damage. Further studies are warranted to compare the sensitivity and specificity of kinetic and fluorometric methods in other experimental models and in human diseases that involve renal dysfunction.

7.1. Aminopeptidases in Urinary Vesicles and Exosomes

Extracellular vesicles (EVs) released by the renal epithelium into the tubular fluid are excreted and may be detected in urine samples [115,116]; they include microvesicles and exosomes. Exosomes are nanovesicles (30–120 nm) released by epithelial cells throughout the urinary tract [117,118]. Thus, the exosomic fraction of urine contains potential biomarkers of various renal diseases. Since exosomes secrete mRNAs, miRNAs, and proteins that affect the function of recipient cells [119], it has been proposed that the biological role of exosomes in the kidney is to regulate the co-functionality of different sections of the nephron.

However, the content of biomarkers in urinary microvesicles has not been fully elucidated. The release of microvesicles into the urine has been studied in some renal diseases [120], and their content can also transmit biological signals within the kidney [121–124].

Our group therefore investigated whether the microvesicular and exosomic content of APA in urine was related to cisplatin-induced renal dysfunction in rats [125]. An increased APA content was observed in microvesicular and exosomic fractions at the peak of toxicity, 3 days post-cisplatin injection, and it showed a significant predictive correlation with serum creatinine, regardless of the method of normalization used for APA values (Figure 6). It was concluded that APA content and activity in urinary microvesicles and exosomes may serve as renal dysfunction biomarkers in this nephrotoxicity model.

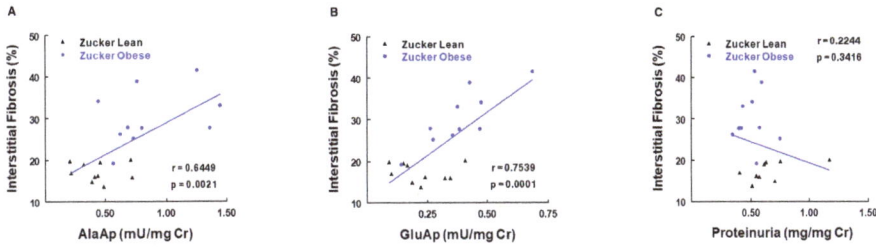

Figure 6. Correlations of urinary activities of APN (AlaAp) (**A**), APA (GluAp) (**B**), and proteinuria (**C**) with percentage of renal interstitial fibrosis in urine samples of Zucker lean and obese rats ($n = 10$ each group). Cr = creatinine (adapted from reference [126]).

Thus, the determination of GluAp in microvesicular and exosomic fractions can be useful to study proximal tubular lesions independently of the glomerular filtration rate. From a technical viewpoint, it is interesting to note that the microvesicular fraction can be obtained more rapidly than can the exosomic fraction. In addition, the analysis of these fractions can avoid interference due to urea content, ionic strength, or other components of urine, because the samples are centrifuged and dissolved in a buffer. According to these observations, examination of the content of the microvesicular fraction can also be a relevant diagnostic tool in nephropathies.

7.2. AKI Induced by Surgical Procedures

Patients undergoing a cardiopulmonary bypass (CPB) can develop AKI as a post-surgical complication. The diagnosis of AKI in these patients is based on an increase in serum creatinine (SCr) concentration over baseline values during the 48 h postoperative period; however, the slow progressive rise of SCr can delay the detection of renal dysfunction. Kim et al. [127] analyzed the serum and urinary enzymatic activity of vasopressinase and SCr in 31 patients at different time points after CPB surgery. Results showed maximum serum and urine activity of vasopressinase at intensive care unit (ICU) admission in patients developing AKI as a complication of CPB earlier than the peak of SCr activity, which is usually observed at 48 h post-surgery. The authors therefore proposed vasopressinase (cystil AP, CAP) activity as an early biomarker for AKI. Animal models of renal ischemia also showed that AKI was related to vasopressinase activity [128].

In a similar study of 103 patients, our group observed a significant increase in urinary APA activity at ICU admission in patients who developed persistent AKI in comparison to those who did not experience AKI or developed only transient AKI. Urinary APA activity showed a higher sensitivity than SCr at this time point, obtaining a higher total number of correctly diagnosed cases in comparison to the application of criteria published by the Acute Kidney Injury Network [129]. These observations also indicate that tubular injury increases the risk of post-surgery AKI.

7.3. Urinary Aminopeptidases as Biomarkers of Renal Dysfunction in Chronic Diseases

7.3.1. Obesity

Obesity and hypertension are chronic diseases that can ultimately lead to renal failure. Experimental models of these diseases have been used for long-term evaluation of the usefulness of urinary APs as renal injury biomarkers.

The obese Zucker rat is an animal model of human type II diabetes [130] characterized by obesity, dyslipidemia, insulin resistance, and kidney damage. Male obese (ZO) and lean (ZL) Zucker rats were studied for 6 months (age of 2–8 months) [131]. At the age of 8 months, ZO rats exhibited various renal lesions, including mild focal and segmental glomerulosclerosis and moderate tubulointerstitial damage. Urinary GluAp (APA) and AlaAp (APN) activities were measured monthly and were increased in ZO rats. Both APA and APN activities correlated with renal lesions and can be considered early diagnostic biomarkers of these lesions (Figure 6). AP activities also showed predictive correlations with the level of interstitial fibrosis in the kidney and with the amount of hydroxyproline accumulated in renal tissue at the age of 8 months. Hence, the early excretion of these markers also serves to evaluate the development of fibrosis in this experimental model.

7.3.2. Hypertension

The SHR model of essential hypertension in humans is widely used [132,133] and is characterized by an increase in BP and development of renal injury as age advances [126,133]. This model has been used to analyze the urinary enzymatic activities of APA, APN, and dipeptidyl peptidase-4 (DPP4) as biomarkers of renal injury in hypertension. These activities were measured in male SHR and WKY rats from the age of 2 to 8 months [134]. The SHR animals did not develop relevant signs of histopathological kidney alterations at the end of the study, but they showed increased glomerular area and cellularity. These activities were increased in monthly-collected urine samples from SHR rats and were correlated with systolic blood pressure throughout the study. Their increased activity in SHR animals indicate that a certain degree of tubular injury can be detected before the appearance of all histopathological manifestations of renal disease. These markers can therefore be used for the diagnosis of renal disease in early stages of hypertension and offer a non-invasive method to follow the progression of renal dysfunction in hypertension and other diseases.

7.3.3. Hyperthyroidism

In rats, hyperthyroidism is an endocrine disease associated with hypertension and renal abnormalities, accelerating the course of experimental hypertension, whereas hypothyroidism is associated with hypotension, preventing the development of hypertension and protecting against renal injury [135]. Ethanol-binding protein and N-acetyl-β-D-glycosaminidase, urinary biomarkers of tubular damage, are increased in hyperthyroid humans [136] and cats [137].

Our group studied the urinary excretion of APN, APA, CAP, and AspAp in control, hyperthyroid, and hypothyroid rats receiving a normal- or high-sodium diet. All APs were augmented in hyperthyroid rats, whereas their levels were similar between hypothyroid and control rats [138]. Hyperthyroid rats receiving a high sodium diet showed increased hypertension, cardiac/renal hypertrophy, albuminuria, and oxidative stress and a marked rise in urinary AP activities. AP activity was modestly elevated in the controls on a high-sodium diet but did not differ between hypothyroid rats on a high- versus normal-sodium diet. According to these results, the combination of T4 treatment and salt exert additive effects on the production of tubular damage, whereas hypothyroidism confers resistance to the effects of high salt intake on urinary AP activities. These findings support previous descriptions of hypothyroid status as beneficial in chronic kidney diseases [139]. It can be concluded that urinary AP activities are diagnostic biomarkers of renal injury in this experimental model. Our group [140] also determined APA activities in renal tissue and plasma samples from adult male euthyroid, hyperthyroid, and hypothyroid rats, and found a significantly higher expression of renal APA in hyperthyroid versus control or hypothyroid rats. However, plasma APA activity was lower in hyperthyroid versus control rats, indicating that the increased APA in these animals is focalized in renal tissue.

7.3.4. Diabetes Mellitus

In a study of urinary levels of enzymes and low-molecular-mass proteins as indicators of diabetes nephropathy, Jung et al. [141] observed an increase in urinary alanine aminopeptidase in diabetic patients and an even greater increase in diabetic patients with proteinuria. However, a study by Lazarevic et al. [106] on the impact of aerobic exercise on microalbuminuria and enzymuria in type II diabetic patients found no significant difference in urinary or plasma APN activities over the study period between patients with and without diabetes or within the diabetes group. Numerous factors may be implicated in these discrepancies between studies.

7.3.5. Urinary APs in Other Chronic Diseases

Sorokman et al. [142] measured urinary levels of renal-specific enzymes (neutral α-glucosidase, L-alanine aminopeptidase, and γ-glutamyltranspeptidase) as markers of proximal tubule damage in children with pyelonephritis, the most common cause of fever in patients with urinary system disorders. They observed an increase in urinary levels of these enzymes during the active phase of pyelonephritis, which correlated with leukocyturia and C-Reactive Protein levels. Finally, Spasovski et al. [143] studied urinary levels of brush border enzymes of the proximal renal tubules (e.g., APN, gamma-glutamyl transferase, and beta2 microglobulin) in patients with untreated rheumatoid arthritis to explore the possible relationship between this disease and dysfunction of the brush border of proximal tubules. They found that urinary APN activity was a superior indicator of asymptomatic renal lesions in untreated rheumatoid arthritis patients compared with measurements of gamma-GT or beta2m.

Author Contributions: All authors have contributed to the review and have read and agreed to the published version of the manuscript.

Funding: This research received no external funding.

Conflicts of Interest: The authors declare no conflict of interest.

Abbreviations

ACE	Angiotensin converting enzyme
AKI	Acute kidney injury
AngI	Angiotensin I
AngII	Angiotensin II
AngIII	Angiotensin III
AngIV	Angiotensin IV
APs	Aminopeptidases
APA	Aminopeptidase A
APN	Aminopeptidase N
AT1	Angiotensin receptor type 1
AT2	Angiotensin receptor type 2
BP	Blood pressure
CAP	Cystinil AP
DOCA	Deoxycorticosterone
L-NAME	N(ω)-nitro-L-arginine methyl ester
RAS	Renin–angiotensin system
SHR	Spontaneous hypertensive rat
WKY	Wistar Kyoto rat
ZO	Zucker obese rats

References

1. Johnston, C.I. Biochemistry and pharmacology of the renin-angiotensin system. *Drugs* **1990**, *39*, 21–31. [CrossRef] [PubMed]
2. Reudelhuber, T.L. The renin-angiotensin system: Peptides and enzymes beyond angiotensin II. *Curr. Opin. Nephrol. Hypertens.* **2005**, *14*, 155–159. [CrossRef] [PubMed]
3. Ferrario, C.M.; Chappell, M.C. Novel Angiotensin peptides. *Cell. Mol. Life. Sci.* **2004**, *61*, 2720–2727. [CrossRef]
4. Vauquelin, G.; Michotte Smolders, Y.I.; Sarre, S.; Ebinger, G.; Dupont, A.; Vanderheyden, P. Cellular targets for angiotensin II fragments: Pharmacological and molecular evidence. *J. Renin Angiotensin Aldosterone Syst.* **2002**, *3*, 195–204. [CrossRef] [PubMed]
5. Enzyme Nomenclature. Recommendations of the Nomenclature Committee of the International Union of Biochemistry and Molecular Biology on the Nomenclature and Classification of Enzymes by the Reactions they Catalyse. Available online: https://www.qmul.ac.uk/sbcs/iubmb/enzyme/ (accessed on 18 June 2020).
6. De Gasparo, M.; Catt, K.J.; Inagami, T.; Wright, J.W.; Unger, T. International union of pharmacology. XXIII. The angiotensin II receptors. *Pharmacol. Rev.* **2000**, *52*, 415–472. [PubMed]
7. Dinh, D.T.; Frauman, A.G.; Johnston, C.I.; Fabiani, M.E. Angiotensin receptors: Distribution, signalling and function. *Clin. Sci.* **2001**, *100*, 481–492. [CrossRef]
8. Chappell, M.C. Nonclassical renin-angiotensin system and renal function. *Compr. Physiol.* **2012**, *2*, 2733–2735. [PubMed]
9. Prieto, I.; Villarejo, A.B.; Segarra, A.B.; Banegas, I.; Wangensteen, R.; Martinez-Cañamero, M.; de Gasparo, M.; Vives, F.; Ramírez-Sánchez, M. Brain, heart and kidney correlate for the control of blood pressure and water balance: Role of angiotensinases. *Neuroendocrinology* **2014**, *100*, 198–208. [CrossRef]
10. Ramírez, M.; Prieto, I.; Alba, F.; Vives, F.; Banegas, I.; de Gasparo, M. Role of central and peripheral aminopeptidase activities in the control of blood pressure: A working hypothesis. *Heart Fail. Rev.* **2008**, *13*, 339–353. [CrossRef]
11. Ramírez, M.; Prieto, I.; Martinez, J.M.; Vargas, F.; Alba, F. Renal aminopeptidase activities in animal models of hypertension. *Regul. Pept.* **1997**, *72*, 155–159. [CrossRef]
12. Prieto, I.; Martinez, A.; Martinez, J.M.; Ramírez, M.J.; Vargas, F.; Alba, F.; Ramírez, M. Activities of aminopeptidases in a rat saline model of volume hypertension. *Horm. Metab. Res.* **1998**, *30*, 246–248. [CrossRef] [PubMed]
13. Tsujimoto, M.; Goto, Y.; Maruyama, M.; Hattori, A. Biochemical and enzymatic properties of the m1 family of aminopeptidases involved in the regulation of blood pressure. *Heart Fail. Rev.* **2008**, *13*, 285–291. [CrossRef] [PubMed]
14. Hattori, A.; Kitatani, K.; Matsumoto, H.; Miyazawa, S.; Rogi, T.; Tsuruoka, N.; Mizutani, S.; Natori, Y.; Tsujimoto, M. Characterization of recombinant human adipocyte-derived leucine aminopeptidase expressed in Chinese hamster ovary cells. *J. Biochem.* **2000**, *128*, 755–762. [CrossRef] [PubMed]
15. Tanioka, T.; Hattori, A.; Masuda, S.; Nomura, Y.; Nakayama, H.; Mizutani, S.; Tsujimoto, M. Human leukocytederived arginine aminopeptidase. The third member of the oxytocinase subfamily of aminopeptidases. *J. Biol. Chem.* **2003**, *278*, 32275–32283. [CrossRef] [PubMed]
16. Hisatsune, C.; Ebisui, E.; Usui, M.; Ogawa, N.; Suzuki, A.; Mataga, N.; Hiromi Takahashi-Iwanaga, H.; Katsuhiko Mikoshiba, K. ERp44 exerts redox dependent control of blood pressure at the ER. *Mol. Cell* **2015**, *58*, 1015–1027. [CrossRef] [PubMed]
17. Yamamoto, N.; Nakayama, J.; Yamakawa-Kobayashi, K.; Hamaguchi, H.; Miyazaki, R.; Arinami, T. Identification of 33 polymorphisms in the adipocyte-derived leucine aminopeptidase (ALAP) gene and possible association with hypertension. *Hum. Mutat.* **2002**, *19*, 251–257. [CrossRef]
18. Robert, Y.; Zee, L.; Rivera, A.; Inostroza, Y.; Ridker, P.M.; Daniel, I.; Chasman, D.I.; Romero, J.R. Gene variation of endoplasmic reticulum aminopeptidases 1 and 2, and risk of blood pressure progression and incident hypertension among 17,255 initially healthy women. *Int. J. Genom.* **2018**, *2018*, 2308585.
19. Hallberg, P.; Lind, L.; Michaelsson, K.; Kurland, L.; Kahan, T.; Malmqvist, K.; Ohman, K.P.; Nystrom, F.; Liljedahl, U.; Syvanen, A.C.; et al. Adipocyte-derived leucine aminopeptidase genotype and response to antihypertensive therapy. *BMC Cardiovasc. Disord.* **2003**, *3*, 11. [CrossRef]

20. Johnson, M.P.; Roten, L.T.; Dyer, T.D.; East, C.E.; Forsmo, S.; Blangero, J.; Brennecke, S.P.; Austgulen, R.; Moses, E.K. The ERAP2 gene is associated with preeclampsia in Australian and Norwegian populations. *Hum. Genet.* **2009**, *126*, 655–666. [CrossRef]
21. Taranta, A.; Gianviti, A.; Palma, A.; De Luca, V.; Mannucci, L.; Procaccino, M.A.; Ghiggeri, G.M.; Caridi, G.; Fruci, D.; Ferracuti, S.; et al. Genetic risk factors in typical haemolytic uraemic syndrome. *Nephrol. Dial. Transplant.* **2009**, *24*, 1851–1857. [CrossRef]
22. Banegas, I.; Ramírez, M.; Vives, F.; Alba, F.; Segarra, A.B.; Duran, R.; De Gasparo, M.; Prieto, I. Aminopeptidase activity in the nigrostriatal system and prefrontal cortex of rats with experimental hemiparkinsonism. *Horm. Metab. Res.* **2005**, *37*, 53–55. [CrossRef] [PubMed]
23. Prieto, I.; Segarra, A.B.; de Gasparo, M.; Martínez-Cañamero, M.; Ramírez-Sánchez, M. Divergent profile between hypothalamic and plasmatic aminopeptidase activities in WKY and SHR. Influence of beta-adrenergic blockade. *Life Sci.* **2018**, *192*, 9–17. [CrossRef] [PubMed]
24. Prieto, I.; Segarra, A.B.; Villarejo, A.B.; de Gasparo, M.; Martínez-Cañamero, M.M.; Ramírez-Sánchez, M. Neuropeptidase activity in the frontal cortex of Wistar-Kyoto and spontaneously hypertensive rats treated with vasoactive drugs: A bilateral study. *J. Hypertens.* **2019**, *37*, 612–628. [CrossRef] [PubMed]
25. Villarejo, A.B.; Ramírez-Sánchez, M.; Segarra, A.B.; Martínez-Cañamero, M.; Prieto, I. Influence of extra virgin olive oil on blood pressure and kidney angiotensinase activities in spontaneously hypertensive rats. *Planta Med.* **2015**, *81*, 664–669. [CrossRef]
26. Wright, J.W.; Mizutani, S.; Harding, J.W. Focus on Brain Angiotensin III and Aminopeptidase A in the Control of Hypertension. *Int. J. Hypertens.* **2012**, *2012*, 124758. [CrossRef]
27. Wright, J.W.; Mizutani, S.; Murray, C.E.; Amir, H.Z.; Harding, J.W. Aminopeptidase-induced elevations and reductions in blood pressure in the spontaneously hypertensive rat. *J. Hypertens.* **1990**, *8*, 969–974. [CrossRef]
28. Jensen, L.L.; Harding, J.W.; Wright, J.W. Increased blood pressure induced by central application of aminopeptidase inhibitors is angiotensinergic-dependent in normotensive and hypertensive rat strains. *Brain Res.* **1989**, *490*, 48–55. [CrossRef]
29. Wright, J.W.; Roberts, K.A.; Cook, V.I.; Murray, C.E.; Sardinia, M.F.; Harding, J.W. Intracerebroventricularly infused [D-Arg1]angiotensin III, is superior to [D-Asp1]angiotensin II, as a pressor agent in rats. *Brain Res.* **1990**, *514*, 5–10. [CrossRef]
30. Wright, J.W.; Tamura-Myers, E.; Wilson, W.L.; Roques, B.P.; Llorens-Cortes, C.; Speth, R.C.; Harding, J.W. Conversion of brain angiotensin II to angiotensin III is critical for pressor response in rats. *Am. J. Physiol. Regul. Integr. Comp. Physiol.* **2003**, *284*, R725–R733. [CrossRef]
31. Lodja, Z.; Gossrau, R. Study on aminopeptidase A. *Histochemistry* **1980**, *67*, 237–290.
32. Wright, J.W.; Harding, J.W. Brain angiotensin receptor subtypes AT1, AT2 and AT4 and their functions. *Regul. Pept.* **1995**, *59*, 269–295. [CrossRef]
33. Speth, R.C.; Thompson, S.M.; Johns, S.J. Angiotensin II receptors: Structural and functional considerations. *Adv. Exp. Med. Biol.* **1995**, *377*, 169–192. [PubMed]
34. Mizutani, S.; Akiyama, H.; Kurauchi, O.; Taira, H.; Narita, O.; Tomoda, Y. In vitro degradation of angiotensin II (A-II) by human placental subcellular fractions, pregnancy sera and purified placental aminopeptidases. *Acta Endocrinol.* **1985**, *110*, 135–139. [CrossRef]
35. Yamada, R.; Mizutani, S.; Kurauchi, O.; Okano, K.; Imaizumi, H.; Narita, O.; Tomoda, Y. Purification and characterization of human placental aminopeptidase A. *Enzyme* **1988**, *40*, 223–230. [CrossRef]
36. Chauvel, E.N.; Llorens-Cortes, C.; Coric, P.; Wilk, S.; Roques, B.P.; Fournie-Zaluski, M.C. Differential inhibition of aminopeptidase A and aminopeptidase N by new-amino thiols. *J. Med. Chem.* **1994**, *37*, 2950–2957. [CrossRef] [PubMed]
37. Mitsui, T.; Nomura, S.; Okada, M.; Ohno, Y.; Kobayashi, H.; Nakashima, Y.; Murata, Y.; Takeuchi, M.; Kuno, N.; Nagasaka, T.; et al. Hypertension and Angiotensin II hypersensitivity in aminopeptidase A-deficient mice. *Mol. Med.* **2003**, *9*, 57–62. [CrossRef]
38. Mizutani, S.; Furuhashi, M.; Imaizumi, H.; Ito, Y.; Kurauchi, O.; Tomoda, Y. Effects of human placental aminopeptidases in spontaneously hypertensive rats. *Med. Sci. Res.* **1987**, *15*, 1203–1204.
39. Goto, Y.; Hattori, A.; Ishii, Y.; Mizutani, S.; Tsujimoto, M. Enzymatic properties of aminopeptidase A: Regulation of its enzymatic activity by calcium and angiotensin IV. *J. Biol. Chem.* **2006**, *281*, 23503–23513. [CrossRef]

40. Bivol, L.M.; Vagnes, O.B.; Iversen, B.M. The renal vascular response to ANG II injection is reduced in the nonclipped kidney of two-kidney, one-clip hypertension. *Am. J. Physiol. Ren. Physiol.* **2005**, *289*, F393–F400. [CrossRef]
41. Prieto, I.; Hermoso, F.; Gaspara, M.; Vargas, F.; Alba, F.; Segarra, A.B.; Banegas, I.; Ramirez, M. Angiotensinase activities in the kidney of renovascular hypertensive rats. *Peptides* **2003**, *24*, 755–760. [CrossRef]
42. Kobori, H.; Nishiyama, A.; Abe, Y.; Navar, G. Enhancement of intrarenal angiotensinogen in Dahl salt-sensitive rats on high salt diet. *Hypertension* **2003**, *41*, 592–597. [CrossRef] [PubMed]
43. Nomura, M.; Nomura, S.; Mitsui, T.; Suzuki, T.; Kobayashi, H.; Ito, T.; Itakura, A.; Kikkawa, F.; Mizutani, S. (2005) Possible involvement of aminopeptidase A in hypertension and renal damage in Dahl saltsensitive rats. *Am. J. Hypertens.* **2005**, *18*, 538–543. [CrossRef] [PubMed]
44. Martinez, J.M.; Prieto, I.; Ramirez, M.J.; de Gasparo, M.; Hermoso, F.; Arias, J.M.; Alba, F.; Ramirez, M. Sex differences and agerelated changes in human serum aminopeptidase A activity. *Clin. Chim. Acta* **1998**, *274*, 53–61. [CrossRef]
45. Baylis, C.; Engels, K.; Hymel, A.; Navar, L.G. Plasma rennin activity and metabolic rate of angiotensin II in the unstressed aging rat. *Mech. Aging Dev.* **1997**, *97*, 163–172. [CrossRef]
46. Velez, J.C.; Arif, E.; Rodgers, J.; Hicks, M.P.; Arthur, J.M.; Nihalani, D.; Bruner, E.T.; Budisavljevic, M.N.; Atkinson, C.; Fitzgibbon, W.R.; et al. Deficiency of the Angiotensinase Aminopeptidase A Increases Susceptibility to Glomerular Injury. *J. Am. Soc. Nephrol.* **2017**, *28*, 2119–2132. [CrossRef] [PubMed]
47. Sjostrom, H.; Noren, O.; Olsen, J. Structure and function of aminopeptidase N. *Adv. Exp. Med. Biol.* **2000**, *477*, 25–34.
48. Paul, M.; Poyan, M.A.; Kreutz, R. Physiology of local renin-angiotensin systems. *Physiol. Rev.* **2006**, *86*, 747–803. [CrossRef]
49. Robert, S.D. Aminopeptidase N in arterial hypertension. *Heart Fail. Rev.* **2008**, *13*, 293–298.
50. Amin, S.A.; Adhikari, N.; Jha, T. Design of aminopeptidase N inhibitors as anti-cancer agents. *J. Med. Chem.* **2018**, *61*, 6468–6490.
51. Dan, H.; Tani, K.; Hase, K.; Shimizu, T.; Tamiya, H.; Biraa, Y.; Huang, L.; Yanagawa, H.; Sone, S. CD13/aminopeptidase N in collagen vascular diseases. *Rheumatol. Int.* **2003**, *23*, 271–276. [CrossRef]
52. Khatun, A.; Kang, K.H.; Ryu, D.Y.; Rahman, M.S.; Kwon, W.S.; Pang, M.G. Effect of Aminopeptidase N on functions and fertility of mouse spermatozoa in vitro. *Theriogenology* **2018**, *118*, 182–189. [CrossRef] [PubMed]
53. Mina-Osorio, P. The moonlighting enzyme CD13: Old and new functions to target. *Trends Mol. Med.* **2008**, *14*, 361–371. [CrossRef]
54. Banegas, I.; Prieto, I.; Vives, F.; Alba, F.; de Gasparo, M.; Segarra, A.B.; Hermoso, F.; Durán, R.; Ramírez, M. Brain aminopeptidases and hypertension. *J. Renin Angiotensin Aldosterone Syst.* **2006**, *7*, 129–134. [CrossRef] [PubMed]
55. Wright, J.W.; Jensen, L.L.; Cushing, L.L.; Harding, J.W. Leucine aminopeptidase M-induced reductions in blood pressure in spontaneously hypertensive rats. *Hypertension* **1989**, *13*, 910–915. [CrossRef] [PubMed]
56. Batt, C.M.; Jensen, L.L.; Harding, J.W.; Wright, J.W. Microinfusion of aminopeptidase M into the paraventricular nucleus of the hypothalamus in normotensive and hypertensive rats. *Brain Res. Bull.* **1996**, *39*, 235–240. [CrossRef]
57. Abhold, R.H.; Sullivan, M.J.; Wright, J.W.; Harding, J.W. Binding, degradation and pressor activity of angiotensins II and III after aminopeptidase inhibition with amastatin and bestatin. *J. Pharmacol. Exp. Ther.* **1987**, *242*, 957–962.
58. Kenny, A.J.; Maroux, S. Topology of microvillar membrane hydrolases of kidney and intestine. *Physiol. Rev.* **1982**, *62*, 91–128. [CrossRef]
59. Albiston, A.L.; McDowall, S.G.; Matsacos, D.; Sim, P.; Clune, E.; Mustafa, T.; Lee, J.; Mendelsohn, F.A.; Simpson, R.J.; Connolly, L.M.; et al. Evidence that the angiotensin IV [AT(4)] receptor is the enzyme insulin-regulated aminopeptidase. *J. Biol. Chem.* **2001**, *276*, 48623–48626. [CrossRef]
60. Chai, S.Y.; Fernando, R.; Peck, G.; Ye, S.Y.; Mendelsohn, F.A.; Jenkins, T.A.; Albiston, A.L. The angiotensin IV/AT4 receptor. *Cell. Mol. Life Sci.* **2004**, *61*, 2728–2737. [CrossRef]
61. Hamilton, T.A.; Handa, R.K.; Harding, J.W.; Wright, J.W. A role for the angiotensin IV/AT4 system in mediating natriuresis in the rat. *Peptides* **2001**, *22*, 935–944. [CrossRef]
62. Handa, R.K.; Krebs, L.T.; Harding, J.W.; Handa, S.E. Angiotensin IV AT4-receptor system in the rat kidney. *Am. J. Physiol. Ren. Physiol.* **1998**, *274*, F290–F299. [CrossRef] [PubMed]

63. Kotlo, K.; Shukla, S.; Tawar, U.; Skidgel, R.A.; Danziger, R.S. Aminopeptidase N reduces basolateral Na_-K_-ATPase in proximal tubule cells. *Am. J. Physiol. Ren. Physiol.* **2007**, *293*, F1047–F1053. [CrossRef] [PubMed]
64. Farjah, M.; Roxas, B.; Danziger, R.S. Dietary NaCl regulates in renal APN transcript/protein abundance and activity: Relevance to hypertension in the Dahl rat. *Hypertension* **2004**, *43*, 282–285. [CrossRef]
65. Williams, J.S.; Raji, A.; Williams, G.H.; Conlin, P.R. Nonmodulating hypertension is associated with insulin resistance and the Lys528Arg variant human adipocyte-derived leucine aminopeptidase. *Hypertension* **2006**, *48*, 331–336.
66. Ogimoto, G.; Yudowski, G.A.; Barker, C.J.; Kohler, M.; Katz, A.I.; Feraille, E.; Pedemonte, C.H.; Berggren, P.O.; Bertorello, A.M. G protein-coupled receptors regulate Na,K-ATPase activity and endocytosis by modulating the recruitment of adaptor protein 2 and clathrin. *Proc. Natl. Acad. Sci. USA* **2000**, *97*, 3242–3247. [CrossRef] [PubMed]
67. Periyasamy, S.M.; Liu, J.; Tanta, F.; Kabak, B.; Wakefield, B.; Malhotra, D.; Kennedy, D.J.; Nadoor, A.; Fedorova, O.V.; Gunning, W.; et al. Salt loading induces redistribution of the plasmalemmal Na-K-ATPase in proximal tubule cells. *Kidney Int.* **2005**, *67*, 1868–1877. [CrossRef]
68. Linardi, A.; Panunto, P.C.; Ferro, E.S.; Hyslop, S. Peptidase activities in rats treated chronically with N (omega)-nitro-L-arginine methyl ester (L-NAME). *Biochem. Pharmacol.* **2004**, *68*, 205–214. [CrossRef]
69. Röhnert, P.; Schmidt, W.; Emmerlich, P.; Goihl, A.; Wrenger, S.; Bank, U.; Nordhoff, K.; Täger, M.; Ansorge, S.; Reinhold, D.; et al. Dipeptidyl peptidase IV, aminopeptidase N and DPIV/APN-like proteases in cerebral ischemia. *J. Neuroinflamm.* **2012**, *9*, 44. [CrossRef]
70. Pereira, F.E.; Cronin, C.; Ghosh, M.; Zhou, S.Y.; Agosto, M.; Subramani, J.; Wang, R.; Shen, J.B.; Schacke, W.; Liang, B.; et al. CD13 is essential for inflammatory trafficking and infarct healing following permanent coronary artery occlusion in mice. *Cardiovasc. Res.* **2013**, *100*, 74–83. [CrossRef]
71. Khakoo, A.Y.; Sidman, R.L.; Pasqualini, R.; Arap, W. Does the renin-angiotensin system participate in regulation of human vasculogenesis and angiogenesis? *Cancer Res.* **2008**, *68*, 9112–9115. [CrossRef]
72. Pasqualini, R.; Koivunen, E.; Kain, R.; Lahdenranta, J.; Sakamoto, M.; Stryhn, A.; Ashmun, R.A.; Shapiro, L.H.; Arap, W.; Ruoslahti, E. Aminopeptidase N is a receptor for tumor-homing peptides and a target for inhibiting angiogenesis. *Cancer Res.* **2000**, *60*, 722–727.
73. Rangel, R.; Sun, Y.; Guzman-Rojas, L.; Ozawa, M.G.; Sun, J.; Giordano, R.J.; Van Pelt, C.S.; Tinkey, P.T.; Behringer, R.R.; Sidman, R.L.; et al. Impaired angiogenesis in aminopeptidase N-null mice. *Proc. Natl. Acad. Sci. USA* **2007**, *104*, 4588–4593. [CrossRef] [PubMed]
74. Schreiber, C.L.; Smith, B.D. Molecular Imaging of Aminopeptidase N in Cancer and Angiogenesis. *Contrast Media Mol. Imaging* **2018**, *2018*, 5315172. [CrossRef] [PubMed]
75. Marc, Y.; Llorens-Cortes, C. The role of the brain renin-angiotensin system in hypertension: Implications for new treatment. *Prog. Neurobiol.* **2011**, *95*, 89–103. [CrossRef] [PubMed]
76. Morton, J.J.; Casals-Stenzel, J.; Lever, A.F. Inhibitors of the renin-angiotensin system in experimental hypertension, with a note on the measurement of angiotensin I, II and III during infusion of converting-enzyme inhibitor. *Br. J. Clin. Pharmacol.* **1979**, *2*, 233S–241S. [CrossRef]
77. Fournie-Zaluski, M.C.; Fassot, C.; Valentin, B.; Djordjijevic, D.; Reaux-Le Goazigo, A.; Corvol, P.; Roques, B.P.; Llorens-Cortes, C. Brain renin-angiotensin system blockade by systemically active aminopeptidase A inhibitors: A potential treatment of salt-dependent hypertension. *Proc. Natl. Acad. Sci. USA* **2004**, *101*, 7775–7780. [CrossRef]
78. Song, L.; Wilk, S.; Healy, D.P. Aminopeptidase A antiserum inhibits intracerebroventricular angiotensin II induced dipsogenic and pressor responses. *Brain Res.* **1997**, *744*, 1–6. [CrossRef]
79. Bodineau, L.; Frugière, A.; Marc, Y.; Inguimbert, N.; Fassot, C.; Balavoine, F.; Roques, B.; Llorens-Cortes, C. Orally active aminopeptidase A inhibitors reduce blood pressure: A new strategy for treating hypertension. *Hypertension* **2008**, *51*, 1318–1325. [CrossRef]
80. Wright, J.W.; Harding, J.W. Brain renin-angiotensin-A new look at an old system. *Prog. Neurobiol.* **2011**, *95*, 49–67. [CrossRef]
81. Goto, Y.; Hattori, A.; Ishii, Y.; Tsujimoto, M. Reduced activity of the hypertension-associated Lys528Arg mutant of human adipocyte-derived leucine aminopeptidase (ALAP)/ ER-aminopeptidase-1. *FEBS Lett.* **2006**, *580*, 1833–1838. [CrossRef]

82. Ishii, M.; Hattori, A.; Numaguchi, Y.; Tsujimoto, M.; Ishiura, S.; Kobayashi, H.; Murohara, T.; Wrght, J.W.; Mizutani, S. The effect of recombinant aminopeptidase a on hypertension in spontaneously hypertensive rats: Its effect in comparison with candesartan. *Horm. Metab. Res.* **2008**, *40*, 887–891. [CrossRef] [PubMed]
83. Mizutani, S.; Okano, K.; Hasegawa, E. Human placental leucine aminopeptidase (P-LAP) as a hypotensive agent. *Experientia* **1982**, *38*, 821–822. [CrossRef] [PubMed]
84. Nakashima, Y.; Ohno, Y.; Itakura, A.; Takeuchi, M.; Murata, Y.; Kuno, N.; Mizutani, S. Possible involvement of aminopeptidase A in hypertension in spontaneously hypertensive rats (SHRs) and change of refractoriness in response to angiotensin II in pregnant SHRs. *J. Hypertens.* **2002**, *20*, 2233–2238. [CrossRef] [PubMed]
85. Mizutani, S.; Wright, J.; Kobayashi, H. A new approach regarding the treatment of preeclampsia and preterm labor. *Life Sci.* **2011**, *88*, 17–23. [CrossRef]
86. Kobayashi, H.; Mizutani, S.; Wright, J.W. Placental leucine aminopeptidase- and aminopeptidase A-deficient mice offer insight concerning the mechanisms underlying preterm labor and preeclampsia. *J. Biomed. Biotechnol.* **2011**, *2011*, 286947.
87. Carey, R.M.; Padia, S.H. Role of angiotensin at2 receptors in natriuresis: Intrarenal mechanisms and therapeutic potential. *Clin. Exp. Pharmacol. Physiol.* **2013**, *40*, 527–534. [CrossRef]
88. Padia, S.H.; Howell, N.L.; Kemp, B.A.; Fournie-Zaluski, M.C.; Roques, B.P.; Carey, R.M. Intrarenal aminopeptidase N inhibition restores defective angiotensin II type 2-mediated natriuresis in spontaneously hypertensive rats. *Hypertension* **2010**, *55*, 474–480. [CrossRef]
89. Padia, S.H.; Kemp, B.A.; Howell, N.L.; Gildea, J.J.; Keller, S.R.; Carey, R.M. Intrarenal angiotensin III infusion induces natriuresis and angiotensin type 2 receptor translocation in Wistar-Kyoto but not in spontaneously hypertensive rats. *Hypertension* **2009**, *53*, 338–343. [CrossRef]
90. Vaidya, V.S.; Ferguson, M.A.; Bonventre, J.V. Biomarkers of acute kidney injury. *Annu. Rev. Pharmacol. Toxicol.* **2008**, *48*, 463–493. [CrossRef]
91. Bonventre, J.V.; Vaidya, V.S.; Schmouder, R.; Feig, P.; Dieterle, F. Nextgeneration biomarkers for detecting kidney toxicity. *Nat. Biotechnol.* **2010**, *28*, 436–440. [CrossRef]
92. Devarajan, P. Emerging biomarkers of acute kidney injury. *Contrib. Nephrol.* **2007**, *156*, 203–212. [PubMed]
93. Lisowska-Myjak, B. Serum and urinary biomarker of acute kidney injury. *Blood. Purif.* **2010**, *29*, 357–365. [CrossRef] [PubMed]
94. Holdt, B.; Peters, E.; Nagel, H.R.; Steiner, M. An automated assay of urinary alanine aminopeptidase activity. *Clin. Chem. Lab. Med.* **2008**, *46*, 537–540. [CrossRef] [PubMed]
95. Song, L.; Ye, M.; Troyanovskaya, M.; Wilk, E.; Wilk, S.; Healy, D.P. Rat kidney glutamyl aminopeptidase (aminopeptidase A): Molecular identity and cellular localization. *Am. J. Physiol.* **1994**, *267*, F546–F557. [CrossRef] [PubMed]
96. Segarra, A.B.; Ramírez, M.; Banegas, I.; Hermoso, F.; Vargas, F.; Vives, F.; Alba, F.; de Gasper, M.; Prieto, I. Influence of thyroid disorders on kidney angiotensinase activity. *Horm. Metab. Res.* **2006**, *38*, 48–52. [CrossRef]
97. Peters, J.E.; Mampel, E.; Schneider, I.; Burchardt, U.; Fukala, E.; Ahrens, I.; Haschen, R.J. Alanine aminopeptidase in urine in renal diseases. *Clin. Chim. Acta* **1972**, *37*, 213–224. [CrossRef]
98. Marchewka, Z.; Długosz, A.; Kúzniar, J. Diagnostic application of AAP isoenzyme separation. *Int. Urol. Nephrol.* **1999**, *31*, 409–416. [CrossRef]
99. Marchewka, Z.; Kúzniar, J.; Długosz, A. Enzymuria and β2-Mikroglobulinuria in the assessment of the influence of proteinuria on the progression of glomerulopathies. *Int. Urol. Nephrol.* **2001**, *33*, 673–676. [CrossRef]
100. Idasiak-Piechocka, I.; Krzymánski, M. The role of tubulointerstitial changes in progression of chronic glomerulonephritis (GN). *Przegl. Lek.* **1996**, *53*, 443–453.
101. Naghibi, B.; Ghafghazi, T.; Hajhashemi, V.; Talebi, A. Vancomycin-induced nephrotoxicity in rats: Is enzyme elevation a consistent finding in tubular injury? *J. Nephrol.* **2007**, *20*, 482–488.
102. Jung, K.; Hempel, A.; Grutzmann, K.D.; Hempel, R.D.; Schreiber, G. Age-dependent excretion of alanine aminopeptydase, alkaline phosphatase, γ-glutamyltransferase and N-acetyl-β-D-glucosaaminidase in human urine. *Enzyme* **1990**, *43*, 10–16. [CrossRef] [PubMed]
103. Inselmann, G.; Balaschke, M.; Heidemann, H.T. Enzymuria following amphotericin B application in the rat. *Mycoses* **2003**, *46*, 169–173. [CrossRef] [PubMed]

104. Mitic, B.; Lazarevic, G.; Vlahovic, P.; Rajic, M.; Stefanovic, V. Diagnostic value of the aminopeptidase N, N-acetyl-beta-D-glucosaminidase and dipeptidylpeptidase IV in evaluating tubular dysfunction in patients with glomerulopathies. *Ren. Fail.* **2008**, *30*, 896–903. [CrossRef] [PubMed]
105. Moon, P.G.; Lee, J.E.; You, S.; Kim, T.K.; Cho, J.H.; Kim, I.S.; Kwon, T.H.; Kim, C.D.; Park, S.H.; Hwang, D.; et al. Proteomic analysis of urinary exosomes from patients of early IgA nephropathy and thin basement membrane nephropathy. *Proteomics* **2011**, *11*, 2459–2475. [CrossRef] [PubMed]
106. Lazarevic, G.; Antic, S.; Vlahovic, P.; Djordjevic, V.; Zvezdanovic, L.; Stefanovic, V. Effects of aerobic exercise on microalbuminuria and enzymuria in type 2 diabetic patients. *Ren. Fail.* **2007**, *29*, 199–205. [CrossRef] [PubMed]
107. Kuzniar, J.; Marchewka, Z.; Krasnowski, R.; Boratynska, M.; Długosz, A.; Klinger, M. Enzymuria and low molecular weight protein excretion as the differentiating marker of complications in the early post kidney transplantation period. *Int. Urol. Nephrol.* **2006**, *38*, 753–758. [CrossRef]
108. Marchewka, Z.; Kuzniar, J.; Zynek-Litwin, M.; Falkiewicz, K.; Szymanska, B.; Roszkowska, A.; Klinger, M. Kidney graft function in long-term cyclosporine and tacrolimus treatment: Comparative study with nephrotoxicity markers. *Transplant. Proc.* **2009**, *41*, 1660–1665. [CrossRef]
109. Molitoris, B.A.; Levin, A.; Warnock, D.G.; Joannidis, M.; Mehta, R.L.; Kellum, J.A.; Ronco, C.; Shah, S. Improving outcomes from acute kidney injury. *J. Am. Soc. Nephrol.* **2007**, *18*, 1992–1994. [CrossRef]
110. Safirstein, R.; Winston, J.; Moel, D.; Dikman, S.; Guttenplan, J. Cisplatin nephrotoxicity-insights into mechanism. *Int. J. Androl.* **1987**, *10*, 325–346. [CrossRef]
111. Winston, J.A.; Safirstein, R. Reduced renal blood-flow in early cisplatin induced acute renal failure in the rat. *Am. J. Physiol.* **1985**, *249*, F490–F496. [CrossRef]
112. Yao, X.; Panichpisal, K.; Kurtzman, N.; Nugent, K. Cisplatin nephrotoxicity: A review. *Am. J. Med. Sci.* **2007**, *334*, 115–124. [CrossRef] [PubMed]
113. Quesada, A.; Vargas, F.; Montoro-Molina, S.; O'Valle, F.; Rodríguez-Martínez, M.D.; Osuna, A.; Prieto, I.; Ramírez, M.; Wangensteen, F. Urinary Aminopeptidase Activities as Early and Predictive Biomarkers of Renal Dysfunction in Cisplatin-Treated Rats. *PLoS ONE* **2012**, *7*, e40402. [CrossRef] [PubMed]
114. Montoro-Molina, S.; Quesada, A.; Zafra-Ruiz, P.V.; O'Valle, F.; Vargas, F.; de Gracia, M.C.; Osuna, A.; Wangensteen, F. Immunological detection of glutamyl aminopeptidase in urine samples from cisplatin-treated rats. *Proteom. Clin. Appl.* **2015**, *9*, 630–635. [CrossRef] [PubMed]
115. Salih, M.; Zietse, R.; Hoorn, E.J. Urinary extracellular vesicles and the kidney: Biomarkers and beyond. *Am. J. Physiol. Ren. Physiol.* **2014**, *306*, 1251–1259. [CrossRef] [PubMed]
116. Gámez-Valero, A.; Lozano-Ramos, S.I.; Bancu, I.; Lauzurica-Valdemoros, R.; Borras, F.E. Urinary extracellular vesicles as source of biomarkers in kidney diseases. *Front. Inmunol.* **2015**, *6*, 6.
117. Pisitkun, T.; Johnstone, R.; Knepper, M.A. Discovery of urinary biomarkers. *Mol. Cell. Proteom.* **2006**, *5*, 1760–1771. [CrossRef]
118. Ohno, S.; Ishikawa, A.; Kuroda, M. Roles of exosomes and microvesicles in disease pathogenesis. *Adv. Drug. Deliv. Rev.* **2013**, *65*, 398–401. [CrossRef]
119. Dimov, I.; Jankovic, V.L.; Stefanovic, V. Urinary exosomes. *Sci. World J.* **2009**, *9*, 1107–1118. [CrossRef]
120. Jayachandran, M.; Lugo, G.; Heiling, H.; Miller, V.M.; Rule, A.D.; Lieske, J.C. Extracellular vesicles in urine of women with but not without kidney stones manifest patterns similar to men: A case control study. *Biol. Sex. Differ.* **2015**, *6*, 2. [CrossRef]
121. Lv, L.L.; Cao, Y.; Liu, D.; Xu, M.; Liu, H.; Tang, R.N.; Ma, K.L.; Liu, B.C. Isolation and quantification of microRNAs from urinary exosomes/microvesicles for biomarker discovery. *Int. J. Biol. Sci.* **2013**, *9*, 1021–1031. [CrossRef]
122. Murakami, T.; Oakes, M.; Ogura, M.; Tovar, V.; Yamamoto, C.; Mitsuhashi, M. Development of glomerulus-, tubule-, and collecting duct-specific mRNA assay in human urinary exosomes and microvesicles. *PLoS ONE* **2014**, *2*, e109074. [CrossRef] [PubMed]
123. Álvarez, S.; Suazo, C.; Boltansky, A.; Ursu, M.; Carvajal, D.; Innocenti, G.; Vukusich, A.; Hurtado, M.; Villanueva, S.; Carreño, J.E. Urinary exosomes as a source of kidney dysfunction biomarker in renal transplantation. *Transplant. Proc.* **2013**, *45*, 3719–3723. [CrossRef] [PubMed]
124. Dear, J.W.; Street, J.M.; Bailey, M.A. Urinary exosomes: A reservoir for biomarker discovery and potential mediators of intrarenal signalling. *Proteomics* **2013**, *13*, 1572–1580. [CrossRef] [PubMed]

125. Quesada, A.; Segarra, A.B.; Montoro-Molina, S.; de Gracia, M.D.C.; Osuna, A.; O'Valle, F.; Gómez-Guzmán, M.; Vargas, F.; Wangensteen, R. Glutamyl aminopeptidase in microvesicular and exosomal fractions of urine is related with renal dysfunction in cisplatin-treated rats. *PLoS ONE* **2017**, *12*, e0175462. [CrossRef]
126. Hultström, M. Development of structural kidney damage in spontaneously hypertensive rats. *J. Hypertens.* **2012**, *30*, 1087–1091. [CrossRef]
127. Kim, N.; Dai, S.Y.; Pang, V.; Mazer, C.D. Vasopressinase Activity: A Potential Early Biomarker for Detecting Cardiopulmonary Bypass-Associated Acute Kidney Injury? *Thorac. Cardiovasc. Surg.* **2016**, *64*, 555–560. [CrossRef]
128. Munshi, R.; Hsu, C.; Himmelfarb, J. Advances in understanding ischemic acute kidney injury. *BMC Med.* **2011**, *9*, 11. [CrossRef]
129. Osuna, A.; de Gracia, M.C.; Quesada, A.; Manzano, F.; Wangensteen, R. Alanil aminopeptidase como marcador temprano del daño renal agudo persistente en pacientes sometidos a cirugía cardíaca. In Proceedings of the XLIX Congreso de la Soc Esp Nefrol, A Coruña, España, 5 October 2019.
130. de Artinano, A.A.; Castro, M.M. Experimental rat models to study the metabolic syndrome. *Br. J. Nutr.* **2009**, *102*, 1246–1253. [CrossRef]
131. Montoro-Molina, S.; López-Carmona, A.; Quesada, A.; O'Valle, F.; Martín-Morales, N.; Osuna, A.; Vargas, F.; Wangensteen, R. Klotho and Aminopeptidases as Early Biomarkers of Renal Injury in Zucker Obese Rats. *Front. Physiol.* **2018**, *9*, 1599. [CrossRef]
132. Llorens, S.; Fernandez, A.P.; Nava, E. Cardiovascular and renal alterations on the nitric oxide path way in spontaneous hypertension and ageing. *Clin. Hemorheol. Microcirc.* **2007**, *37*, 149–156.
133. Sun, Z.J.; Zhang, Z.E. Historic perspectives and recent advances in major animal models of hypertension. *Acta Pharmacol. Sin.* **2005**, *26*, 295–301. [CrossRef] [PubMed]
134. Montoro-Molina, S.; Quesada, A.; O'Valle, F.; Osuna, A.; de Gracia, M.C.; Vargas, F.; Wangensteen, R. Urinary aminopeptidase activities in spontaneously hypertensive rats. In Proceedings of the Physiology 2016, Dublin, Ireland, 39–31 July 2016. PCA320.
135. Vargas, F.; Moreno, J.M.; Rodríguez-Gómez, I.; Wangensteen, R.; Osuna, A.; Alvarez-Guerra, M.; García-Estañ, J. Vascular and renal function in experimental thyroid disorders. *Eur. J. Endocrinol.* **2006**, *154*, 197–212. [CrossRef] [PubMed]
136. Nakamura, S.; Ishiyama, M.; Kosaka, J.; Mutoh, J.; Umemura, N.; Harase, C. Urinary N-acetyl-beta-D-glucosaminidase (NAG) activity in patients with Graves' disease, subacute thyroiditis, and silent thyroiditis: A longitudinal study. *Endocrinol. Jpn.* **1991**, *38*, 303–308. [CrossRef] [PubMed]
137. Van Hoek, I.; Meyer, E.; Duchateau, L.; Peremans, K.; Smets, P.; Daminet, S. Retinol-binding protein in serum and urine of hyperthyroid cats before and after treatment with radioiodine. *J. Vet. Intern. Med.* **2009**, *23*, 1031–1037. [CrossRef]
138. Pérez-Abud, R.; Rodríguez-Gómez, I.; Villarejo, A.B.; Moreno, J.M.; Wangensteen, R.; Tassi, M.; O'Valle, F.; Osuna, A.; Vargas, F. Salt sensitivity in experimental thyroid disorders in rats. *Am. J. Physiol. Endocrinol. Metab.* **2011**, *301*, E281–E287. [CrossRef]
139. Conger, J.D.; Falk, S.A.; Gillum, D.M. The protective mechanism of thyroidectomy in a rat model of chronic renal failure. *Am. J. Kidney Dis.* **1989**, *13*, 217–225. [CrossRef]
140. Wangensteen, R.; Segarra, A.B.; Ramirez-Sanchez, M.; Gasparo, M.D.; Dominguez, G.; Banegas, I.; Vargas, F.; Vives, F.; Prieto, I. Influence of thyroid disorders on the kidney expression and plasma activity of aminopeptidase A. *Endocr. Regul.* **2015**, *49*, 68–72. [CrossRef]
141. Jung, K.; Pergande, M.; Schimie, E.; Ratzmann, K.P.; Illus, A. Urinary enzymes and low-molecular-mass proteins as indicator of diabetes nephropathy. *Clin. Chem.* **1988**, *34*, 544–547. [CrossRef]
142. Sorokman, T.; Sokolnyk, S.; Popelyuk, O.; Makarova, O.; Kopchuk, T. Biomarkers of renal injury risk in children with pyelonephritis. *Georgian Med. News* **2018**, *280–281*, 98–103.
143. Spasovski, D.; Masin-Spasovska, J.; Nada, M.; Calovski, J.; Sandevska, E.; Osmani, B.; Sotirova, T.; Balkanov, S.; Dukovski, D.; Ljatifi, A.; et al. Diagnostic value of brush border enzymes of the proximal renal tubules in rheumatoid arthritis. *Clin. Lab.* **2011**, *57*, 305–314.

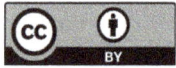

© 2020 by the authors. Licensee MDPI, Basel, Switzerland. This article is an open access article distributed under the terms and conditions of the Creative Commons Attribution (CC BY) license (http://creativecommons.org/licenses/by/4.0/).

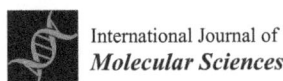

International Journal of
Molecular Sciences

Review

Changes in Novel AKI Biomarkers after Exercise. A Systematic Review

Wojciech Wołyniec [1,*], Wojciech Ratkowski [2], Joanna Renke [3] and Marcin Renke [1]

[1] Department of Occupational, Metabolic and Internal Diseases, Institute of Maritime and Tropical Medicine, Medical University of Gdańsk, 9b Powstania Styczniowego Street, 81-519 Gdynia, Poland; mrenke@gumed.edu.pl
[2] Department of Athletics, Gdańsk University of Physical Education and Sport, 1 Górskiego Street, 80-336 Gdańsk, Poland; maraton1954@o2.pl
[3] Department of General and Medical Biochemistry, University of Gdansk, 59 Wita Stwosza Street, 80-308 Gdańsk, Poland; joanna.renke@biol.ug.edu.pl
* Correspondence: wolyniecwojtek@gmail.com; Tel.: +48-58-7260490

Received: 28 June 2020; Accepted: 4 August 2020; Published: 7 August 2020

Abstract: More than 100 substances have been identified as biomarkers of acute kidney injury. These markers can help to diagnose acute kidney injury (AKI) in its early phase, when the creatinine level is not increased. The two markers most frequently studied in plasma and serum are cystatin C and neutrophil gelatinase-associated lipocalin (NGAL). The former is a marker of kidney function and the latter is a marker of kidney damage. Some other promising serum markers, such as osteopontin and netrin-1, have also been proposed and studied. The list of promising urinary markers is much longer and includes cystatin C, NGAL, kidney injury molecule-1 (KIM-1), liver-type fatty-acid-binding protein (L-FABP), interleukin 18, insulin-like growth factor binding protein 7 (IGFBP-7), tissue inhibitor of metalloproteinases-2 (TIMP-2) and many others. Although these markers are increased in urine for no longer than a few hours after nephrotoxic agent action, they are not widely used in clinical practice. Only combined IGFBP-7/TIMP-2 measurement was approved in some countries as a marker of AKI. Several studies have shown that the levels of urinary AKI biomarkers are increased after physical exercise. This systematic review focuses on studies concerning changes in new AKI biomarkers in healthy adults after single exercise. Twenty-seven papers were identified and analyzed in this review. The interpretation of results from different studies was difficult because of the variety of study groups, designs and methodology. The most convincing data concern cystatin C. There is evidence that cystatin C is a better indicator of glomerular filtration rate (GFR) in athletes after exercise than creatinine and also at rest in athletes with a lean mass lower or higher than average. Serum and plasma NGAL are increased after prolonged exercise, but the level also depends on inflammation and hypoxia; therefore, it seems that in physical exercise, it is too sensitive for AKI diagnosis. It may, however, help to diagnose subclinical kidney injury, e.g., in rhabdomyolysis. Urinary biomarkers are increased after many types of exercise. Increases in NGAL, KIM-1, cystatin-C, L-FABP and interleukin 18 are common, but the levels of most urinary AKI biomarkers decrease rapidly after exercise. The importance of this short-term increase in AKI biomarkers after exercise is doubtful. It is not clear if it is a sign of mild kidney injury or physiological metabolic adaptation to exercise.

Keywords: urinary biomarkers; markers of AKI; cystatin-C; NGAL; KIM-1; exercise; acute kidney injury

1. Introduction

The analysis of human urine has been a part of medical practice for 6000 years. Uroscopy was "the mirror of medicine" or, in more ordinary terms, the first additional test in medicine, and was widely used to diagnose almost all medical conditions [1]. Now, urinalysis is one of the most common laboratory tests in medical practice.

Two-hundred years ago, the father of modern nephrology, Dr Richard Bright, discovered that patients with dropsy had albuminuria and structural changes in the kidneys. Dr Bright first described the classical nephrological triad and found a correlation between changes in urine (albuminuria) and diseased kidneys at autopsy [2]. Sixty-six years ago, Kenneth D. Gardner Jr. first described changes in urine after physical exercise. The proteinuria and hematuria were found in healthy subjects after relatively gentle exercise, therefore Gardner called these conditions "athletic pseudo-nephritis", assuming that it is a physiological, transient and benign condition [3]. Those two observations defined the limits of our understanding of the significance of proteinuria. On the one hand, albuminuria is one of the most important markers of severe and sometimes fatal kidney diseases with well-described structural changes. But on the other hand, the list of physiological conditions in which transient proteinuria is observed is quite long. Protein in urine is found after exercise, exposure to cold or heat and protein-rich food (alimentary proteinuria), and proteinuria can also occur in pregnancy, fever, heart failure and in a vertical position (orthostatic, postural proteinuria) [4].

In recent decades, new methods of urine examination have been proposed: tubular enzymes, novel biomarkers of acute kidney injury (AKI), metabolomics, proteomics, transcriptomics and genomics [5–7]. The very promising new AKI biomarkers were called "kidney troponins" and hinted at the possibility of early diagnosis of kidney diseases. Some of the markers showed high sensitivity in AKI diagnosis. Numerous studies concerned urinary neutrophil gelatinase-associated lipocalin (NGAL), kidney injury molecule-1 (KIM-1), cystatin C (Cyst-C), liver-type fatty-acid-binding protein (L-FABP), interleukin 18, insulin-like growth factor binding protein 7 (IGFBP-7) and tissue inhibitor of metalloproteinases-2 (TIMP-2) [5,8,9]. Nevertheless, the only AKI biomarker test which is currently FDA (Food and Drug Administration)-approved for clinical use in the USA, and which is also used in some European countries, is NephroCheck, which combines TIMP-2 and IGFBP-7 [10].

The history of serum examination in kidney diseases is relatively short. In the last 100 years, creatinine established its position as the best marker of glomerular filtration rate (GFR) [11,12]. 22 years ago, Cyst-C was considered as an equal or even better marker of GFR than creatinine. Due to its higher price and lower availability, it is not widely used. Interestingly, although serum concentrations of both substances correlate strictly, they are eliminated by kidneys in two different ways. Both are freely filtered in the glomeruli, but creatinine is never reabsorbed and secreted, while cystatin C in healthy individuals is reabsorbed and metabolized in the proximal tubule. Therefore, in normal conditions, excretion of Cyst-C is very low [13]. Some other novel biomarkers of AKI, like NGAL and osteopontin, can be measured in serum [5].

The serum and urine markers of kidney injury were mainly studied in AKI. The aim of this review was to analyze changes of those markers after physiological condition—exercise. All but one of the studies analyzed were conducted in the last 10 years. The high number of proposed markers of AKI is sometimes confusing. Consequently, this review was ordered according to the classification suggested by Oh in a state-of-the-art review published this year (Table 1) [5]. The purpose of this review was to describe the newest markers of AKI, which is why conventional markers—creatinine, albuminuria, tubular enzymes—were not in the scope of the paper.

Table 1. Biomarkers of acute kidney injury (AKI) studied in exercise discussed in this review—classification according to Oh et al. [5].

Functional Biomarkers	Damage Biomarkers	Pre-Injury Phase Biomarkers
sCyst-C	uCyst-C uNGAL, sNGAL, pNGAL uKIM-1 uL-FABP uIL-6, uIL-8, uIL-18, uTTF uCalbindin uTNFα uYKL-40 uMCP-1	uIGFBP-7 uTIMP-2

Abbreviations: u—urinary, s—serum, p—plasma, Cyst-C—cystatin C, NGAL—neutrophil gelatinase-associated lipocalin, KIM-1—kidney injury molecule-1, L-FABP—liver-type fatty-acid-binding protein, IL—interleukin, TTF3—trefoil factor-3, TNFα—tumor necrosis factor α, YKL-40—chitinase 3-like protein 1, MCP-1—monocyte chemoattractant protein-1, IGFBP-7—insulin-like growth factor binding protein 7, TIMP-2—tissue inhibitor of metalloproteinases-2.

Repeated episodes of acute kidney failure may lead to chronic kidney disease (CKD); therefore, proper diagnosis of AKI is important [14]. There is no evidence that sport practicing can lead to chronic kidney problems; nevertheless, after marathon run and other endurance events, an acute renal failure requiring renal replacement therapy was observed [15]. The possible factors causing post-exercise AKI are dehydration, sub-clinical rhabdomyolysis, inflammation, increased energy demanding renal sodium uptake, reduced renal perfusion and nonsteroidal anti-inflammatory drugs (NSAIDs) frequently used by runners [16,17]. There is evidence that dehydration and soft drink intake during and following exercise may lead to acute kidney dysfunction [18] and that physical work in heat is leading to chronic kidney disease [19].

2. Results: Studies Concerning Novel Biomarkers of AKI after Exercise

2.1. Functional Biomarker—Serum Cystatin C

Cystatin C is a non-glucosylated 13 kD basic protein which belongs to the cysteine protein inhibitors family and is produced at a constant rate by all nucleated cells. Cystatin C is an inhibitor of lysosomal proteinases and one of the most important extracellular inhibitors of cysteine proteases [5,9]. Cystatin C is freely filtered in glomeruli and then reabsorbed and metabolized in the proximal tubule. Studies on diabetes, protein-induced glomerular hyperfiltration and extreme exercise demonstrated that acute changes in serum (s)Cyst-C provide a better approximation of GFR than serum creatinine (sCr). sCyst-C is affected by sex and race and to a small degree, by inflammation [20]. In clinical studies on acute kidney injury, an increase in serum and urine cystatin C levels is observed earlier than an increase in creatinine [5,9,20,21].

2.1.1. Changes in sCyst-C after a Marathon

There were several studies dedicated to study changes in sCyst-C level after exercise. The increase in sCyst-C after a marathon was first noticed by Mingels et al. In this study of 70 recreational runners, the authors showed that the increase in sCyst-C is lower than the increase in sCr after exercise. This increase after a marathon was half that of creatinine (34% vs 53% increase, and after correction for the effect of dehydration, 21% vs 42%). Serum Cyst-C was increased above the upper reference limit in 46% of runners (in 26% after correction) [20]. Very similar changes—a significant increase in the sCyst-C level immediately after a marathon run—were observed by Scherr [22], McCullough [23] and Hewing [24] (Table 2).

Table 2. Changes in sCyst-C level after a marathon.

Study	sCyst-C Before a Marathon (mg/L)	sCyst-C after a Marathon (mg/L)	The Relative Increase in sCyst-C (%)	sCyst-C in Follow-Up (mg/L)
Mingels et al. [20]	0.71 (0.56–0.95)	0.95 (0.63–1.45)	34% (21% after correction of effect of dehydration)	0.73 (0.6–0.93) (day after, measured only in 18/70 subjects)
Scherr et al. [22]	0.77 (0.71–0.85)	0.94 (0.86–1.01)	22%	0.9 (0.81–1.00) (24 h after the race) 0.81 (0.72–0.86) (72 h after the race)
McCullough et al. [23]	0.8 ± 0.1	1.0 ± 0.2	25%	0.8 ± 0.1 (24 h after the race)
Hewing et al. [24]	0.68 (0.75–0.93)	0.85 (0.69–0.99)	25%	0.66 (0.59–0.78) (14 days after the race)

Abbreviations: sCyst-C—serum cystatin-C.

The main differences in these studies concerned changes in the follow-up, but the time of the follow-up was defined in different ways. Therefore, it is difficult to compare those data. Nevertheless, all studies showed a rapid decrease in sCyst-C at rest.

2.1.2. Changes in sCyst-C after Exercises Shorter than a Marathon

Poortmans et al. found that after a 30-min treadmill test at 80% of the maximal oxygen capacity, sCyst-C increased significantly by 13% (from 0.91 ± 0.06 to 1.03 ± 0.09 mg/L) and eGFR -Cyst-C decreased significantly by 19.8% [25]. Another study concerning subjects performing a submaximal test on a cycle ergometer at an exercise intensity of 80% of the maximal heart rate was performed by Bongers et al. In contrast to Poortmans, they did not find any changes in eGFR -Cyst-C after 30 min of exercise (eGFR 118 vs. 116 mL/min/1.73 m^2), but after 150 min of exercise, a significant decrease in eGFR -Cyst-C to 103 mL/min/1.73 m^2 was observed [26]. In Poortmans' and Bongers' studies, only males of the similar age (25 and 23 years) were studied. The difference between these two studies can be related to the type of exercise—in Poortmans' study, a run on a treadmill, and in Bongers' study, cycling on an ergometer [25,26].

2.1.3. Changes in sCyst-C after Longer Exercise than a Marathon

Serum cystatin C was also measured after very long exercise—a 120 km "Infernal trail" race. Surprisingly, there was no change in sCyst-C (0.8 vs. 0.8 mg/L) and eGFR Cyst-C value even increased after the race—from 113.5 to 118.5 mL/min (p = 0.04). This could be due to the very low intensity of physical activity. The exercise was very long—a 120 km race with 5700 m positive elevation. The speed was very low (5.2 km/h) and the median time was 23.1 h [27].

2.1.4. sCyst-C is a Better Marker of eGFR than sCr

Interesting observations were made in nine professional cyclists during the Giro d'Italia. In this study, blood was taken before, on the 12th and on the 22nd day of the race. The mean sCyst-C remained very stable: 0.61 ± 0.06 vs 0.62 ± 0.07 vs. 0.63 ± 0.06 mg/L. In this very interesting study, which is described in detail in two papers [28,29], blood was not taken immediately after the single race. Therefore, the study is not exactly in the scope of this review. Nevertheless, it provided evidence that even one of the most exhausting multistage efforts does not lead to an eGFR decrease in healthy, well-trained sportsmen [28,29]. Studies published by Banfi and Colombini showed that in athletes, sCyst-C is a better marker of eGFR than serum creatinine (sCr), also at rest. Some athletes, like cyclists, have a creatinine level that is lower than the reference values, due to a low lean mass (e.g., 9/9 cyclists taking part in the Giro d'Italia), while 12/15 professional rugby players had serum creatinine above the reference values due to their high body mass. In both of these studies, athletes had levels of serum Cyst-C in the normal range [28–30].

sCyst-C is also more precise than a sCr marker of eGFR in studies in which lean body mass is changing. In a study of a 6-month physical activity program in obese boys, serum creatinine increased, but sCyst-C remained unchanged. In the subjects, the lean mass and height increased, while their weight did not change [31].

2.1.5. Summary of Changes in sCyst-C

In summary, the main advantages of sCyst-C over creatinine in studies concerning exercise is that sCyst-C is not correlated with lean mass [28–30,32]. Therefore, sCyst-C may be more suitable for assessing renal function in individuals with a higher muscle mass when mild kidney impairment is suspected [33]. The studies performed after single exercise may suggest that sCyst-C elevation is dependent on intensity and duration. Long and intensive exercises such as a marathon will cause an increase [20,22–24], while short exercises or exercises with lower intensity will not [26,27].

2.2. Plasma and Serum Damage Markers

Damage markers can help in early AKI diagnosis even before elevation of sCr and sCyst-C levels [5]. Only a few damage markers are measured in serum or plasma: NGAL, KIM-1, osteopontin and netrin-1. The most studies concerned changes in NGAL.

NGAL, also known as siderocalin or lipocalin 2, is a member of the lipocalin superfamily of carrier proteins, which are approximately 25 kDa in size. NGAL has a bacteriostatic function related to its ability to bind iron-siderophore complexes and thereby prevents iron uptake by bacteria. NGAL also provides an antiapoptotic effect and enhances proliferation of renal tubular cells [8]. It is produced by activated neutrophils in the proximal tubules. NGAL is filtered in the glomerulus and reabsorbed in the proximal tubule. After ischemic, septic or toxic kidney injury, NGAL is dramatically upregulated at the transcript and protein level. Plasma and urinary NGAL levels are significantly increased in those with early structural renal tubular damage caused by various factors [5,8,9].

2.2.1. Changes in Plasma NGAL (pNGAL) after Short Exercises

Changes in pNGAL after exercise were first investigated by Junglee et al. in 2012. In this study dedicated to AKI in exercise, after relatively short exercise (an 800 m run), pNGAL was decreased, which was interpreted by the authors as an effect of increased NGAL renal clearance [34].

In another study performed by Junglee, the pNGAL level increased after a 40-min heat stress run (running on a treadmill on a 1% gradient for 40 min at 65% VO_{2max} (maximal oxygen consumption) in an environmental chamber maintained at a dry bulb temperature of 33 °C with 50% relative humidity (RH)). In this study, the heat stress run was preceded by a 60-min downhill muscle-damaging run (EIMD group) or a 60-min flat run (CON group) and a 30-min seated rest. pNGAL increased in both groups, but the increase was greater in the EIMD group [35].

There were also three studies dedicated to investigating a pNGAL as a marker of inflammation, neutrophil degranulation and organ damage, but not an AKI biomarker [36–38].

Bender et al. studied pNGAL as an inflammatory marker of hand osteoarthiritis (OA) after mechanical exercise of the OA hand. pNGLA increased during the first 15 min after exercising the index hand within the venous blood of the ipsilateral forearm [36]. Kanda et al. studied 9 untrained men during a one leg, calf-rise exercise. pNGAL was studied as a marker of organ damage, muscle disruption and neutrophil mobilization and migration. The authors did not find any changes in pNGAL [37]. Rullman et al., found no significant changes in pNGAL after 27 and 57 min of cycle exercise. During the first 20 min, the subjects exercised at 50% of VO_{2max} and during the next 40 min, at 65% VO_{2max}. In the Rullman study, pNGAL was investigated as a marker of neutrophil degranulation [38].

2.2.2. Changes in pNGAL or Serum NGAL (sNGAL) Levels after Long Exercises

Chapman et al. studied the impact of soft drink consumption during long exercise in heat. Twelve healthy subjects drank two liters of a beverage (soft drink or water) during four hours of exercise in 35.1 °C heat. pNGAL increased post-exercise in both groups [18].

McDermott et al. found a 2-fold significant increase in sNGAL (from 68.51 to 139.12 ng/mL) after a 6-h endurance cycling event during heat (33.2 ± 5.0 °C, 38.4 ± 10.7% RH). Moderate ibuprofen ingestion of 600 mg ibuprofen had no influence on the sNGAL level [39]. Moreover, Lippi et al., found a significant 1.6-fold increase in sNGAL (from 105 to 196 ng/mL) after a 60-km run in a group of trained male athletes [40].

Furthermore, Andrezzoli et al. found only a mild increase in pNGAL in a group of professional cyclists after the mountain stages of two major European professional cycling competitions (Giro D'Italia and Tour de France). Post-competition NGAL values of all the variables investigated remained within the physiological range. The results suggest that even if NGAL values rose slightly and not significantly after competition, no kidney injury occurred in these highly trained athletes during the mountain stages of professional competitions [41].

NGAL, which is an acute phase protein and is upregulated in the lungs during inflammation, was also studied as a marker of inflammation and oxidative stress after long exercise. Mellor et al. found a non-significant NGAL rise after an ascent from sea level to 1085 m over 6 h [42]. In this study, two other cohorts were also studied. There were no changes in NGAL after 3 h exposure to normobaric hypoxia with a 5-min step test, but there was an increase in NGAL after trekking in Nepal [42].

2.2.3. Changes in pNGAL after Work in Heat

Chapman et al. analyzed changes in pNGAL and other biomarkers in two interesting studies. In the first, the impact of different beverage consumption (soft drink or water) during exercise in heat was studied. Twelve healthy subjects drank two liters of fluid during four hours of exercise in 35.1 °C heat [18]. In the second study, thirteen healthy adults (3 women, 10 men, age 23 ± 2 years) exercised for 2 h in a 39.7 ± 0.6 °C, 32% ± 3% relative humidity environmental chamber. In four trials, the subjects received water to remain hydrated (*Water group*), were exposed to continuous upper-body cooling (*Cooling group*), a combination of both (*Water + Cooling group*), or no intervention (*Control group*) [43]. In the first study, in both groups, pNGAL was increased post-exercise and returned to pre-exercise levels after 24 h [18]. In the second study, an increase in pNGAL was also observed and was greater in the control group (without hydration and cooling) compared with the other conditions [43].

2.2.4. Summary of Changes in s/pNGAL

The importance of s/pNGAL in the diagnosis of AKI in exercise is questionable. NGAL is released by respiratory epithelium, liver and heart, and therefore changes in the s/pNGAL level could be caused by inflammation, hypoxia or muscle damage, conditions which are integral to exercise [35,42]. Therefore, it is unclear to which degree, if any, an increase in NGAL after exercise is related to kidney injury. The methodological problem is that a huge difference between athletes is observed [40].

2.3. Urinary Damage Markers

2.3.1. Urinary Cystatin C (uCyst-C)

Since Cyst-C is freely filtered by the glomerulus, reabsorbed and metabolized in the renal tubule, even a small elevation of urinary Cyst-C (uCyst-C) reflects proximal tubule injury [13].

Bongers et al. studied subjects performing submaximal exercise at an 80% HR rate and found a significant increase in uCyst-C with higher values after prolonged exercise (150 min) compared to acute (30 min) exercise [26]. In 2012, the same authors studied urinary markers after single and repetitive bouts of exercise. They examined participants of the International Four Day Marches Nijmegen. Subjects walked at 70% intensity over 30, 40 or 50 km for 3 consecutive days. Bongers studied several urinary markers and found that uCyst-C increased 1.8 times after the first day (from 0.05 to 0.09 mg/L), but this effect disappeared on day 3 (uCyst-C = 0.06 mg/L) [44]. Interestingly, in these studies, uCyst-C was measured mainly to normalize uKIM-1 and uNGAL levels [26,44]. The increase in uCyst-C was also found by Wolyniec after 10 and 100 km runs. There was a 2.56-fold increase after 10 km and a 4.96-fold increase after 100 km. When normalized to creatinine, these increases were 1.39- and 1.95-fold, respectively [45].

The number of studies coming from only two centers is small, but it seems that uCyst-C is a very sensitive marker of proximal tubule dysfunction after exercise.

2.3.2. Changes in uNGAL and uKIM-1 after a Marathon

KIM-1 is a 38.7 kDa type 1 transmembrane glycoprotein member of the TIM family of immunoglobulin superfamily molecules. KIM-1 plays a role in kidney recovery and tubular regeneration because it acts as a phosphatidylserine receptor and thereby mediates the phagocytosis of apoptotic cells. KIM-1 protects kidney against ischemic-reperfusion injury [8]. KIM-1 was found to be expressed at low to undetectable levels in normal kidney tissue but is markedly expressed after ischemic or toxic injury in proximal tubule cells. KIM-1 can serve as a urine and blood AKI biomarker. KIM is elevated in early stages of AKI and its urinary concentration is closely related to the severity of renal damage [5,8,9].

The first study concerning changes in urinary NGAL and KIM-1 after a marathon was performed by McCullough and published in 2010 [23]. The authors showed a 5.7-fold increase in uNGAL and a minor rise in uKIM-1 after a marathon [23]. According to the authors, those were changes "supporting a pathobiologic case for AKI" [23]. Changes in uKIM-1 and uNGAL levels after a marathon were also studied by Mansour et al. [46] The results concerning uNGAL were very similar to these from McCullough's study (a 4.71-fold increase in uNGAL), but the increase in uKIM-1 was much higher. The decrease in uKIM-1 was slower than the other markers studied (uNGAL, uTNF-alfa [tumor necrosis factor α], uIL-18, uIL6, uIL8, uYKL-40, uMCP-1) and 24 h after a marathon, the level was still increased (Table 3) [46].

Table 3. Changes in uNGAL and uKIM-1 after a marathon.

Study	uNGAL before a Marathon (ng/mL)	uNGAL after a Marathon	Fold Increase	KIM-1 before a Marathon	uKIM-1 after a Marathon	Fold Increase
McCullough et al. [23]	8.2 ± 4.0	47.0 ± 28.6 (10.6 ± 7.2 after 24 h)	5.73× (1.29×)	2.6 ± 1.6 ng/mL	3.5 ± 1.6 (2.7 ± 1.6 after 24 h) ng/mL	1.35× (1.03×)
Mansour et al. [46]	8.00 (4.15–30.48)	37.64 (19.03–84.61) (day 2: 18.49 (9.25–33.69))	4.71× (2.31×)	132.59 (67.61–219.98) pg/mL	723.32 (459.36–1970.64) (day 2: 702.42 (123.27–1098.67)) pg/mL	5.46× (5.3×)

Abbreviations: uNGAL—urinary neutrophil gelatinase-associated lipocalin, uKIM-1—urinary kidney injury molecule-1.

2.3.3. Changes in uNGAL after Exercises Shorter than a Marathon

No changes were found in the uNGAL level in Kanda's study on 9 untrained males during a one leg calf-rise exercise [37] and in the Wołyniec study of amateur runners after a submaximal test on a treadmill [47]. In contrast, in two other studies, uNGAL was increased after very short exercise. Junglee et al. noticed an increase in uNGAL and uNGAL/uCr immediately and 25 min after an 800 m run. The uNGAL level returned to the baseline levels after two hours [34]. Spada et al. also noticed an increase in uNGAL after 4 min of an high-intensity interval resistance training (HIIT) session (eight sets of squats performed with the fastest speed and the highest number of repetitions achievable in 20 s with 10 s of rest between sets). In this study, uNGAL was increased in women 2 after exercise and returned to values similar to the baseline 24 h after exercise. In 5/29 females, uNGAL/uCr exceeded 100 ng/mgCr, the value of which is compatible with clinical AKI. In men, the increase in uNGAL and uNGAL/uCr was not statistically significant [48].

Junglee et al. found an 8-fold uNGAL increase after a 40-min heat stress run (65% VO_{2max}, 33 °C): 80% of subjects from the muscle-damaging group and 30% from the flat-run group had uNGAL above the normal range after exercise [35]. Bongers, who studied uNGAL after 30 and 150 min of exercise, found that uncorrected uNGAL and uNGAL corrected to osmolality were increased, while there were no changes in uNGAL corrected to creatinine and cystatin-C [26]. After a 10-km run, both uNGAL and uNGAL/Cr increased significantly (3.9- and 2.9-fold, respectively) in the Wołyniec study [45]. Otherwise, in Semen et al.'s study, a 10 km run caused an increase in uNGAL only when combined with ibuprofen/naproxen use [49]. In the same study, a significant increase in uNGAL was observed in the half-marathon runners [49].

In another study, Semen et al. found that completion of a half marathon after use of a 400 mg single dose ibuprofen led to a 2-fold increase in uNGAL. However, this increase was smaller and not significant in the group supplemented with monomeric and oligomeric flavanols (MOF-VVPP) [50]. In the Wolyniec study, the increase in uNGAL was higher than in Semen's study, although the exercise was shorter. This difference could be partially explained by the higher intensity of a 10-km run but could also be related to the methodology. In the first study, urine samples were collected immediately after the run and in the second, urine samples were collected within 2 h after the run [45,50].

2.3.4. Changes in uNGAL after Exercises Longer than a Marathon

The uNGAL level was elevated after all exercises longer than a marathon run. Bongers found that prolonged walking exercise at 70% intensity caused a 2.25-fold increase in uNGAL on day 1, and a 1.54-fold increase on day 3 compared to the baseline levels [44]. An uNGAL increase was also found by Lippi et al. after a 60-km run (7.7- fold increase in uNGAL) [40], by Jouffroy et al. after an 80-km run (5-fold increase after 53 km, and 2.5-fold after 80 km, without significant changes in uNGAL/uCr) [51], by Wolyniec et al. after 100 km (6.82-fold increase in uNGAL, and only a 2.94-fold increase in uNGAL/uCr) [45] and by Poussel el al. after a 120-km run (2.6-fold increase in uNGAL and a 1.5-fold in uNGAL/uCr) [27]. Only 6.25% of the participants in the Wołyniec study and 12.5 % in the Poussel study had uNGAL/uCr above the reference value [27,45].

2.3.5. Changes in uNGAL after Exercise in Heat

Chapmen et al., performed two exciting studies, as mentioned above [18,43]. In the first, they found that 24 h after exercise in heat, uNGAL was elevated above the pre-exercise level in subjects drinking soft drinks, although uNGAL corrected to uCr osmolality did not produce any changes [18]. In the second study, uNGAL was elevated after 2 h of exercise in heat, and this increase was greater in the control group compared with the other conditions (hydration or/and cooling) [43].

2.3.6. Summary of Changes in uNGAL

Changes in uNGAL were typically found after long exercise. It seems that uNGAL is frequently increased, but rarely exceeds normal values when normalized to creatinine. Some factors, like environmental temperature, type of cooling and hydration, are related to changes in uNGAL. Interpreting these changes is difficult. Machado found elevated levels of uNGAL in endurance cycling athletes 48 h after exercise and suggested that the increase in uNGAL is related to metabolic adaptation to endurance exercise, or possibly predisposition to acute kidney injury over time [52]. In Bongers' study, uNGAL was elevated after the first day of marching and then decreased, which also suggested some kind of kidney adaptation to exercise [44].

2.3.7. Changes in Urinary KIM

Except for the two studies after a marathon mentioned above [23,46], uKIM was studied only in 5 studies coming from 3 centers. In all these studies, uKIM-1 was increased.

Bongers et al. found an increase in uKIM-1 after 30- and 150-min submaximal exercise [26] and after one day of walking, with a subsequent decrease in its level after 3 consecutive days of marching [44]. In the first study, the uKIM-1 corrected to uCr, uCyst-C and urine osmolality showed no significant changes [26]. In the second study, uKIM- 1 corrected to osmolality was increased, while uKIM-1/uCr and uKIM/uCyst-C ratios were unchanged [44]. Wolyniec found an increase in uKIM-1 but not in the uKIM/uCr ratio after a treadmill test, 10 and 100 km runs [45,47]. Jouffroy found a significant increase in uKIM-1 but not in uKIM/uCr during an 80-km run. Interestingly, nine days after the race, uKIM-1 remained significantly higher than the baseline level [51].

2.3.8. Summary of Changes in uKIM-1

uKIM-1 was increased after all exercises, but when normalized to uCr, it was unchanged. The changes in uKIM-1 were long-lasting, uKIM-1 was elevated 2 days after a marathon [46] and 9 days after an 80 km run [51]. At the same time, uNGAL decreased more rapidly.

2.3.9. Changes in Urinary L-FABP after Exercise

L-FABP belongs to the fatty acid-binding protein superfamily and has a molecular mass of about 14 kDa. The function of the members of the FABP family is the regulation of fatty acids uptake and the intracellular transport. L-FABP binds fatty acids and transports them to the mitochondria and peroxisomes. L-FABP also protects renal cells from oxidative stress [8]. The urinary L-FABP level is correlated with the peritubular capillary flow and ischemia. It appears to be a promising biomarker for both the diagnosis and prediction of AKI and its outcomes among critically ill patients [5,8,9]. L-FABP is localized in the proximal tubule and secreted into urine in response to a number of different intrarenal stresses, such as proteinuria, hypoxia, hyperglycemia, hypertension and oxidative stress [37,53,54].

Only two studies in healthy populations concerning changes in uL-FABP after exercise have been published. uL-FABP was significantly increased after incremental short maximal exercise on a cycling ergometer in a group of 116 adults of variable age (24–83 years) in a study published by Kosaki et al. In this experiment, uL-FABP/uCr changes were independently correlated with albuminuria, which supported previous observations that protein overload in the proximal tubule may cause an increase in uL-FABP [53]. After short exercise (one leg calf-rise exercise), Kanda et al. did not find any changes in uL-FABP [37].

2.3.10. Other Studies Concerning Changes in uL-FABP

Hiraki showed that after a single case of a 20-min moderate intensity exercise (20-min treadmill walking, 40–60% exercise intensity) session in 31 adults with chronic kidney disease (CKD), there was no change in uL-FABP. This exercise was rather gentle and even albuminuria was not increased [55]. Kosaki studied individuals aged 50–83 without CKD and found that uL-FABP was the lowest in participants with a higher level of aerobic fitness and muscular strength [56,57] and that 12-week aerobic exercise training significantly decreases uL-FABP levels [57]. Relative changes in uFABP were significantly correlated with the relative changes in physical activity and the mean arterial pressure after intervention. The authors concluded that "habitual exercise appears to be associated with the degree of several stresses on the proximal tubule and to be beneficial for kidney health in middle-aged and older adults" [57]. Uchiyama et al. found a decrease in uL-FABP after a 12-week, home-based exercise program involving 47 patients undergoing peritoneal dialysis [58].

2.3.11. Urinary Interleukins

Urinary interleukins, Il-1, Il-6, IL-8 and Il-18, were proposed as markers of AKI. Interleukins are important mediators of the immune reaction in the innate immune system response and adaptive immunity [8]. All these cytokines are freely filtered and then reabsorbed and metabolized in the proximal tubule; therefore, tubular injury leads to an elevation in their levels in urine [5,6,8,9,48].

Manosur et al. studied changes in urinary interleukins after a marathon and found a 19.2-fold increase in uIL-6, a 9.13-fold increase in uIL-8 and a 7.13-fold increase in uIL-18 [46]. Similarly, Semen et al. observed significant increases of urinary interleukins after a half marathon and the use of 400 mg ibuprofen. There was a 10-fold increase in uIL-6, a 2.87-fold increase in uIL-8 and a non-significant increase in IL-18. The elevations of uIL-6 and uIL-8 were smaller in runners supplemented with MOF-VVPP (5.8- and 1.49-fold, respectively) [50]. Elevation of uIL-6 and uIL-8 was also found by Sugama et al. after a duathlon [59]. Spada et al. found an increase in uIL-18 after a HIIT session [48]. Dutheil et al. found an increase in uIL-8 after a 24 h work shift and, according to the author, this elevation was related to stress [60].

2.4. Pre-Injury Phase Biomarkers IGFBP-7/TIMP-2

Insulin-like growth factor binding protein 7 (IGFBP-7) is a 29 kDa protein, a member of IGFBPs. It is a kind of glycoprotein with a molecular weight of 30 kDa. IGFBP-7 is known to bind and inhibit signaling through IGF-1 receptors [8]. Urinary IGFBP-7 is increased in kidney damage caused by sepsis or ischemia [8,9].

TIMP-2 is a 21 kDa protein, a member of the TIMP family. TIMP2 is a member of the tissue inhibitor of matrix metalloproteinase family. TIMP2 is an endogenous inhibitor of metalloproteinase activities and participates in the regulation of cell growth and apoptosis [8,9].

Combined urinary IGFBP-7 and TIMP-2 predict the occurrence of AKI better than other markers (NGAL KIM, IL19) [8,9]. NephroCheck, which combines TIMP-2 and IGFBP-7, is the only FDA-approved AKI biomarker test for use in the USA and is also used in some European countries [10].

Surprisingly, IGFBP-7 and TIMP-2 were studied only in one study after exercise. Chapman et al. studied thirteen healthy adults exercising in heat (the study is described above) and found elevated levels of uIGFBP-7 and uTIMP-2. There was a greater increase in the urinary biomarkers of AKI in the *Control* group. The differential findings between IGFBP7 (preferentially secreted in the proximal tubules) and TIMP-2 (secreted in the distal tubules) suggested that the proximal tubules are the location of potential renal injury [43].

2.5. Other Promising Markers of AKI (YKL-40, MCP-1 and TNF-alfa, Trefoil Factor 3 (TTF3), Calbindin)

There are over 100 biomarkers of AKI [61]. The urinary biomarkers which have been assessed in numerous studies are: chitinase 3-like protein 1 (YKL-40), MCP-1, TNF-alfa, osteopontin, DKK-1, micro RNAs, hemojuvelin, clusterin, CYR-61, cytochrome-C, epidermal growth factor, malondialdehyde, calprotectin, urine AGT angiotensinogen, matrix metalloproteinase 9, urine cysteine-rich 61, Na^+/H^+ exchanger isoform 3 protein, netrin-1, fetuin-A and trefoil factor 3 (TFF3) [5,8,9]. Most of these markers were not studied after exercise.

In one of the most interesting and largest studies concerning AKI biomarkers after exercise, Mansour et al. found increases in several urinary markers: a 4.5-fold increase in TNFα, a 6.69-fold increase in MCP-1 and an 8.99-fold increase in YKL-40 after a marathon [46]. Sugama et al. found increased uMCP-1 after a duathlon, but this change was not significant when normalized to uCr [59]. Semen et al. found a significant uTNFα increase after a half marathon [50]. Calbindin and TTF3 were studied in one study, and both of these markers increased after HIIT training [48]. The TTF3 family is a group of small molecule polypeptides, and uTTF3 was significantly reduced following renal tubular damage [9]; therefore, the increase in uTTF3 after exercise was surprising.

3. Discussion

Studies concerning new markers of AKI after physical exercise combine two different entities. Markers of AKI were introduced to diagnose the early phase of kidney injury in critically ill patients with sepsis or shock [5,6,8,9], but in these studies, they were measured in healthy subjects during physical activity, like walking, running or cycling. The increase in new AKI biomarkers was anticipated in these studies, because even much less sensitive markers, like serum creatinine and urinalysis, show changes after exercise [3,23].

Although many markers of AKI were described, only a minority were studied after exercise. Some markers are classified as injury markers (e.g., uKIM-1, uTNFalfa, uIL-6, uIL-8, uIL-18, uNGAL) and others as repair biomarkers (e.g., uYKL-40, uMCP-1) [46]. Another classification is based on the site of injury. There are markers of tubular (e.g., NGAL, IL-18, L-FABP, KIM-1, IGFBP-7) and glomerular (e.g., matrix metallopeptidase 9 [MMP-9]) injury [9]. The authors of this review used the classification proposed by Oh et al. [5] (Table 1), which has practical implications.

3.1. Limitations of the Studies Presented

There are several limitations to the studies presented in this review. Twenty-seven studies were analyzed. All but one were published during the last 10 years and 15/27 in the last 5 years. The number of subjects studied ranged from 9 to 167, although most of the studies had a small number of participants: in 16 studies, fewer than 30 participants were investigated and only in 3 studies were there more than 100 participants studied. In 12 studies, only males were analyzed, and only in 7 studies were both sexes represented to the same or very similar degree. In three studies, all concerning marathons, more females were analyzed. The mean age of the participants differed greatly, ranging from 20 to 60 years. There were many different study designs proposed by the researchers, although the most common was a marathon (distance 42,195 m), which was used in 5 studies (Figure 1, Table 4).

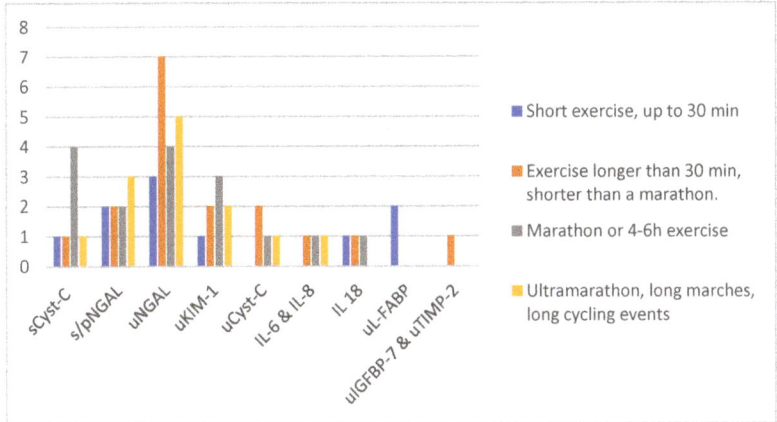

Figure 1. Number of studies in different types of exercise. Abbreviations: u—urinary, s—serum, p—plasma, Cyst-C—cystatin C, NGAL—neutrophil gelatinase-associated lipocalin, KIM-1—kidney injury molecule-1, L-FABP—liver-type fatty-acid-binding protein, IL—interleukin, IGFBP-7—insulin-like growth factor binding protein 7, TIMP-2—tissue inhibitor of metalloproteinases-2.

Table 4. Studies on changes in new AKI markers after single exercise in healthy subjects—ordered according to the year of publication.

Author (Year of Publication)	Study Group	Exercise/Study Design	Markers
Mingels et al. (2009) [20]	70 recreational male runners age 47 (range 30–68) years	marathon	sCyst-C
Scherr et al. (2011) [22]	102 healthy male runners age 42 ± 9.5 y	Marathon	sCyst-C
McCullough et al. (2011) [23]	25 healthy runners age 38.7 ± 9.0 years (13 females, 12 males)	Marathon	sCyst-C uNGAL uKIM-1
Poortmans et al. (2012) [25]	12 male physical educators age 25 ± 5 years	30-min treadmill exercise at 80% of VO_2max	sCyst-C
Junglee et al. (2012) [34]	20 healthy active adults age 24 ± 4 years (7 females, 13 males)	800-m sprint	pNGAL uNGAL uNGAL/uCr
Rullman et al. (2012) [38]	10 healthy men age 25 (range 18–37) years	60-min cycle ergometer test (20 min at 50% of VO_2max; +40 min at 65% of VO_2max)	pNGAL
Lippi et al. (2012) [40]	16 trained male athletes age 42 (range 34–52) years	60-km ultramarathon	sNGAL, uNGAL, uNGAl/uCr
Junglee et al. (2013) [35]	10 active healthy men age 20 ± 2 years	1. 60-min running downhill at a −10% gradient + 40-min run on the treadmill at a 1% gradient at 65% VO_2max in a temp. of 33 °C with 50% RH 2. 60-min flat run + 40-min run on the treadmill at a 1% gradient at 65% VO_2max in a temp. of 33 °C with 50% RH	pNGAL uNGAL uNGLA/u.f.
Mellor et al. (2013) [42]	22 subjects age 36 ± 2.4 years (7 females, 15 males)	ascent from sea level to 1085 m over 6 h	pNGAL
Sugama et al. (2013) [59]	14 male triathletes age 28.7 ± 7.9 years	duathlon race: 5 km of running + 40 km of cycling + 5 km of running	uIL-6 uIL-8
Kanda et al. (2014) [37]	9 untrained healthy men age 24.8 ± 1.3 years	One leg calf-raise exercise 10 sets of 40 repetitions of exercise at 0.5 Hz with 3 min rest between sets	pNGAL uNGAL uFABP
Hewing et al. (2015) [24]	167 recreational runners age 50.3 ± 11.4 years (89 females, 78 males)	marathon	sCyst-C
Andreazzoli et al. (2017) [41]	18 professional male cyclists age 31.5 ± 4 years	mountain stage of one of the major European professional cycling competitions	pNGAL uNGAL
Mansour et al. (2017) [46]	22 heathy amateur runners age 44 (range 22–63) years (13 females, 9 males)	marathon	uNGAL uKIM-1 uIL-6, uIL-8, uIL-18, uTNFα, uYKL-40, uMCP-1
Bongers et al. (2017) [44]	60 marchers age 29 ± 78 years (30 females, 30 males)	30, 40 or 50 km for three consecutive days	uCyst-C, uNGAL, uNGAL/uCyst-C, uNGAL/Cr, uNGAL/uOsm uKIM-1, uKIM-1/uCyst-C, uKIM-1/uCr, uKIM-1/uOsm

Table 4. Cont.

Author (Year of Publication)	Study Group	Exercise/Study Design	Markers
Bongers et al. (2018) [26]	35 active healthy males age 23 ± 3 years	150-min cycle ergometer test at 80% of HRmax until 3% hypohydration (samples taken after 30 and 50 min)	sCyst-C, uCyst-C uNGAL, uNGAL/uCyst-C, uNGAL/uCr, uNGAL/uOsm uKIM-1, uKIM/uCyst-C, uKIM-1/uCr, uKIM-1/uOsm
Spada et al. (2018) [48]	58 healthy volunteers age 24 (range 21–28) years (29 males, 29 females)	4 min of HIIRT	uNGAL, uNGAL/uCr uIL-18, uIL-18/uCr uCalbindin, uCalbindin/uCr uTTF, uTTF/uCr
Wołyniec et al. (2018) [47]	19 healthy amateur runners age 35.74 ± 6.99 years (9 females, 10 males)	treadmill run test	uNGAL, uNGAL/uCr uKIM-1, uKIM-1/uCr
McDermott et al. (2018) [39]	40 healthy cyclists age 52 ± 9 years	endurance cycling event (5.7 ± 1.2 h) in heat (33.2 ± 5.0 °C, 38.4 ± 10.7% RH)	sNGAL
Chapman et al. (2019) [18]	12 healthy adults age 24 ± 5 years (3 females, 9 males)	4 h exercise in heat (35,1 °C, 61% RH)	pNGAL uNGAL, uNGAL/u.f.
Wolyniec et al. (2019) [45]	16 Healthy amateur runners age 36.7 ± 8.2 years (2 females, 14 males)	10- and 100-km runs	uCyst-C uNGAL, uNGAL/uCr uKIM-1, uKIM-1/uCr
Jouffroy et al. (2019) [51]	47 healthy males age 43 ± 7 years	80-km ultramarathon	uNGAL, uNGAL/uCr uKIM-1, uKIM-1/uCr
Poussel et al. (2020) [27]	24 healthy runners age 36.5 (range 24–57) years (1 female, 23 males)	120-km ultramarathon with 5700 m of positive elevation gain	sCyst-C uNGAL, uNGAL/uCr
Chapman et al. (2020) [43]	13 healthy adults age 23 ± 2 years (3 females, 10 males)	2 h exercise in a heat (temp 39 °C, 32 % RH)	uNGAL uIGFBP-7 uTIMP-2
Kosaki et al. (2020) [53]	116 adults without chronic kidney disease age 62 (range 24–83) years (31 females, 85 males)	incremental short maximal exercise using a cycling ergometer	uL-FABP/uCr
Semen et al. (2020) [50]	54 healthy runners age 47 ± 15 years (21 females, 33 males)	half marathon after use of 400 mg single-dose ibuprofen: two groups: 1. supplemented with MOF-VVPP 2. Control	uNGAL, uCyst-C uIL-6, uIL-8, uIL-18, uTNFα
Semen et al. (2020) [49]	1. 35 runners age 44 ± 2 years (17 females, 18 males) 2. 45 runners age 55 ± 2 years (24 females, 21 males)	1. 10 km run 2. half marathon	uNGAL

Abbreviations: u—urinary, s—serum, p—plasma, Cyst-C—cystatin C, NGAL—neutrophil gelatinase-associated lipocalin, KIM-1—kidney injury molecule-1, L-FABP—liver-type fatty-acid-binding protein, Il—interleukin, TTF3—trefoil factor-3, TNFα—tumor necrosis factor α, YKL-40—chitinase 3-like protein 1, MCP-1—monocyte chemoattractant protein-1, IGFBP-7—insulin-like growth factor binding protein 7, TIMP-2—tissue inhibitor of metalloproteinases-2, Cr—creatinine, Osm—osmolality, u.f.—urine flow, uMarker/uCyst-C—urinary marker normalized to cystatin C, uMarker/uCr—urinary marker normalized to creatinine, uMarker/uOsm—urinary marker normalized to osmolality, uMarker/u.f.—urinary marker normalized to urine flow, HIIRT—high-intensity interval resistance training, VO$_2$max—maximal oxygen consumption, HRmax—maximal heart rate, RH—relative humidity, monomeric and oligomeric flavanols (MOF-VVPP).

The diagnosis of AKI was never confirmed by kidney biopsy, which is completely understandable. The studies were performed in relatively small groups and no cases of AKI requiring HD or rhabdomyolysis were observed, because both of these severe complications are extremely rare after exercise. There is insufficient data to describe changes in AKI biomarkers in such severe complications of exercise.

The follow-up was defined in a different way in the studies presented, and in some, there was no follow-up at all.

Suggestions: Studies in larger groups, preferably multicenter, are needed. It could be reasonable to study all markers after a marathon, which is the classical distance, relatively long and intensive. Indeed, it is the most commonly studied type of exercise. More studies in females are also required. Studies with a precisely defined follow-up with several time points, as well as observational case studies on changes in AKI biomarkers in subjects with severe complications could be very interesting.

3.2. Serum or Plasma Markers

Reasonable data only concern cystatin C and NGAL. The results of the studies presented provided enough information to consider cystatin C as a better marker of eGFR than creatinine after exercise and at rest in athletes with high or low lean mass [28–30]. The information concerning plasma or serum NGAL is more questionable. In fact, after some exercises, NGAL is elevated. However, NGAL is also a marker of inflammation, organ damage and hypoxia, and in exercise, it seems to have low specificity for AKI. One practical problem is the huge variability of levels between studies and subjects. One of the possible implications of p/sNGAL measurement is diagnosis of subclinical AKI in uncomplicated rhabdomyolysis, when creatinine and cystatin levels are within the normal range [62].

The general problem with serum measurement after exercise is hemoconcentration. In many publications, the authors used a correction of the effect of dehydration according to Dill and Costill's method [63], on the basis of changes in pre- and post-blood morphology. This approach is reasonable in experimental studies, but in clinical practice, it is difficult to use, because pre-injury blood morphology results are unknown.

Suggestion: We suggest measuring sCyst-C instead of creatinine in future studies of kidney function in exercise. It is reasonable to check sNGAL in the risk group with rhabdomyolysis.

3.3. Urinary Markers

The urinary markers are increased after almost every exercise. The increment is rather small but consistent with individuals. The changes are dependent on the duration and intensity of exercise. Most studies investigated changes in uKIM-1 and uNGAL. After short exercise, an increase in uKIM-1, but not uNGAL, was observed. Elevated uKIM-1 was observed 2 and even 9 days after prolonged exercise. It is difficult to discuss the utility of uL-FABP, uCyst-C and other markers, because only few studies were performed. L-FABP is a marker of hypoxia, therefore it could be an ideal marker for studies in exercise but was used only in very few studies from one study group. What is also surprising is that uIGFBP-7 and uTIMP-2 were only analyzed in one study, and were the only markers approved for early diagnosis of AKI. The methodological problem with interpreting the changes in urinary markers is normalization. It is known that all urinary markers can be diluted, and, e.g., normalization of albuminuria is a standard procedure. In some studies, un-normalized values are used, but most authors normalized AKI markers to creatinine, osmolality, urine flow or cystatin C [18,23,26,27,34,35,40,44–48,51,53]. All these approaches had some limits. The most common was normalization to creatinine.

Suggestion: There is a need for studies on follow-up. Studies showing changes in urine markers shortly after exercise are interesting but have little practical value. In clinical practice, AKI is suspected and diagnosed several hours after exercise. What is most important is what levels of markers are typical for AKI 3, 6, 12 or 24 h after exercise. Although normalization to creatinine has some limits, it is the most common approach, and therefore it is reasonable to use this kind of normalization in subsequent studies.

There is no biomarker specific enough to assess AKI as a single biomarker. There is also no panel assessment using a couple of biomarkers, except combined urinary IGFBP-7 and TIMP-2. Taking into account the results presented in this review, combined uKIM-1/uCr and uNGAL/uCr could be the best to exclude or diagnose AKI after exercise.

3.4. Interpretation

In the presented studies, changes in AKI biomarkers were common. The main problem is how to implement the knowledge from these studies in clinical practice. There are several facts concerning AKI biomarkers, AKI and CKD in athletes:

1. Exercise-induced renal impairment is commonly present but temporary,
2. Severe complications of exercise, like AKI requiring hemodialysis, are rare,
3. Repeated episodes of AKI lead to CKD,
4. There is no data showing that CKD could be related to sports activity,
5. There is a growing body of evidence that exhausting work in heat leads to CKD [19,58–64] and the same risk factors—dehydration and muscle damage, soft drink consumption—are present, for example, in marathon runners.

Suggestion: We suggest that further studies on the physiological role of biomarkers are needed. Epidemiological studies and studies on athletes who have completed several dozen marathons or other long forms of exercise and studies on the impact of work and soft drinks on kidney function are awaited.

4. Materials and Methods

The authors researched the PubMed/MEDLINE electronic database by using terms consisting of the following: (AKI biomarker or cystatin C or NGAL or KIM-1 or urinary interleukin-18 or urinary interleukin or urinary liver-type fatty acid-binding protein or urinary L-FABP or urinary insulin-like growth factor-binding protein 7 or urinary IGFBP7 or urinary tissue inhibitor of metalloproteinases-2 or urinary TIMP-2 or nephrocheck or urinary osteopontin or urinary calbindin or urinary TTF) (nordic walking or physical activity or exercise or marathon or ultramarathon or swimming or cycling or games or football). The search was repeated regularly, and the database was updated until the last update on 13 July 2020, prior to manuscript submission. An additional search was conducted according to a reference list of read papers and by using investigators' names. As the initial selection was done through titles and abstracts, it is possible that some important papers might have been omitted, although the authors tried to identify all that were important. A total of 27 papers were retrieved from 629 titles and abstracts identified in the PubMed database (Figure 2).

In this review, results of 13 additional studies were also shortly discussed. These papers did not consider single exercise in healthy subjects, but revealed important information, and the authors decided to present their results. There was no possibility to perform any statistical analysis because of the high variability of schedules, experimental conditions and different study groups described in the papers cited. Ethical approval was not necessary, because the study did not involve participants.

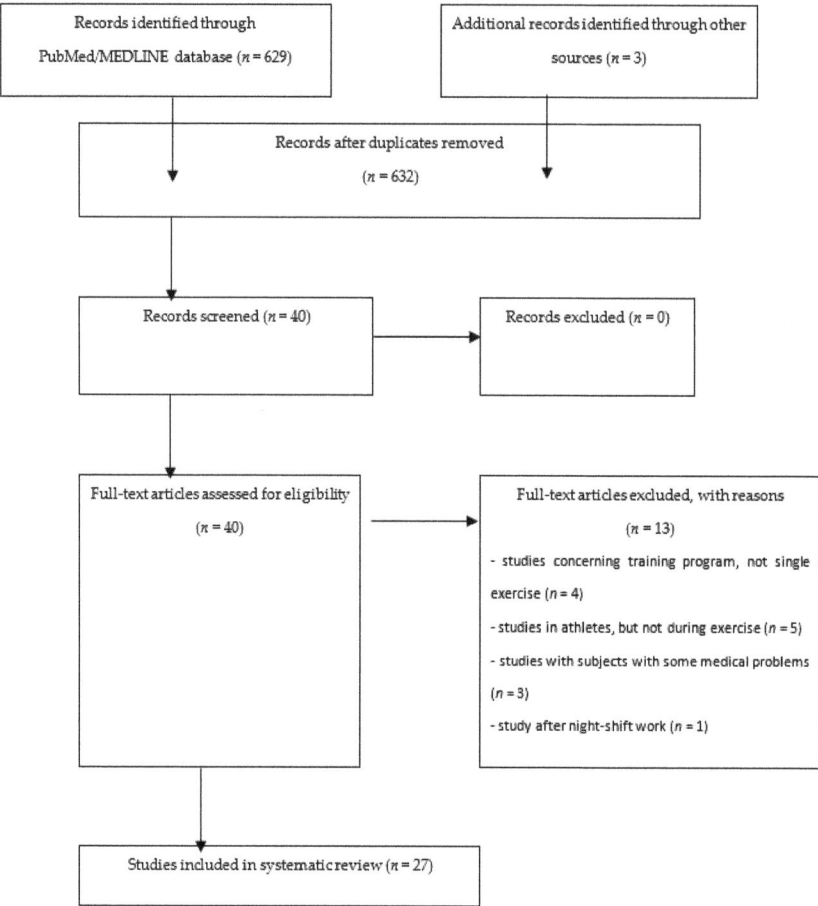

Figure 2. Flow chart illustrating the procedure for article inclusion and exclusion in a systematic review of changes in AKI biomarkers after exercise.

Author Contributions: Conceptualization, W.W. and W.R.; resources W.W., W.R. and J.R.; writing—original draft preparation, W.W.; writing—review and editing, W.R., M.R. and J.R.; visualization W.W.; supervision, M.R. All authors have read and agreed to the published version of the manuscript.

Funding: This research received no external funding.

Conflicts of Interest: The authors declare no conflict of interest.

Abbreviations

AKI	acute kidney injury
u	urinary
s	serum
p	plasma
NGAL	neutrophil gelatinase-associated lipocalin
KIM-1	kidney injury molecule-1
Cyst-C	cystatin C
Cr	creatinine
L-FABP	liver-type fatty-acid-binding protein

IL	interleukin
TTF3	trefoil factor-3
TNFα	tumor necrosis factor α
YKL-40	chitinase 3-like protein 1
MCP-1	monocyte chemoattractant protein-1
IGFBP7	insulin-like growth factor binding protein 7
TIMP-2	tissue inhibitor of metalloproteinases-2
uMarker/uCyst-C	urinary marker normalized to cystatin C
uMarker/uCr	urinary marker normalized to creatinine
uMarker/uOsm	urinary marker normalized to osmolality
uMarker/u.f.	urinary marker normalized to urine flow
eGFR	estimated glomerular filtration rate
CKD EPI	Chronic Kidney Disease Epidemiology Collaboration equation
HIIRT	high-intensity interval resistance training
VO_2max	maximal oxygen consumption
HRmax	maximal heart rate
RH	relative humidity
OA	osteoarthiritis
MOF-VVPP	monomeric and oligomeric flavanols
VO_{2max}	maximal oxygen consumption
MMP-9	matrix metallopeptidase 9

References

1. Armstrong, J.A. Urinalysis in Western culture: A brief history. *Kidney Int.* **2007**, *71*, 384–387. [CrossRef] [PubMed]
2. MacKenzie, J.C. Dr Richard Bright—A man of many parts. His bicentenary year—1789–1858. *Bristol Med. Chir. J.* **1989**, *104*, 63–67. [PubMed]
3. Gardner, K.D. Athletic pseudonephritis; alteration of urine sediment by athletic competition. *J. Am. Med. Assoc.* **1956**, *161*, 1613–1617. [CrossRef] [PubMed]
4. Floege, J.; Feehally, J. Introduction to Glomerular Disease: Clinical Presetation. In *Comprehensive Clinical Nephrology*, 4th ed.; Floege, J., Johnson, R.J., Feehally, J., Eds.; Elsevier Inc.: New York, NY, USA, 2010; pp. 15–28. ISBN 978-0-323-05876-6.
5. Oh, D.J. A long journey for acute kidney injury biomarkers. *Ren. Fail.* **2020**, *42*, 154–165. [CrossRef]
6. Wasung, M.E.; Chawla, L.S.; Madero, M. Biomarkers of renal function, which and when? *Clin. Chim. Acta* **2015**, *438*, 350–357. [CrossRef]
7. Rhee, E.P. How omics data can be used in nephrology. *Am. J. Kidney Dis.* **2018**, *72*, 129–135. [CrossRef]
8. Kashani, K.; Cheungpasitporn, W.; Ronco, C. Biomarkers of acute kidney injury: The pathway from discovery to clinical adoption. *Clin. Chem. Lab. Med.* **2017**, *55*, 1074–1089. [CrossRef]
9. Liu, X.; Guan, Y.; Xu, S.; Li, Q.; Sun, Y.; Han, R.; Jiang, C. Early Predictors of Acute Kidney Injury: A Narrative Review. *Kidney Blood Press Res.* **2016**, *41*, 680–700. [CrossRef]
10. Guzzi, L.M.; Bergler, T.; Binnall, B.; Engelman, D.T.; Forni, L.; Germain, M.J.; Gluck, E.; Göcze, I.; Joannidis, M.; Koyner, J.L.; et al. Clinical use of [TIMP-2]•[IGFBP7] biomarker testing to assess risk of acute kidney injury in critical care: Guidance from an expert panel. *Crit. Care* **2019**, *23*, 225. [CrossRef]
11. Jamieson, H.C. Some newer tests of renal function. *Can. Med. Assoc. J.* **1933**, *29*, 598–604.
12. Narayanan, S.; Appleton, H.D. Creatinine: A review. *Clin. Chem.* **1980**, *26*, 1119–1126. [CrossRef] [PubMed]
13. Randers, E.; Kristensen, J.H.; Erlandsen, E.J.; Danielsen, H. Serum cystatin C as a marker of the renal function. *Scand. J. Clin. Lab. Investig.* **1998**, *58*, 585–592. [CrossRef] [PubMed]
14. Rangaswamy, D.; Sud, K. Acute kidney injury and disease: Long-term consequences and management. *BMJ Open Sport Exerc. Med.* **2017**, *3*, e000093. [CrossRef] [PubMed]
15. Hodgson, L.E.; Walter, E.; Venn, R.M.; Galloway, R.; Pitsiladis, Y.; Sardat, F.; Forni, L.G. Acute kidney injury associated with endurance events-is it a cause for concern? A systematic review. *Nephrology* **2018**, *23*, 969–980. [CrossRef] [PubMed]

16. Lima, R.S.A.; Junior, G.B.D.S.; Liborio, A.B.; Daher, E.D.F. Acute kidney injury due to rhabdomyolysis. *Saudi J. Kidney Dis. Transplant.* **2008**, *19*, 721–729.
17. Lipman, G.S.; Shea, K.; Christensen, M.; Phillips, C.; Burns, P.; Higbee, R.; Koskenoja, V.; Eifling, K.; Krabak, B.J. Ibuprofen versus placebo effect on acute kidney injury in ultramarathons: A randomized controlled trial. *Emerg. Med. J.* **2017**, *34*, 637–642. [CrossRef] [PubMed]
18. Chapman, C.L.; Johnson, B.D.; Sackett, J.R.; Parker, M.D.; Schlader, Z.J. Soft drink consumption during and following exercise in the heat elevates biomarkers of acute kidney injury. *Am. J. Physiol. Integr. Comp. Physiol.* **2019**, *316*, R189–R198. [CrossRef]
19. Kupferman, J.; Ramírez-Rubio, O.; Amador, J.J.; López-Pilarte, D.; Wilker, E.H.; Laws, R.L.; Sennett, C.; Robles, N.V.; Lau, J.L.; Salinas, A.J.; et al. Acute Kidney Injury in Sugarcane Workers at Risk for Mesoamerican Nephropathy. *Am J Kidney Dis.* **2018**, *72*, 475–482. [CrossRef]
20. Mingels, A.; Jacobs, L.; Kleijnen, V.; Wodzig, W.; Dieijen-Visser, M. Cystatin C a marker for renal function after exercise. *Int. J. Sports Med.* **2009**, *30*, 668–671. [CrossRef]
21. Odutayo, A.; Cherney, D. Cystatin C and acute changes in glomerular filtration rate. *Clin. Nephrol.* **2012**, *78*, 64–75. [CrossRef]
22. Scherr, J.; Braun, S.; Schuster, T.; Hartmann, C.; Moehlenkamp, S.; Wolfarth, B.; Pressler, A.; Halle, M. 72-h kinetics of high-sensitive troponin T and inflammatory markers after marathon. *Med. Sci. Sports Exerc.* **2011**, *43*, 1819–1827. [CrossRef] [PubMed]
23. McCullough, P.A.; Chinnaiyan, K.M.; Gallagher, M.J.; Colar, J.M.; Geddes, T.; Gold, J.M.; Trivax, J.E. Changes in renal markers and acute kidney injury after marathon running. *Nephrology* **2011**, *16*, 194–199. [CrossRef] [PubMed]
24. Hewing, B.; Schattke, S.; Spethmann, S.; Sanad, W.; Schroeckh, S.; Schimke, I.; Halleck, F.; Peters, H.; Brechtel, L.; Lock, J.; et al. Cardiac and renal function in a large cohort of amateur marathon runners. *Cardiovasc. Ultrasound* **2015**, *13*, 13. [CrossRef] [PubMed]
25. Poortmans, J.R.; Gulbis, B.; De Bruyn, E.; Baudry, S.; Carpentier, A. Limitations of serum values to estimate glomerular filtration rate during exercise. *Br. J. Sports Med.* **2013**, *47*, 1166–1170. [CrossRef] [PubMed]
26. Bongers, C.C.W.G.; Alsady, M.; Nijenhuis, T.; Tulp, A.D.M.; Eijsvogels, T.M.H.; Deen, P.M.T.; Hopman, M.T.E. Impact of acute versus prolonged exercise and dehydration on kidney function and injury. *Physiol. Rep.* **2018**, *6*, e13734. [CrossRef] [PubMed]
27. Poussel, M.; Touzé, C.; Allado, E.; Frimat, L.; Hily, O.; Thilly, N.; Rousseau, H.; Vauthier, J.C.; Chenuel, B. Ultramarathon and Renal Function: Does Exercise-Induced Acute Kidney Injury Really Exist in Common Conditions? *Front. Sports Act. Living* **2020**, *1*, 17. [CrossRef]
28. Colombini, A.; Corsetti, R.; Machado, M.; Graziani, R.; Lombardi, G.; Lanteri, P.; Banfi, G. Serum creatine kinase activity and its relationship with renal function indices in professional cyclists during the Giro d'Italia 3-week stage race. *Clin. J. Sport Med.* **2012**, *22*, 408–413. [CrossRef]
29. Colombini, A.; Corsetti, R.; Graziani, R.; Lombardi, G.; Lanteri, P.; Banfi, G. Evaluation of creatinine, cystatin C and eGFR by different equations in professional cyclists during the Giro d'Italia 3-weeks stage race. *Scand. J. Clin. Lab. Investig.* **2012**, *72*, 114–120. [CrossRef]
30. Banfi, G.; Del Fabbro, M.; D'Eril, G.M.; Melegati, G. Reliability of cystatin C in estimating renal function in rugby players. *Ann. Clin. Biochem.* **2009**, *46*, 428. [CrossRef]
31. Lousa, I.; Nascimento, H.; Rocha, S.; Catarino, C.; Reis, F.; Rêgo, C.; Santos-Silva, A.; Seabra, A.; Ribeiro, S.; Belo, L. Influence of the 6-month physical activity programs on renal function in obese boys. *Pediatr. Res.* **2018**, *83*, 1011–1015. [CrossRef]
32. Beetham, K.S.; Howden, E.J.; Isbel, N.M.; Coombes, J.S. Agreement between cystatin-C and creatinine based eGFR estimates after a 12-month exercise intervention in patients with chronic kidney disease. *BMC Nephrol.* **2018**, *18–19*, 366. [CrossRef] [PubMed]
33. Baxmann, A.C.; Ahmed, M.S.; Marques, N.C.; Menon, V.B.; Pereira, A.B.; Kirsztajn, G.M.; Heilberg, I.P. Influence of muscle mass and physical activity on serum and urinary creatinine and serum cystatin C. *Clin. J. Am. Soc. Nephrol.* **2008**, *3*, 348–354. [CrossRef] [PubMed]
34. Junglee, N.A.; Lemmey, A.B.; Burton, M.; Searell, C.; Jones, D.; Lawley, J.S.; Jibani, M.M.; Macdonald, J.H. Does proteinuria-inducing physical activity increase biomarkers of acute kidney injury? *Kidney Blood Press Res.* **2012**, *36*, 278–289. [CrossRef] [PubMed]

35. Junglee, N.A.; Di Felice, U.; Dolci, A.; Fortes, M.B.; Jibani, M.M.; Lemmey, A.B.; Walsh, N.P.; Macdonald, J.H. Exercising in a hot environment with muscle damage: Effects on acute kidney injury biomarkers and kidney function. *Am. J. Physiol. Ren. Physiol.* **2013**, *305*, F813–F820. [CrossRef] [PubMed]
36. Bender, A.; Kaesser, U.; Eichner, G.; Bachmann, G.; Steinmeyer, J. Biomarkers of Hand Osteoarthritis Are Detectable after Mechanical Exercise. *J. Clin. Med.* **2019**, *8*, 1545. [CrossRef] [PubMed]
37. Kanda, K.; Sugama, K.; Sakuma, J.; Kawakami, Y.; Suzuki, K. Evaluation of serum leaking enzymes and investigation into new biomarkers for exercise-induced muscle damage. *Exerc. Immunol. Rev.* **2014**, *20*, 39–54. [PubMed]
38. Rullman, E.; Olsson, K.; Wågsäter, D.; Gustafsson, T. Circulating MMP-9 during exercise in humans. *Eur. J. Appl. Physiol.* **2013**, *113*, 1249–1255. [CrossRef] [PubMed]
39. McDermott, B.P.; Smith, C.R.; Butts, C.L.; Caldwell, A.R.; Lee, E.C.; Vingren, J.L.; Munoz, C.X.; Kunces, L.J.; Williamson, K.; Ganio, M.S.; et al. Renal stress and kidney injury biomarkers in response to endurance cycling in the heat with and without ibuprofen. *J. Sci. Med. Sport* **2018**, *21*, 1180–1184. [CrossRef]
40. Lippi, G.; Sanchis-Gomar, F.; Salvagno, G.L.; Aloe, R.; Schena, F.; Guidi, G.C. Variation of serum and urinary neutrophil gelatinase associated lipocalin (NGAL) after strenuous physical exercise. *Clin. Chem. Lab. Med.* **2012**, *50*, 1585–1589. [CrossRef]
41. Andreazzoli, A.; Fossati, C.; Spaccamiglio, A.; Salvo, R.; Quaranta, F.; Minganti, C.; Di Luigi, L.; Borrione, P. Assessment of pN-GAL as a marker of renal function in elite cyclists during professional competitions. *J. Biol. Regul. Homeost. Agents* **2017**, *31*, 829–835.
42. Mellor, A.; Boos, C.; Stacey, M.; Hooper, T.; Smith, C.; Begley, J.; Yarker, J.; Piper, R.; O'Hara, J.; King, R.; et al. Neutrophil gelatinase-associated lipocalin: Its response to hypoxia and association with acute mountain sickness. *Dis. Markers* **2013**, *35*, 537–542. [CrossRef] [PubMed]
43. Chapman, C.L.; Johnson, B.D.; Vargas, N.T.; Hostler, D.; Parker, M.D.; Schlader, Z.J. Both hyperthermia and dehydration during physical work in the heat contribute to the risk of acute kidney injury. *J. Appl. Physiol.* **2020**, *128*, 715–728. [CrossRef] [PubMed]
44. Bongers, C.C.W.G.; Alsady, M.; Nijenhuis, T.; Hartman, Y.A.W.; Eijsvogels, T.M.H.; Deen, P.M.T.; Hopman, M.T.E. Impact of acute versus repetitive moderate intensity endurance exercise on kidney injury markers. *Physiol. Rep.* **2017**, *5*. [CrossRef] [PubMed]
45. Wołyniec, W.; Kasprowicz, K.; Giebułtowicz, J.; Korytowska, N.; Zorena, K.; Bartoszewicz, M.; Rita-Tkachenko, P.; Renke, M.; Ratkowski, W. Changes in Water Soluble Uremic Toxins and Urinary Acute Kidney Injury Biomarkers After 10- and 100-km Runs. *Int. J. Environ. Res. Public Health* **2019**, *16*, 4153. [CrossRef] [PubMed]
46. Mansour, S.G.; Verma, G.; Pata, R.W.; Martin, T.G.; Perazella, M.A.; Parikh, C.R. Kidney Injury and Repair Biomarkers in Marathon Runners. *Am. J. Kidney Dis.* **2017**, *70*, 252–261. [CrossRef]
47. Wołyniec, W.; Ratkowski, W.; Urbański, R.; Bartoszewicz, M.; Siluk, D.; Wołyniec, Z.; Kasprowicz, K.; Zorena, K.; Renke, M. Urinary Kidney Injury Molecule-1 but Not Urinary Neutrophil Gelatinase Associated Lipocalin Is Increased after Short Maximal Exercise. *Nephron* **2018**, *138*, 29–34. [CrossRef]
48. Spada, T.C.; Silva, J.M.R.D.; Francisco, L.S.; Marçal, L.J.; Antonangelo, L.; Zanetta, D.M.T.; Yu, L.; Burdmann, E.A. High intensity resistance training causes muscle damage and increases biomarkers of acute kidney injury in healthy individuals. *PLoS ONE* **2018**, *13*, e0205791. [CrossRef]
49. Semen, K.O.; van der Doelen, R.H.A.; van der Lugt, M.; van Dam, D.; Reimer, J.; Stassen, F.R.M.; Janssen, L.; Janssen, P.; Janssen, M.J.W.; Bast, A.; et al. Non-steroidal anti-inflammatory drugs increase urinary neutrophil gelatinase-associated lipocalin in recreational runners. *Scand. J. Med. Sci. Sports* **2020**. [CrossRef]
50. Semen, K.O.; Weseler, A.R.; Janssen, M.J.W.; Drittij-Reijnders, M.J.; le Noble, J.L.M.L.; Bast, A. Effects of Monomeric and Oligomeric Flavanols on Kidney Function, Inflammation and Oxidative Stress in Runners: A Randomized Double-Blind Pilot Study. *Nutrients* **2020**, *12*, 1634. [CrossRef]
51. Jouffroy, R.; Lebreton, X.; Mansencal, N.; Anglicheau, D. Acute kidney injury during an ultra-distance race. *PLoS ONE* **2019**, *14*, e0222544. [CrossRef]
52. Machado, J.C.Q.; Volpe, C.M.O.; Vasconcellos, L.S.; Nogueira-Machado, J.A. Quantification of NGAL in Urine of Endurance Cycling Athletes. *J. Phys. Act. Health* **2018**, *15*, 679–682. [CrossRef] [PubMed]
53. Kosaki, K.; Kamijo-Ikemori, A.; Sugaya, T.; Kumamoto, S.; Tanahashi, K.; Kumagai, H.; Kimura, K.; Shibagaki, Y.; Maeda, S. Incremental short maximal exercise increases urinary liver-type fatty acid-binding protein in adults without CKD. *Scand. J. Med. Sci. Sports* **2020**, *30*, 709–715. [CrossRef] [PubMed]

54. Yamamoto, T.; Noiri, E.; Ono, Y.; Doi, K.; Negishi, K.; Kamijo, A.; Kimura, K.; Fujita, T.; Kinukawa, T.; Taniguchi, H.; et al. Renal L-type fatty acid—Binding protein in acute ischemic injury. *J. Am. Soc. Nephrol.* **2007**, *18*, 2894–2902. [CrossRef] [PubMed]
55. Hiraki, K.; Kamijo-Ikemori, A.; Yasuda, T.; Hotta, C.; Izawa, K.P.; Watanabe, S.; Sugaya, T.; Kimura, K. Moderate-intensity single exercise session does not induce renal damage. *J. Clin. Lab. Anal.* **2013**, *27*, 177–180. [CrossRef]
56. Kosaki, K.; Kamijo-Ikemori, A.; Sugaya, T.; Tanahashi, K.; Kumagai, H.; Sawano, Y.; Akazawa, N.; Ra, S.G.; Kimura, K.; Shibagaki, Y.; et al. Relationship between exercise capacity and urinary liver-type fatty acid-binding protein in middle-aged and older individuals. *Clin. Exp. Nephrol.* **2017**, *21*, 810–817. [CrossRef]
57. Kosaki, K.; Kamijo-Ikemori, A.; Sugaya, T.; Tanahashi, K.; Sawano, Y.; Akazawa, N.; Ra, S.G.; Kimura, K.; Shibagaki, Y.; Maeda, S. Effect of habitual exercise on urinary liver-type fatty acid-binding protein levels in middle-aged and older adults. *Scand. J. Med. Sci. Sports* **2018**, *28*, 152–160. [CrossRef]
58. Uchiyama, K.; Washida, N.; Morimoto, K.; Muraoka, K.; Nakayama, T.; Adachi, K.; Kasai, T.; Miyashita, K.; Wakino, S.; Itoh, H. Effects of exercise on residual renal function in patients undergoing peritoneal dialysis: A post-hoc analysis of a randomized controlled trial. *Ther. Apher. Dial.* **2020**. [CrossRef]
59. Sugama, K.; Suzuki, K.; Yoshitani, K.; Shiraishi, K.; Kometani, T. Urinary excretion of cytokines versus their plasma levels after endurance exercise. *Exerc. Immunol. Rev.* **2013**, *19*, 29–48.
60. Dutheil, F.; Trousselard, M.; Perrier, C.; Lac, G.; Chamoux, A.; Duclos, M.; Naughton, G.; Mnatzaganian, G.; Schmidt, J. Urinary interleukin-8 is a biomarker of stress in emergency physicians, especially with advancing age—The JOBSTRESS* randomized trial. *PLoS ONE* **2013**, *8*, e71658. [CrossRef]
61. Pryor, R.R.; Pryor, J.L.; Vandermark, L.W.; Adams, E.L.; Brodeur, R.M.; Schlader, Z.J.; Armstrong, L.E.; Lee, E.C.; Maresh, C.M.; Casa, D.J. Acute Kidney Injury Biomarker Responses to Short-Term Heat Acclimation. *Int. J. Environ. Res. Public Health* **2020**, *17*, 1325. [CrossRef]
62. Apeland, T.; Danielsen, T.; Staal, E.M.; Åsberg, A.; Thorsen, I.S.; Dalsrud, T.O.; Ørn, S. Risk factors for exertional rhabdomyolysis with renal stress. *BMJ Open Sport Exerc. Med.* **2017**, *3*, e000241. [CrossRef] [PubMed]
63. Matomäki, P.; Kainulainen, H.; Kyröläinen, H. Corrected whole blood biomarkers—The equation of Dill and Costill revisited. *Physiol. Rep.* **2018**, *6*, e13749. [CrossRef] [PubMed]
64. Yang, X.; Wu, H.; Li, H. Dehydration-associated chronic kidney disease: A novel case of kidney failure in China. *BMC Nephrol.* **2020**, *21*, 159. [CrossRef] [PubMed]

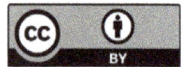

© 2020 by the authors. Licensee MDPI, Basel, Switzerland. This article is an open access article distributed under the terms and conditions of the Creative Commons Attribution (CC BY) license (http://creativecommons.org/licenses/by/4.0/).

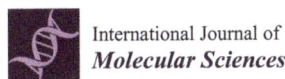

Review

New Biomarkers in Acute Tubulointerstitial Nephritis: A Novel Approach to a Classic Condition

Laura Martinez Valenzuela [1,2], **Juliana Draibe** [1,2], **Xavier Fulladosa** [1,2] **and Juan Torras** [1,2,3,*]

1. Bellvitge University Hospital, Nephrology Department, Hospitalet de Llobregat, 08907 Barcelona, Spain; lmartinezv@bellvitgehospital.cat (L.M.V.); jbordignon@bellvitgehospital.cat (J.D.); xfulladosa@bellvitgehospital.cat (X.F.)
2. IDIBELL Biomedical Research Institute, Hospitalet de Llobregat, 08907 Barcelona, Spain
3. Clinical Sciences Department, Campus de Bellvitge, Barcelona University, Hospitalet de Llobregat, 08907 Barcelona, Spain
* Correspondence: 15268jta@comb.cat

Received: 10 June 2020; Accepted: 29 June 2020; Published: 30 June 2020

Abstract: Acute tubulointerstitial nephritis (ATIN) is an immunomediated cause of acute kidney injury. The prevalence of ATIN among the causes of acute kidney injury (AKI) is not negligible, especially those cases related to certain drugs. To date, there is a lack of reliable non-invasive diagnostic and follow-up markers. The gold standard for diagnosis is kidney biopsy, which shows a pattern of tubulointerstitial leukocyte infiltrate. The urinalysis findings can aid in the diagnosis but are no longer considered sensitive or specific. At the present time, there is a rising attentiveness to finding trustworthy biomarkers of the disease, with special focus in urinary cytokines and chemokines that may reflect kidney local inflammation. Cell-based tests are of notable interest to identify the exact drug involved in hypersensitivity reactions to drugs, manifesting as ATIN. Certain single-nucleotide polymorphisms in HLA or cytokine genes may confer susceptibility to the disease according to pathophysiological basis. In this review, we aim to critically examine and summarize the available evidence on this topic.

Keywords: acute tubulointerstitial nephritis; immunology; biomarkers

1. Introduction

Acute tubulointerstitial nephritis (ATIN) is an immunomediated disease affecting the tubulointerstitial area of the kidneys. The tubulointerstitium comprises 80% of the kidney surface and is composed of cellular and extracellular matrix components [1]. The specific and identifying pathological picture consists of a cellular infiltrate composed by leukocytes, primarily lymphocytes, but also including eosinophils, macrophages, or plasma cells. A myriad of etiologies can lead to ATIN, although drug-induced ATIN is the most common, accounting for 3–14% of biopsy-proven acute kidney injury (AKI) [2] and 70–90% of ATIN cases [3]. Also, of note, ATIN is related to autoimmune and inflammatory diseases—systemic lupus erythematosus, IgG-4 related disease, and tubulointerstitial nephritis with uveitis (TINU) syndrome, among others—or infectious diseases, such as cytomegalovirus or adenovirus infections.

Type IV hypersensitivity reactions are the underlying pathomechanisms of drug-induced ATIN. The kidneys are adapted to filter a high rate of blood flow that contains proteins and potential antigens, thus leaving them exposed to drugs and their metabolites [4]. Tubular epithelial cells (TECs) are able to process and present these antigens from tubular lumen, working as non-professional antigen-presenting cells (APCs). TECs present antigens to dendritic cells, which in turn migrate to regional lymph nodes, activate specific T cells, and integrate innate and adaptive immune responses [5]. Those activated T cells infiltrate the renal parenchyma and amplify inflammation through increased secretion of cytokines and the recruitment of other inflammatory cells [4].

The involvement of necroinflammation pathways has been recently described to collaborate in the pathogenesis of drug induced ATIN. It has been hypothesized that drugs can directly damage TECs and induce necroptosis. This is a recently-described form of cell death, halfway between necrosis and apoptosis, leading to the release of proinflammatory cytokines and the recruitment of innate immune system cells. After necroptosis of TECs, intracellular molecules are dropped to the interstitial space and bind to several receptors that recognize danger signals, such as toll-like receptors (TLRs), expressed by immune cells. Signal–receptor interaction leads to the release of proinflammatory cytokines that, in turn, magnify the immune response, triggering further direct TEC necroptosis [6]. A role for necroinflammation has been confirmed in a murine model of cisplatin-induced AKI, but further research is required to confirm the participation of these pathways in human ATIN [7].

Inflammatory phenomena and cellular infiltration lead to tubular dysfunction and (AKI). It is usually difficult for the clinician to distinguish between ATIN and acute tubular necrosis (ATN) in this setting. ATIN may be accompanied by fever, skin rash, arthralgias, or flank pain, contrarily to ATN, and this picture can help guide the diagnosis, but those are not universal findings. The presence of known previous autoimmune conditions, concomitant infections, or recently-administered drugs can also support the hypothesis of ATIN of a specific etiology. The gold standard in ATIN diagnosis is kidney biopsy. Based on the predominance of an inflammatory component in the kidneys of ATIN, some classical and novel biomarkers, reviewed hereunder, may serve in the diagnosis, prognosis, and follow-up of this disease.

2. ATIN Classical Biomarkers

Urine cellularity and casts have been used classically to find evidence of localized inflammation in the kidneys. Routine optical microscopy examination of the urine samples requires trained personnel and is time-consuming. In recent decades, automated cytometric urinalysis has replaced provider-performed urine microscopy. The information obtained here may guide the diagnosis but has limitations. Occasionally, urine sediment can be negative despite the existence of inflammatory kidney disease, and the presence of cells and crystals is not always specific to a certain pathology. Also, automated examination is less precise for diagnosis than laboratory-based microscopy examination. Thus, although useful, urine sediment examination should always be accompanied by knowledge of the clinical context [8].

Sterile leukocyturia is a common finding in ATIN patients. Depending on the series, the prevalence of leukocyturia ranges within 50–70% of all-cause-ATIN cases [9,10]. Interestingly, leukocyturia is an almost universal finding in drug-related and especially in antibiotic-related ATIN, while it is found merely in about 50% of ATIN patients related to autoimmune diseases [11].

Due to the Type IV hypersensitivity basis of drug-induced ATIN and the usual presence of eosinophils in kidney biopsy specimens [6]., eosinophiluria was considered a classical biomarker in ATIN. The belief inthe utility of this parameter is based on a small-case series. Although the increased sensitivity was noted using Hansel stain instead of Wright stain [12], eosinophiluria is no longer considered sensitive or specific. In the largest cohort studied, Muriithi et al. found 31% sensitivity and 68% specificity for the diagnosis of ATIN among 566 patients with AKI, and found no utility of eosinophiluria in the distinction between ATIN and ATN [13]. Patients with urinary tract abnormalities, urinary tract infections, acute tubular necrosis, and glomerulonephritis also exhibit eosinophiluria [14].

Other findings from urine microscopic examination are white blood cell (WBC) casts, which are either not sensitive and not specific for ATIN diagnosis. WBC casts are found in urine from patients with inflammatory kidney diseases, not only ATIN. They have also been seen in other conditions such as glomerulonephritis and pyelonephritis. Surprisingly, less than 14% of ATIN patients present WBC in urine microscopy according to the published series. Red blood cell (RBC) casts were once thought to be specific for glomerular disease, however up to one third of ATIN patients exhibit RBC, probably related to disruption of interstitial blood vessels and leakage of erythrocytes to the tubular lumen [15]. Granular casts are the most frequent casts seen in ATIN, up to 95% [16]. depending on the series, but they are also very common in ATN.

3. Novel Biomarkers

ATIN involves cell immunity rather than humoralmechanisms, as suggested by the extensive and pleiomorphic inter-tubular cell infiltrate in ATIN kidney biopsies, with lack of immune deposits in most of the cases. Rarely anti-tubular basal membrane (TMB) antibodies and immune complexes can be noticed. The presence of this immune cell infiltration can damage TECs due to direct cytotoxicity or local cytokine release. At the same time, TECs acquire an active role in inflammation by orchestrating the immune response and directly producing diverse cytokines. In the same line, cell infiltrates together with activated TECs also produce signaling molecules that promote matrix deposition and remodeling, thus promoting fibrosis [17].

Identification of the differential nature of the tubulointerstitial infiltrates in ATIN and the cytokines produced by this infiltrate—in comparison to other inflammatory kidney diseases—and their detection in serum or urine, can be useful as biomarkers of the disease.

4. Serum and Urine Cytokines and Chemokines

In the recent years, there has been a rise in the number of studies published in the field of urinary biomarkers, seizing the non-invasive nature of the sampling. The introduction and spread of novel multiplex assays that allow multiple simultaneous cytokine measurements in the same procedure has become a valuable tool in this kind of research. The presence in urine of the different chemokines and cytokines evaluated isillustrative of the pathophysiologic processes occurring in this disease.

Monocyte chemoattractant protein-1 (MCP-1) has a key role in the recruitment of monocytes, neutrophils, and lymphocytes in tissue inflammation processes. In the kidney, it is produced by TECs, endothelial cells of the peritubular capillaries, and macrophages themselves. MCP-1 has been identified as a chemokine involved in autoimmune diseases [18]. Wu et al. found higher MCP-1 levels in a cohort of 40 patients with drug-induced ATIN compared to controls. Urinary MCP-1 correlated and predicted the severity of the acute lesions in kidney biopsies from these patients [19]. In the same line, Yun et al. described higher MCP-1 serum and urine concentration among 113 ATIN patients from different causes in their bead-based multiplex assay [20]. Interestingly, Dantas et al. found that urinary MCP-1 concentration finely correlated with the amount of tubulointerstitial infiltrate but not with the glomerular infiltrate in a cohort of patients with glomerular autoimmune diseases [21]. Other authors also reported higher urinary levels of MCP-1 in patients with systemic lupus erythematosus (SLE) that correlated with the extension of the tubulointerstitial infiltrate, thus confirming the utility of MCP-1 in urine as a biomarker of acute infiltration of kidneys with dense affectation of this compartment [22].

Tumor necrosis factor alpha (TNF-α) is a proinflammatory cytokine produced by macrophages and monocytes. It participates in signaling cascades that lead to cell apoptosis or necrosis. Several authors reported higher levels of TNF-α in serum and urine samples from ATIN patients. Moledina et al. reported a higher urinary TNF-α in patients with ATIN that helped in the differential diagnosis of patients with ATN [23]. The same group showed that urinary TNF-α was also higher in a large series of ATIN cases compared to other causes of inflammatory kidney disease, and that urinary TNF-α correlated well with the number of TNF-α-positive cells in the renal biopsy [24]. Aoyagi et al. reported the value of serum TNF-α levels in the follow-up of a case of TINU, which dramatically decreased during the first week after treatment initiation [25]. Moledina et al. found higher urinary IL-9 along with higher TNF-α levels in patients with ATIN. IL-9 is involved in allergic responses and induces mast cell accumulation, which isin turn a source of TNF-α [23,24]. TNF-α inducessecretion of IL-6, among other cytokines. This is a cytokine with a local proinflammatory effect in the early stages of inflammation that also induces acute-phase production of proteins such as CRP [26]. Numerous authors reported elevated IL-6 concentration in urine and plasma from patients with ATIN compared to healthy controls [20,27,28].

Other unspecific tubular AKI biomarkers have also been evaluated in ATIN. N-acetyl-β-D-glucosaminidase (NAG) is a lysosomal enzyme present in TECs which is a marker of proximal renal tubular damage [29]. Neutrophil gelatinase-associated lipocalin (NGAL) is a protein contained in the neutrophil granules but also in other human tissues such as kidney TECs. Some authors have demonstrated NGAL release during inflammatory processes [30]. α1-microglobulin is a low-molecular-weight protein that acts as radical scavenger and reductase [31]. NAG, α1-microglobulin, and NGAL are filtered in the glomeruli and completely reabsorbed by proximal TECs. Thus, urinary presence of these three molecules indicates proximal TEC damage and dysfunction. Many authors have found high levels of these biomarkers in urine and have used combination strategies to increase sensitivity and specificity of ATIN diagnosis [19,32–34]. Figure 1 illustrates the role of the suggested cytokines and chemokines in ATIN.

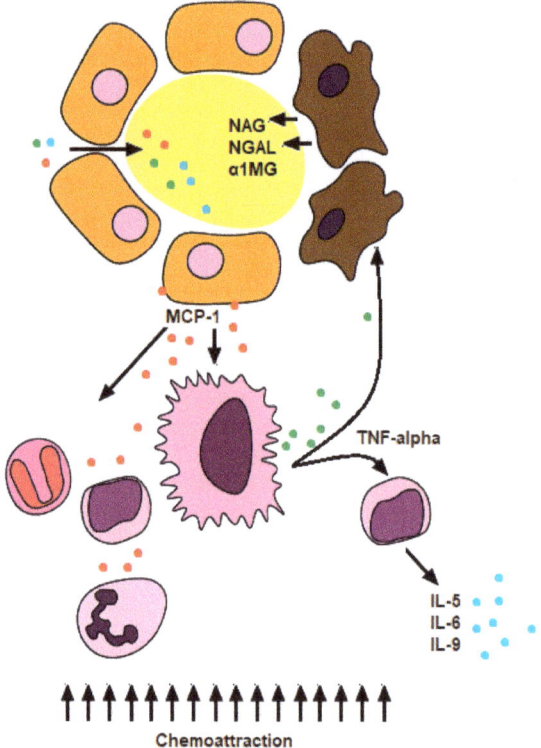

Figure 1. Cytokines and chemokines suggested as biomarkers in acute tubulointerstitial nephritis. Tubular endothelial cells (TECs) secrete MCP-1, which is a powerful chemoattractant for inflammatory cells towards the interstitium. Incoming macrophages release TNF-α, that primes and activates lymphocytes to secrete various proinflammatory interleukins (IL). In parallel, TNF-α can damage TECs inducing acute tubular necrosis (ATN). As a consequence of ATN, some markers of the injury of TECs (NAG, NGAL, and α1MG) are found in urine.MCP-1, monocyte chemoattractant protein-1; TNFα, tumor necrosis factor α; NAG, N-acetyl glucosamidinadase; NGAL, neutrophil gelatinase-associated lipocalin; α1MG, α1 microglobulin.

Renal regional complement activation has been examined as an ATIN biomarker in a study by Zhao et al. Soluble urinary C5b9 was found to correlate with the degree of interstitial inflammatory infiltrates and also with tubular dysfunction in a cohort of 44 patients with ATIN of different etiologies [35].

In addition to the diagnostic value in the acute stage of the disease, urinary biomarkers have been evaluated in other settings. Shi et al. evaluated a panel of biomarkers in the follow-up of 54 patients with ATIN along a median time of 38 months. They found that NAG, matrix metalloproteinase 2 (MMP)2, and MMP9 clearly correlated with the rate of glomerular filtration rate (GFR) decline. The authors performed a multiple linear regression analysis to exclude other factors, and confirmed that higher concentration of these biomarkers at diagnostic was independently associated with faster progression of chronic kidney disease [34]. Table 1 summarizes the published evidence of ATIN serum and urinary cytokines and chemokines as biomarkers.

Table 1. Summary of the main publications related to serum and urinary biomarkers of acute tubulointerstitial nephritis (ATIN).

Reference	Population Samples	Relevant Findings
Dantas et al., Kidney Blood Press Res, 2007	Glomerulopathy $n=37$	Urinary MCP-1 correlated with the extent of tubulointerstitial infiltrate by macrophages but not with the degree of glomerular infiltrate.
Yu et al., Journal of Peking University, 2010	Acute drug-induced TIN $n=28$ Chronic drug-induced TIN $n=12$	The combination of urinary NAG and α1-MG increased sensitivity and specificity for the detection of acute drug-induced tubulointerstitial nephritis (TIN).
Wu et al., Clin J Am SocNephrol, 2010	Drug-induced ATIN $n=40$ Healthy controls $n=20$	MCP-1, α1-MG, NGAL, and NAG urinary levels were higher in ATIN patients compared to controls. MCP-1 urinary levels correlated with the extent and severity of the acute lesions.
Nakashima et al., ClinNephrol, 2010	IgG 4 disease-related ATIN $n=4$ Other cause ATIN $n=16$	IL-4, IL-10, and TGFβ RNA expression in kidney tissue was higher in IgG4 disease related ATIN compared to the rest of ATIN causes.
Shi et al., Am J Med Sci, 2013	Drug-induced ATIN $n=51$	Patients with higher urinary levels of NAG, metalloproteinase 2(MMP2) and MMP9 presented faster GFR decline during follow-up
Wu et al., Am J Med Sci, 2013	ATIN $n=40$ Healthy controls $n=20$	Urinary α1-MG correlated with the degree of interstitial edema and inflammatory infiltrate in kidney biopsy. Urinary NAG correlated with the degree of inflammatory infiltrate. Urinary TGFβ correlated with the presence of fibrosis.
Aoyagi et al., CEN Case Rep, 2014	One case of TINU	Serum TNFα, IL-8 and IFNγ levels decreased during follow up of an episode of TINU.
Chen et al. Braz J Med Biol Res, 2018	ATIN $n=30$ Healthy controls $n=15$	Serum IL-6, IL-10, and TNFα were significantly higher in ATIN patients compared to controls.
Zhao et al., Am J Physiol Renal Physiol, 2019	ATIN $n=44$ Healthy controls $n=24$	Urinary levels of KIM-1 and C5b9 were higher in ATIN patients compared to healthy controls. Urinary C5b9 correlated with the extent of tubulointerstitial infiltrates in kidney biopsy in ATIN patients.
Yun et al., BMC nephrology, 2019	ATIN $n=113$ Healthy controls $n=40$	Serum IL-1β, IFNα2, TNFα, MCP-1, IL-8, IL-17A, IL-18, and IL-23 were higher in ATIN patients compared to healthy controls. Urinary IFNα2, MCP-1, IL-6, IL-8, IL-12p70, and IL-17A were higher in ATIN patients compared to healthy controls
Moledina et al., JCI Insight, 2019	ATIN $n=32$ Other kidney diseases $n=186$	Urinary TNFα and IL-9 were higher in ATIN patients compared to other kidney diseases. Urinary IL-5 was higher among those ATIN patients with prominent eosinophil infiltrates.
Moledina et al., Nephron, 2019	ATIN $n=32$ ATIN $n=41$	Urinary TNFα and IL-9 were higher in ATIN patients.

MCP-1 macrophage chemoattractant protein; NAG N-acetyl-neuraminidase; α1-MG α1-microglobulin; NGAL neutrophil gelatinase-associated lipocalin; IL-4 interleukin-4, IL-10 interleukin-10, transforming growth factor-β; GFR glomerular filtration rate; TNFα Tumor Necrosis Factor α; IL-8 Interleukin-8; IFNγ interferon γ; IL-6 interleukin-6; KIM-1 kidney injury molecule; IL-1β interleukin 1 β, IFNα2 interferon α2; IL-17A interleukin-17A, IL-18 interleukin-18; IL-23 interleukin-23; IL-12p70 interleukin-12p70; IL-9 interleukin-9; IL-5 interleukin-5.

5. Cellular Biomarkers

In the context of drug-induced ATIN, the most common cause of this group of diseases, in vivo cellular assays are key to demonstrate the existence of drug hypersensitivity and identify the offending drug. Throughout their lives, but also during a previous ATIN episode, people are frequently exposed to multiple drugs. Proper identification of which exact medication is the culprit allows for safe discontinuation. Binding of T cells with a drug is a complex process that generates a cascade of events that can be measured in its different steps. These cellular assays are based on the demonstration of the lymphocyte proliferation response and the cytokine secretion response when exposed to the suspected drug.

On the one hand, the activation phenotype of lymphocytes after drug exposure can be assessed using fluorescence cytometry techniques. Detection of activation markers onthe surface of lymphocytes after incubation with the offending drug—such as CD25, CD69, or Human Leukocyte Antigen (HLA)-DR—may indicate hypersensitivity [36,37].

Also, activation of T cells after drug exposure triggers a specific pattern of cytokine secretion. These cytokines can be detected in the supernatant of the stimulated cell cultures using enzyme-linked assays. Many authors have reported the release of high amounts of IL-5 in the setting of hypersensitivity. Mauri-Hellweg et al. reported high IL-5 concentration in supernatant of lymphocyte cultures from patients with known hypersensitivity to diverse antiepileptic drugs after culturing with these drugs[37]. Zanni et al. found a predominant Th2 response with prominent IL-5 release among a cohort of 13 patients affected by lidocaine hypersensitivity [38]. Sachs et al. found higher IL-5 concentration and, to a lesser extent IL-10 and IFN-γ, was even more sensitive for the detection of drug hypersensitivity than lymphocyte proliferation tests [39].

Enzyme-linked immunospot (ELISpot) assay is a sensitive test that allows the ex vivo measurement of the production of cytokines by lymphocytes in response to a certain stimulus. It provides quantitative information of the amount of responder cells. There are some reports of the usefulness of this test in evaluating drug hypersensitivity reactions. Tanvarasethee et al. studied 25 patients with cephalosporin-induced maculopapular exanthema. They found that the combined quantification of INF-γ and IL-5 spots by ELISpot assay was more sensitive than skin tests to diagnose cephalosporin hypersensitivity [40]. Rozieres et al. proved the specificity of the IFN-γELISpot assay for the demonstration of Type IV delayed hypersensitivity reaction (DHR) detecting amoxicillin-specific T cells. Twenty of twenty-two patients with known amoxicillin DHR had detectable amoxicillin-specific T cells. Interestingly, none of the control patients with IgE-mediated amoxicillin hypersensitivity nor the healthy controls presented amoxicillin-specific T cells [41]. At the moment, there is little evidence on the usefulness of ELISpot assays specifically targeting patients with ATIN. Punrin et al., in a cohort of patients with drug-induced ATIN, reported a positive IFN-γELISpot assay in 50% of them [42].

The lymphocyte transformation test (LTT) measures the proliferation of lymphocytes in response to the pure form of a suspicious drug. In vitro, prior to the exposure, lymphocytes are incubated with ^{3}H-thymidine or carboxyfluoresceinsuccinimidyl ester (CFSE). The attenuation of radioactivity incorporation or dilution of CFSE with each cell division after incubation with the offending drug, measured in a β-counter or flow cytometry, is an indicator of cell proliferation. Positive LTT has been reported in the setting of ATIN induced by β-lactams and NSAIDs [43]. Koda et al. described a case of ATIN in the setting of the treatment with nivolumab and lansoprazole [44]. The LTT demonstrated reactivity against lansoprazole and not against nivolumab, indicating which was the culprit drug for ATIN.

6. Genetic Biomarkers

Some descriptions of the association of ATIN, mainly in the setting of TINU, with certain human leukocyte antigen (HLA) or single-nucleotide polymorphisms (SNPs) as markers of disease susceptibility have been published.

To identify genetic markers of TINU, Levinson et al. performed HLA genotyping of 18 American TINU patients. They found that the disease was strongly associated with HLA-DQA1*01, HLA-DQB1*05, and HLA-DRB1*01. The prevalence of these HLA genes was elevated among their cohort of TINU patients, and significantly higher in comparison with the published HLA frequencies in North American whites [45]. A study conducted in a cohort of 154 Chinese patients with ATIN of different causes showed that, similarly to the American study, HLA-DQA1*0104/DQB1*0503/DRB1*1405 are risk haplotypes for the development of ATIN. These studies suggest that these variants may enhance antigen presentation and facilitate renal tubulointerstitial inflammation.

Rytkönen et al. studied IL-10 gene SNPs in a cohort of 30 pediatric cases of TINU or idiopathic TIN. They found a higher prevalence of the IL-10 SNP s3024490 in TINU/ATIN cases compared with its prevalence in a control group of 393 individuals from their own population [46]. IL-10 is an immunoregulatory cytokine that inhibits the synthesis of proinflammatory cytokines and chemokines. Interestingly, IL-10 SNPs have also been linked to susceptibility to recurrent attacks of acute pyelonephritis [47]. Based on these findings, the authors suggested that patients with SNPs in immunoregulatory cytokines and other inflammatory mediators may confer higher susceptibility to TINU/ATIN.

7. Final Remarks

To date, there is no reliable, non-invasive test for the diagnosis and monitoring of ATIN. Classical urine studies have shown poor sensitivity and specificity in ATIN diagnosis. Kidney biopsy is the gold standard for the assessment of ATIN, but there are significant drawbacks in the performance of this procedure in certain settings. First, it is contraindicated in certain patients such as those with uncontrolled hypertension or non-corrigible coagulation disorders, and the indication in the case of mononephric, small-sized kidney, or obese patients may be questionable due to the increased risk of serious complications. Second, although infrequent, variable degrees of bleeding may occur during the procedure or the following hours, especially when inflammation is prominent. Third, kidney biopsy requires trained personnel and a sufficient infrastructure that is not generally available in all hospitals, and a shift to specialized units may cause delays in the diagnosis.

Urinary biomarkers are excellent candidates for the evaluation of kidney diseases. Urine sampling has the advantage of being a non-invasive, immediate, and easy-to-perform procedure and can be repeated over time. The infrastructure required for cytokine quantification is relatively simple and frequently ELISA based, thus its use can be widespread. Urinary molecular content is a valuable live, and direct reflection of the inflammatory reactions occurring locally in the kidney tissue. The selection of novel biomarkers based on the pathophysiology of the disease will, over time, permit refinement in the diagnosis of the disease and the follow-up of the immune activity.

Cell-based assays have an added value because they go beyond the diagnosis of ATIN. They confirm the presence of a DHR against a specific drug in ATIN patients. Genetic biomarkers can help to deepen the knowledge of the pathophysiology of the disease.

Summarizing, novel biomarkers of ATIN are of interest to avoid kidney biopsy and its complications, are based on non-invasive sampling techniques, are low-resource consuming, reflect pathogenic processes ongoing in the kidney tissue, and can help identify the culprit drug in the case of drug-induced ATIN.

Author Contributions: L.M.V. performed a literature review of the topic and elaborated the manuscript. J.T. elaborated the manuscript. J.D. and X.F. critically revised the manuscript. All authors have read and agreed to the published version of the manuscript.

Funding: This research received no external funding.

Acknowledgments: This study has been funded by Instituto de Salud Carlos III through the grant CM19/00107 (co-funded by European Social Fund (ESF investing in your future). We thank CERCA Program /Generalitat de Catalunya for institutional support.

Conflicts of Interest: The authors declare no conflict of interest.

References

1. Tanaka, T.; Nangaku, M. Pathogenesis of tubular interstitial nephritis. *Contrib. Nephrol.* **2011**, *169*, 297–310. [CrossRef] [PubMed]
2. Cruz, D.N.; Perazella, M.A. Drug-induced acute tubulointerstitial nephritis: The clinical spectrum. *Hosp. Pract.* **1998**, *33*, 151–164. [CrossRef] [PubMed]
3. Raghavan, R.; Eknoyan, G. Acute interstitial nephritis-a reappraisal and update. *Clin. Nephrol.* **2014**, *82*, 149–162. [CrossRef]
4. Raghavan, R.; Shawar, S. Mechanisms of Drug-Induced Interstitial Nephritis. *Adv. Chronic Kidney Dis.* **2017**, *24*, 64–71. [CrossRef]
5. Waeckerle-Men, Y.; Starke, A.; Wahl, P.R.; Wüthrich, R.P. Limited costimulatory molecule expression on renal tubular epithelial cells impairs T cell activation. *Kidney Blood Press. Res.* **2007**, *30*, 421–429. [CrossRef]
6. Eddy, A.A. Drug-induced tubulointerstitial nephritis: Hypersensitivity and necroinflammatory pathways. *Pediatr. Nephrol.* **2020**, *35*, 547–554. [CrossRef]
7. Xu, Y.; Ma, H.; Shao, J.; Wu, J.; Zhou, L.; Zhang, Z.; Wang, Y.; Huang, Z.; Ren, J.; Liu, S.; et al. A role for tubular necroptosis in cisplatin-induced AKI. *J. Am. Soc. Nephrol.* **2015**, *26*, 2647–2658. [CrossRef]
8. Cavanaugh, C.; Perazella, M.A. Urine Sediment Examination in the Diagnosis and Management of Kidney Disease: Core Curriculum 2019. *Am. J. Kidney Dis.* **2019**, *73*, 258–272. [CrossRef]
9. Muriithi, A.K.; Leung, N.; Valeri, A.M.; Cornell, L.D.; Sethi, S.; Fidler, M.E.; Nasr, S.H. Biopsy-Proven Acute Interstitial Nephritis, 1993–2011: A Case Series. *Am. J. Kidney Dis.* **2014**, *64*, 558–566. [CrossRef]
10. Wilson, G.J.; Kark, A.L.; Francis, L.P.; Hoy, W.; Healy, H.G.; Mallett, A.J. The increasing rates of acute interstitial nephritis in Australia: A single centre case series. *BMC Nephrol.* **2017**, *18*, 329. [CrossRef]
11. Perazella, M.A. Clinical Approach to Diagnosing Acute and Chronic Tubulointerstitial Disease. *Adv. Chronic Kidney Dis.* **2017**, *24*, 57–63. [CrossRef]
12. Nolan, C.R.; Anger, M.S.; Kelleher, S.P. Eosinophiluria—A New Method of Detection and Definition of the Clinical Spectrum. *N. Engl. J. Med.* **1986**, *315*, 1516–1519. [CrossRef]
13. Muriithi, A.K.; Nasr, S.H.; Leung, N. Utility of urine eosinophils in the diagnosis of acute interstitial nephritis. *Clin. J. Am. Soc. Nephrol.* **2013**, *8*, 1857–1862. [CrossRef]
14. Lusica, M.; Rondon-Berrios, H.; Feldman, L. Urine eosinophils for acute interstitial nephritis. *J. Hosp. Med.* **2017**, *12*, 343–345. [CrossRef]
15. Nussbaum, E.Z.; Perazella, M.A. Diagnosing acute interstitial nephritis: Considerations for clinicians. *Clin. Kidney J.* **2019**, *12*, 808–813. [CrossRef]
16. Fogazzi, G.B.; Ferrari, B.; Garigali, G.; Simonini, P.; Consonni, D. Urinary sediment findings in acute interstitial nephritis. *Am. J. Kidney Dis.* **2012**, *60*, 330–332. [CrossRef]
17. Rossert, J. Drug-induced acute interstitial nephritis. In *Kidney International*; Blackwell Publishing Inc.: Paris, France, 2001; Volume 60, pp. 804–817. [CrossRef]
18. Deshmane, S.L.; Kremlev, S.; Amini, S.; Sawaya, B.E. Monocyte chemoattractant protein-1 (MCP-1): An overview. *J. Interf. Cytokine Res.* **2009**, *29*, 313–325. [CrossRef]
19. Wu, Y.; Yang, L.; Su, T.; Wang, C.; Liu, G.; Li, X.M. Pathological significance of a panel of urinary biomarkers in patients with drug-induced tubulointerstitial nephritis. *Clin. J. Am. Soc. Nephrol.* **2010**, *5*, 1954–1959. [CrossRef]
20. Yun, D.; Jang, M.J.; An, J.N.; Lee, J.P.; Kim, D.K.; Chin, H.J.; Kim, Y.S.; Lee, D.S.; Han, S.S. Effect of steroids and relevant cytokine analysis in acute tubulointerstitial nephritis. *BMC Nephrol.* **2019**, *20*, 1–10. [CrossRef]
21. Dantas, M.; Almeida Romão, E.; Silva Costa, R. Urinary excretion of monocyte chemoattractant protein-1: A biomarker of active tubulointerstitial damage in patients with glomerulopathies. *Kidney Blood Press. Res.* **2007**, *30*, 306–313. [CrossRef]
22. Ding, Y.; Nie, L.M.; Pang, Y.; Wu, W.J.; Tan, Y.; Yu, F.; Zhao, M.H. Composite urinary biomarkers to predict pathological tubulointerstitial lesions in lupus nephritis. *Lupus* **2018**, *27*, 1778–1789. [CrossRef]
23. Moledina, D.G.; Parikh, C.R. Differentiating Acute Interstitial Nephritis from Acute Tubular Injury: A Challenge for Clinicians. *Nephron* **2019**, *143*, 211–216. [CrossRef]
24. Moledina, D.G.; Wilson, F.P.; Pober, J.S.; Perazella, M.A.; Singh, N.; Luciano, R.L.; Obeid, W.; Lin, H.; Kuperman, M.; Moeckel, G.W.; et al. Urine TNF-α and IL-9 for clinical diagnosis of acute interstitial nephritis. *JCI Insight* **2019**, *4*, e127456. [CrossRef]

25. Aoyagi, J.; Kanai, T.; Ito, T.; Odaka, J.; Saito, T.; Momoi, M.Y. Cytokine dynamics in a 14-year-old girl with tubulointerstitial nephritis and uveitis syndrome. *CEN Case Rep.* **2014**, *3*, 49–52. [CrossRef]
26. Tanaka, T.; Narazaki, M.; Kishimoto, T. Il-6 in inflammation, Immunity, And disease. *Cold Spring Harb. Perspect. Biol.* **2014**, *6*, a016295. [CrossRef]
27. Chen, Y.; Zheng, Y.; Zhou, Z.; Wang, J. Baicalein alleviates tubular-interstitial nephritis in vivo and in vitro by down-regulating NF-κB and MAPK pathways. *Braz. J. Med. Biol. Res.* **2018**, *51*, e7476. [CrossRef]
28. Correlation between Urinary Biomarkers and Pathological Lesions in Drug-Induced Tubulointerstitial Nephritis. Available online: https://www.ncbi.nlm.nih.gov/pubmed/20979765 (accessed on 12 May 2020).
29. Mohkam, M.; Ghafari, A. The Role of Urinary N-acetyl-beta-glucosaminidase in Diagnosis of Kidney Diseases. *J. Pediatr. Nephrol.* **2015**, *3*, 84–91. [CrossRef]
30. Shang, W.; Wang, Z. The Update of NGAL in Acute Kidney Injury. *Curr. Protein Pept. Sci.* **2017**, *18*, 1211–1217. [CrossRef]
31. Stefanović, V.; Djukanović, L.; Cukuranović, R.; Bukvić, D.; Ležaić, V.; Marić, I.; Ogrizovic, S.S.; Jovanović, I.; Vlahovic, P.; Pešić, I.; et al. Beta2-Microglobulin and Alpha1-Microglobulin as Markers of Balkan Endemic Nephropathy, a Worldwide Disease. *Ren Fail* **2011**, *33*, 176–183. [CrossRef]
32. [Significance of Urinary Biomarkers in Differential Diagnosis of Acute Tubulointerstitial Nephritis]-PubMed -NCBI. Available online: https://www.ncbi.nlm.nih.gov/pubmed/20396357 (accessed on 19 May 2020).
33. Shi, Y.; Su, T.; Qu, L.; Wang, C.; Li, X.; Yang, L. Evaluation of urinary biomarkers for the prognosis of drug-associated chronic tubulointerstitial nephritis. *Am. J. Med. Sci.* **2013**, *346*, 283–288. [CrossRef]
34. Wu, Y.; Su, T.; Yang, L.; Wang, C.; Liu, G.; Li, X. Correlation between urinary biomarkers and pathological lesions in drug-induced tubulointerstitial nephritis. *Zhonghua nei ke za zhi* **2010**, *49*, 568–571. [PubMed]
35. Zhao, W.T.; Huang, J.W.; Sun, P.P.; Su, T.; Tang, J.W.; Wang, S.X.; Liu, G.; Yang, L. Diagnostic roles of urinary kidney injury molecule 1 and soluble C5b-9 in acute tubulointerstitial nephritis. *Am. J. Physiol. Renal. Physiol.* **2019**, *317*, F584–F592. [CrossRef] [PubMed]
36. Koponen, M.; Pichler, W.J.; de Weck, A.L. T cell reactivity to penicillin: Phenotypic analysis of in vitro activated cell subsets. *J. Allergy Clin. Immunol.* **1986**, *78Pt 1*, 645–652. [CrossRef]
37. Wu, Y.; Farrell, J.; Pirmohamed, M.; Park, B.K.; Naisbitt, D.J. Generation and characterization of antigen-specific CD4+, CD8+, and CD4+CD8+ T-cell clones from patients with carbamazepine hypersensitivity. *J. Allergy Clin. Immunol.* **2007**, *119*, 973–981. [CrossRef] [PubMed]
38. Zanni, M.P.; Mauri-Hellweg, D.; Brander, C.; Wendland, T.; Schnyder, B.; Frei, E.; von Greyerz, S.; Bircher, A.; Pichler, W.J. Characterization of lidocaine-specific T cells. *J. Immunol.* **1997**, *158*, 1139–1148. [PubMed]
39. Sachs, B.; Erdmann, S.; Baron, J.M.; Neis, M.; Al Masaoudi, T.; Merk, H.F. Determination of interleukin-5 secretion from drug-specific activated ex vivo peripheral blood mononuclear cells as a test system for the in vitro detection of drug sensitization. *Clin. Exp. Allergy* **2002**, *32*, 736–744. [CrossRef] [PubMed]
40. Tanvarasethee, B.; Buranapraditkun, S.; Klaewsongkram, J. The potential of using enzyme-linked immunospot to diagnose cephalosporin-induced maculopapular exanthems. *Acta. Derm. Venereol.* **2013**, *93*, 66–69. [CrossRef]
41. A Rozieres, A Hennino, K Rodet, M-C Gutowski, N Gunera-Saad, F Berard, G Cozon, J Bienvenu, J-F Nicolas Detection and quantification of drug-specific T cells in penicillin allergy. *Allergy Eur. J. Allergy Clin. Immunol.* **2009**, *64*, 534–542. [CrossRef]
42. Punrin, S.; Thantiworasit, P.; Mongkolpathumrat, P.; Klaewsongkram, J. Evaluated the Diagnostic Utility of Interferon-Gamma Enzyme-Linked Immunospot (ELISPOT) Assays in 117 Patients with Non-Immediate Drug Hypersensitivity Reactions. *J. Allergy Clin. Immunol.* **2016**, *137*, AB36. [CrossRef]
43. Pichler, W.J.; Tilch, J. Review article The lymphocyte transformation test in the diagnosis of drug hypersensitivity. *Allergy* **2004**, *59*, 809–820. [CrossRef]
44. Koda, R.; Watanabe, H.; Tsuchida, M.; Iino, N.; Suzuki, K.; Hasegawa, G.; Imai, N.; Narita, I. Immune checkpoint inhibitor (nivolumab)-associated kidney injury and the importance of recognizing concomitant medications known to cause acute tubulointerstitial nephritis: A case report. *BMC Nephrol.* **2018**, *19*, 48. [CrossRef] [PubMed]
45. Jia, X.; Horinouchi, T.; Hitomi, Y.; Shono, A.; Khor, S.S.; Omae, Y.; Kojima, K.; Kawai, Y.; Nagasaki, M.; Kaku, Y.; et al. Strong associations between specific HLA-DQ and HLA-DR alleles and the tubulointerstitial nephritis and uveitis syndrome. *Investig. Ophthalmol. Vis. Sci.* **2003**, *44*, 653–657. [CrossRef]

46. Rytkönen, S.; Ritari, J.; Peräsaari, J.; Saarela, V.; Nuutinen, M.; Jahnukainen, T. IL-10 polymorphisms +434T/C, +504G/T, and -2849C/T may predispose to tubulointersititial nephritis and uveitis in pediatric population. *PLoS ONE* **2019**, *14*, 0211915. [CrossRef]
47. Javor, J.; Králinský, K.; Sádová, E.; Červeňová, O.; Bucová, M.; Olejárová, M.; Buc, M.; Liptáková, A. Association of interleukin-10 gene promoter polymorphisms with susceptibility to acute pyelonephritis in children. *Folia Microbiol. (Praha)* **2014**, *59*, 307–313. [CrossRef] [PubMed]

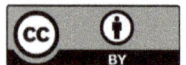

© 2020 by the authors. Licensee MDPI, Basel, Switzerland. This article is an open access article distributed under the terms and conditions of the Creative Commons Attribution (CC BY) license (http://creativecommons.org/licenses/by/4.0/).

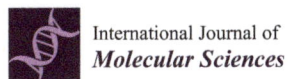

International Journal of
Molecular Sciences

Review

Role of the Furosemide Stress Test in Renal Injury Prognosis

Armando Coca [1], Carmen Aller [1], Jimmy Reinaldo Sánchez [1], Ana Lucía Valencia [1], Elena Bustamante-Munguira [2,†] and Juan Bustamante-Munguira [3,*,†]

1. Department of Nephrology, Hospital Clinico Universitario de Valladolid, 47003 Valladolid, Spain; a.coca.rojo@gmail.com (A.C.); mcaller@saludcastillayleon.es (C.A.); jreinaldo@salud.castillayleon.es (J.R.S.); avalenciape@saludcastillayleon.es (A.L.V.)
2. Department of Intensive Care Medicine, Hospital Clinico Universitario de Valladolid, 47003 Valladolid, Spain; ebustamante@saludcastillayleon.es
3. Department of Cardiac Surgery, Hospital Clinico Universitario de Valladolid, 47003 Valladolid, Spain
* Correspondence: jbustamantemunguira@gmail.com
† These authors contributed equally to this work.

Received: 11 April 2020; Accepted: 24 April 2020; Published: 27 April 2020

Abstract: Risk stratification and accurate patient prognosis are pending issues in the management of patients with kidney disease. The furosemide stress test (FST) has been proposed as a low-cost, fast, safe, and easy-to-perform test to assess tubular integrity, especially when compared to novel plasma and urinary biomarkers. However, the findings regarding its clinical use published so far provide insufficient evidence to recommend the generalized application of the test in daily clinical routine. Dosage, timing, and clinical outcomes of the FST proposed thus far have been significantly different, which further accentuates the need for standardization in the application of the test in order to facilitate the comparison of results between series. This review will summarize published research regarding the usefulness of the FST in different settings, providing the reader some insights about the possible implications of FST in clinical decision-making in patients with kidney disease and the challenges that research will have to address in the near future before widely applying the FST.

Keywords: acute kidney injury; renal biomarkers; furosemide stress test; functional assessment

1. Introduction

Acute kidney injury (AKI) is an intricate clinical syndrome defined by a sudden decrease of kidney function, the accumulation of nitrogen waste products such as urea, electrolyte, and acid-base disturbances and volume overload [1]. The incidence of such complication has been increasing in recent years, affecting 20% of adult and 33% of pediatric patients during hospital admission, especially among subjects with predisposing factors, such as advanced age, diabetes, cardiovascular disease, chronic kidney disease (CKD), or those exposed to nephrotoxins or to cardio-pulmonary bypass. Patients developing AKI have increased morbidity and worse surviving rates than those with normal renal function. In addition, it increases ICU and in-hospital stay, risk of infection, and hospitalization costs. AKI associates a pooled mortality rate of 23.9% in adults and 13.8% in children, rates that increase with higher degrees of severity [1–3].

Diagnosis of AKI should comprise several steps, including a thoughtful clinical evaluation, physical examination, consideration of alternative diagnoses, and laboratory data. An abrupt increase of serum creatinine (≥0.3 mg/dL) is still the laboratory finding most closely associated to AKI [4–6]. Creatinine is an uncharged 113 Da molecule formed in muscles from creatine, freely filtered at the glomerulus and completely eliminated through the kidney in healthy subjects [7]. Although serum creatinine fulfills most requisites of an ideal filtration marker, it is far from being perfect. In healthy individuals approximately 15% of urinary creatinine is secreted in the proximal tubule, a percentage that can be increased in CKD patients [8]. Additionally, as a product of muscular catabolism, serum creatinine is not an adequate marker of kidney function in subjects with extremely high or low muscle mass such as the elderly or children [9]. Certain drugs (i.e., trimethoprim, cimetidine) can also interfere with tubular secretion of creatinine, producing an increase of serum creatinine levels without real kidney function loss [10,11]. Finally, there is a 48–72 h delay between actual kidney injury and the rise of serum creatinine, which limits early diagnosis and initiation of the appropriate therapeutic measures [12].

Several possible solutions have been developed to overcome this issue. Equations that estimate glomerular filtration rate (eGFR) take into account individual characteristics such as age, gender, weight, or ethnicity to better estimate renal function [13,14]. However, serum creatinine-derived eGFR equations should not be used in the AKI setting due high biases and unacceptably poor performance [15]. Moreover, GFR is not a constant parameter; it changes throughout the day and it is modified by protein consumption and other processes [16].

The development of proteomic technology has triggered extensive research in novel protein indicators that may help characterize AKI mechanisms, improve risk stratification, and facilitate clinical decision making and treatment response monitoring [17]. As a result, multiple potential markers have been discovered in recent years, such as kidney injury molecule-1 (KIM-1) [18,19], neutrophil gelatinase-associated lipocalin (NGAL) [20,21], cystatin C [22], N-acetyl-β-D-glucosaminidase (NAG) [23,24], or liver fatty-acid binding protein (L-FABP) [25,26]. However, despite intensive research effort, none of the discovered biomarkers have managed to replace serum creatinine in clinical practice. Timing of sample procurement, differences in urine concentration and flow, inconsistency among laboratory assays, or higher price are some of the barriers that routine application of novel renal biomarkers must overcome [27]. Additional validation studies that may associate biomarker levels to patient-centered clinical outcomes such as dialysis or death are needed [28].

2. Kidney Tubular Stress Test Assessment

Human organ systems have developed the capability to increase their workload in stressful situations. The analysis of this reserve capacity is a useful tool to uncover subclinical disease [16]. Reserve capacity tests are widely applied to study other pathologies, such as coronary artery disease (dobutamine stress echocardiography or exercise electrocardiogram tests). The kidney reserve capacity is built upon two main components, glomerular and tubular (Figure 1). The degree of injury of each component in AKI or CKD can present great variability and be completely independent. Therefore, testing both components could help describe the underlying pathophysiological process with much greater accuracy.

Glomerular reserve testing has been described in detail, but is sparingly used in day-to-day clinical practice. In brief, GFR, which is commonly used as a surrogate of kidney function, depends on age, sex, weight, or diet and presents great fluctuation among individuals. In healthy subjects, a protein load of 1–1.2 g/kg can induce a considerable increase of GFR above its baseline in 60–120 min. The difference between baseline and maximum GFR is considered the renal glomerular function reserve and is directly associated with stress-associated nephron recruitment and increased renal blood flow [16]. However, the lack of large cohort studies that may help describe the population variability of renal glomerular function reserve is an important limitation of this test.

The study of tubular reserve capacity is a relatively new diagnostic tool whose clinical application holds great potential [16,29]. The tubules and tubulointerstitium occupy a significant portion of the kidney and are responsible for a wide variety of functions, such as water and electrolyte handling, secretion of endogenous and exogenous acids, and protein catabolism. Tubular epithelial cells (TECs) regulate tubulointerstitial inflammation and are key mediators of tissue repair and fibrosis processes due to their capability to release cytokines, chemokines, and reactive-oxygen species [16,30]. Damaged TECs facilitate tubulointerstitial inflammation due to their capability to modulate the immune response through the formation of several proinflammatory cytokines such as interleukin-6, interleukin-34, or tumor necrosis factor alpha [30,31]. The consequent macrophage infiltration and neutrophil recruitment can aggravate tubular cell injury and perpetuate the pro-inflammatory response to AKI [32,33]. Furthermore, TECs can endure adaptive changes after kidney injury and modify their structure and phenotype, increasing the production of profibrotic factors that stimulate fibroblast proliferation, tubular cell de-differentiation, and epithelial–mesenchymal transition such as connective tissue growth factor, tubular growth factor beta, or renin-angiotensin components [34–36]. The epithelial–mesenchymal transition of TECs is a potential key point in the progression of renal fibrosis. This phenomenon involves the replacement of epithelial-type markers, such as E-cadherin or cytokeratin, for mesenchymal-type markers such as vimentin, fibronectin, or type I collagen [30,37].

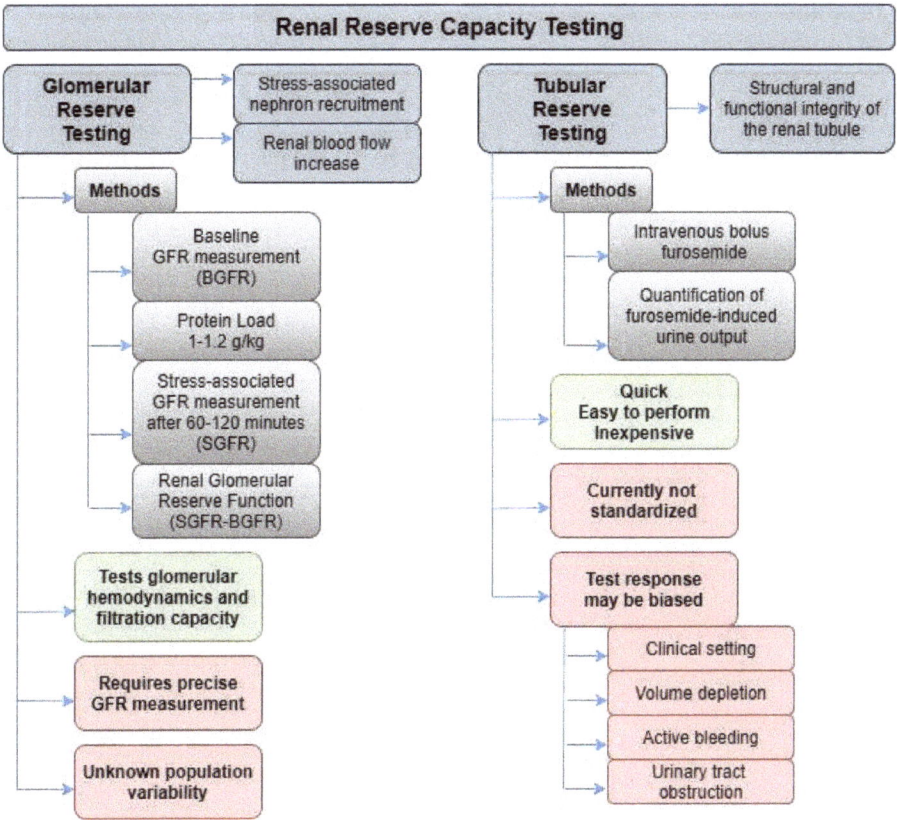

Figure 1. Renal reserve capacity testing.

Recent studies have also described the role of incomplete healing of tubulointerstitial damage as a possible link between AKI and CKD. Although TECs have several repair mechanisms to facilitate full recovery after injury, the repair process can be halted in an intermediate phase, inducing cell atrophy and fibrosis [38]. Mitochondria also play a significant part in AKI associated cell death. The use of SS-31, a drug with mitochondria-protecting effects, has been shown to diminish the development of ischemic damage and interstitial fibrosis in the kidney [39]. Additionally, disturbances of TEC energy-producing pathways, fundamentally fatty acid oxidation, can induce cell death, fibrogenesis, and inflammation [40].

The main tool to assess tubular function is to study tubular secretion of an endogenous or exogenous substance, such as creatinine or furosemide. Salt or acid loading can be used to analyze the efficiency of the tubule to eliminate sodium or acid, while water deprivation or the administration of desmopressin would serve as tests of the concentrating capabilities of the tubule [16].

3. Furosemide Stress Test

Furosemide is a short-acting loop diuretic frequently used to treat hypertension, acute or chronic heart failure, or cirrhosis-associated volume overload [41]. This drug can also be used for diagnostic purposes, which constitutes the fundamental bases of the furosemide stress test (FST). The FST is based on the pharmacokinetic properties of furosemide and is aimed to assess the functional integrity of the renal tubule. The drug is strongly bound to plasma proteins and reaches the proximal tubule lumen through active secretion using the human organic acid transporter (hOAT) pathway present in the proximal tubule [42]. After entering the tubule lumen, furosemide blocks the Na^+-K^+-$2Cl^-$ symporter located in the thick ascending limb of the loop of Henle, preventing Na^+ reabsorption and increasing the urinary volume excreted. Only the protein-bound fraction of the drug is pharmacodynamically active and as such its effect could be reduced in hypoalbuminemia [42]. In patients with CKD, furosemide produces a lower amount of urine despite its prolonged plasma half-life, due to diminished renal blood flow and reduced tubular secretion [42,43]. Furthermore, in the AKI setting, the accumulation of uremic organic acids could reduce the amount of furosemide reaching the lumen of the tubule due to increased competition at the hOAT site [42]. Additional structural modifications of the proximal tubule during AKI, including upregulation of hOAT1 and hOAT3 or reduced expression of several transporters, such as the Na^+-K^+-$2Cl^-$ symporter, the epithelial sodium channel or the Na^+/K^+ ATPase could further modify the urine output induced by furosemide [44,45].

In this setting, furosemide-induced urinary output has been proposed as a surrogate marker of the integrity of renal tubular function which could help clinicians identify patients with tubular injury and at higher risk of AKI or CKD progression. The clinical utility of the FST has been tested in different backgrounds such as AKI in the critically ill, kidney transplantation, or CKD prognosis (Table S1) since its inception in 1973 [46]. Due to the growing relevance of AKI in different clinical settings, such as those undergoing cardiac surgery, the potential application of the FST as a tool to better characterize the degree of tubular injury, achieve an earlier diagnosis of AKI and help initiate the most adequate treatment aimed at minimizing AKI-associated morbidity and mortality and preventing AKI-to-CKD transition deserves further attention.

To perform the present review, we searched the PubMed, Web of Science, and Scopus databases to identify relevant published studies in English. Search terms included a combination of subject headings, abstracts, and keywords (e.g., furosemide stress test, furosemide biomarker). Conference papers were excluded from this review.

4. Critical Care

Baek et al., first described in 1973 the application of a furosemide challenge in critically ill, postoperative patients [46]. The study included 38 patients admitted to intensive care units without a past history of CKD. A subset of 15 adequately hydrated patients without diagnosis of AKI and a free water clearance between +15 and -15 received a furosemide bolus dose ranging from 80 to 400 mg. The inability to produce an adequate response to the furosemide challenge was assumed by the authors as a predictor of imminent AKI in this set of patients.

In 2013, Chawla et al., developed a standardized version of the FST [47]. The authors studied two cohorts of 23 and 54 critically ill patients, respectively. All recruited subjects suffered stage I or II AKI according to the Acute Kidney Injury Network (AKIN) classification [5]. Dosing of furosemide was standardized: loop diuretic naïve patients received an intravenous dose of 1 mg/kg while those previously treated with loop diuretics were administered a dose of 1.5 mg/kg. Urine output during the 6 h after furosemide administration was replaced with either saline or Ringers lactate in a 1:1 ratio. The main outcome of the study was the progression to AKIN stage III within 14 days after furosemide administration. The FST was fairly safe, with no adverse events or episodes of hypotension considered attributable to it. A 2-h urine output cutoff of 200 cc showed the best combination of sensitivity (87.1%) and specificity (84.1%) and was a robust predictor of progression to AKIN stage III. The area under the receiver operator characteristic curves (AUC) for the complete urine output over the first 2 h after the FST to predict the primary outcome was 0.87. Nonetheless, the authors highlight that, for the test to be applied, patients should be euvolemic and any obstruction to urinary flow should have been resolved before the administration of the FST.

A secondary analysis of the same cohort was published in 2017 [48]. In this study, Koyner et al., compared the predictive capacity of FST with that of eight plasma and urinary biomarkers such as NGAL, KIM-1, interleukin-18, uromodulin, tissue inhibitor of metalloproteinases (TIMP-2), IGF-binding protein-7 (IGFBP-7), or albumin-to-creatinine ratio. The 2-h urine output after FST outperformed all studied urinary biomarkers when predicting progression to AKIN stage III with an AUC of 0.87. Furthermore, the FST outperformed most urinary biomarkers when predicting the need of renal replacement therapy (RRT) (AUC: 0.86) or a composite outcome of patient death or progression to AKIN stage III (AUC: 0.81). The combined use of FST and urinary biomarkers to predict outcomes did not significantly improve the performance of FST as a predictor when used alone. Authors concluded that FST was a promising tool that may help clinicians to improve risk stratification in patients with early stages of AKI.

Another approach to test the predictive capacity of the FST was used by van der Voort et al. [49]. In this study, urinary production was measured during a 4-h period after termination of continuous renal replacement therapy (CRRT) in a sample of critically ill patients with AKI. After this period, a subset of patients received either furosemide 0.5 mg/kg/h or placebo with a 4-h urine output repeated measurement after 24 h. In this study, both spontaneous urinary production after CRRT cessation and furosemide-induced urine output were significantly higher in those subjects with immediate recovery of renal function. The AUC for the total urinary output over the first 4 h after the FST to predict in-hospital renal recovery was 0.79. The authors postulated that the FST could be used as a potential predictor to assess renal function recovery after CRRT.

In 2018, Matsuura et al., retrospectively analyzed 95 patients admitted to an intensive care unit and who were treated with bolus furosemide [50]. Authors excluded those patients with AKI stage 3 according to the Kidney Disease: Improving Global Outcomes (KDIGO) AKI classification and those who received a continuous intravenous furosemide infusion. The final sample included 95 subjects with either no AKI or AKI stage 1 or 2. Furosemide responsiveness was defined as the urine output (ml) produced in 2 h divided by the dose of furosemide administered (mg). Urinary biomarkers such as plasma NGAL and urinary L-FABP and NAG were also determined. Main outcomes were progression to AKI stage 3 and a combined outcome of progression to AKI stage 3 or patient death. Furosemide responsiveness was significantly higher among non-progressors, with an AUC for the combined outcome of 0.88, which was higher than that of plasma NGAL (0.81), urinary L-FABP (0.62), or urinary NAG (0.53). Furthermore, the efficacy of furosemide responsiveness was tested in a group of 51 patients with plasma NGAL levels >142 ng/mL at the time of furosemide administration. In this subset, furosemide responsiveness presented an AUC of 0.88 to predict the composite outcome AKI stage 3 progression or patient death.

An alternative clinical use for the FST was tested by Lumlertgul et al., in a prospective, multicenter, randomized controlled trial [51]. In this study, investigators used the FST as an initial triage strategy to identify patients for randomization to different RRT initiation times. Those subjects with poor response after the FST were randomized to either early or standard RRT initiation. Although in this study FST was not assessed as a predictor of clinical outcomes, the test proved to be a safe and effective tool to stratify AKI patients at high risk for RRT.

Recently, Rewa et al., prospectively analyzed the predictive power of FST in a sample of 92 critically ill patients with AKIN stage I or II, recruited from five intensive care units [52]. Patients with evidence of volume depletion, active bleeding, or obstructive uropathy were excluded from the analysis. The dose of intravenous bolus furosemide administered was that proposed by Chawla et al.,: 1 mg/kg for loop diuretic naïve patients and 1.5 mg/kg for those previously treated with loop diuretics. The primary outcome was progression to AKIN stage III within 30 days of FST administration. FST-induced urine output was a significant predictor of the primary outcome, with an AUC of 0.87. However, the FST failed to predict in-hospital patient survival. Moreover, in a multivariate logistic regression model that included the Acute Physiology and Chronic Health Evaluation (APACHE II) score, baseline urine output or serum creatinine at the time of FST, only FST-induced urine output and sex were significant predictors of AKI progression. Authors also registered adverse events that occurred after FST; 9.8% of patients suffered an episode of clinically significant hypotension and 5.4% developed hypokalemia or hypomagenesemia, with no life-threatening events recorded. Authors concluded that FST was a safe and effective predictive tool in patients with mild to moderate AKI.

Sakhuja et al., examined if FST could be used to detect AKI stage 3 patients at risk of needing RRT [53]. Due to the retrospective nature of this study, the furosemide dose was not standardized, but only subjects that received at least 1 mg/kg of intravenous bolus furosemide or its equivalent dose of intravenous bumetanide were included. Patients that had previously received loop diuretics before the FST were excluded from this analysis. Primary and secondary outcomes for Sakhuja et al., were defined as the need for urgent dialysis within 24 or 72 h after the FST. A total of 687 patients were included in the final sample. Dialysis had to be administered to 162 patients (23.6%) during the first 24 h after FST. The 6-h urinary production after FST had only modest discriminative power to predict need of dialysis within the next 24 h, but, according to authors, its application could be useful to evaluate the need for dialysis in critically ill patients with AKI stage 3.

Finally, the usefulness of furosemide response as a predictor of AKI has also been tested in the pediatric critical care setting. Borasino et al., retrospectively examined a sample of 90 infants and neonates younger than 90 days old who received at least one dose of furosemide in the first 24 h after cardiopulmonary bypass surgery [54]. Average furosemide dose was 1.1 ± 0.3 mg/kg. The primary endpoint of the study was the development of cardiac surgery-associated AKI, defined as the doubling of serum creatinine within 72 h of index surgery or a urinary output <0.5 mL/kg/h on average in a 24 h period over the first 72 h after index surgery. Response to furosemide predicted cardiac surgery-associated AKI in this setting, with an AUC of 0.69. Additionally, furosemide response predicted peritoneal dialysis initiation and fluid overload.

5. Kidney Transplantation

There is a paucity of literature regarding the application of FST outside of the intensive care setting. The FST has been tested as a predictive tool after kidney transplantation with different approaches regarding timing of administration and furosemide dosage. McMahon et al. [55] published in 2018 a single-center retrospective analysis of a random sample of 200 deceased-donor kidney transplant recipients who received an intraoperative bolus of 100 mg furosemide. Urinary production was measured 2 and 6 h after furosemide administration. The primary outcome was the development of delayed graft function, defined as the need of dialysis within 7 days of transplantation. Authors included as secondary outcomes safety endpoints such as incidence of hypotension or hypokalemia during the first 24 h after the bolus, graft loss, rejection, death with functioning graft or length of hospital stay. Subjects who developed delayed graft function presented a significantly lower urine output 2 and 6 h after FST. A 6-h urinary output <600 mL (which defined FST non-responders) presented an AUC of 0.85 for the development of DGF. Regarding safety-related outcomes, no episodes of hypotension (defined as mean arterial pressure <60 mmHg) or change in plasma potassium levels were observed in the sample. Although FST non-responders showed longer length of in-hospital stay, the rates of graft loss or death were similar between both groups.

The usefulness of FST after kidney transplantation was also studied by Udomkarnjananun et al. [56]. The authors prospectively studied a sample of 59 adult deceased-donor kidney transplant recipients without hypoalbuminemia or surgical complications that required reoperation during the first 24 h after transplantation. Dry weight adjustment was used to ensure euvolemia prior to transplantation.

An intravenous bolus dose of 1.5 mg/kg furosemide was administered 3 h after allograft reperfusion. Urinary production was registered for 6 h after the bolus. Each mL of urine produced during the first 24 h was replaced by 1 mL of saline to avoid volume depletion. The primary outcome was incidence of DGF, using the same definition applied by McMahon et al. Mean cumulative urine volume was significantly lower in those who developed DGF compared to that of non-DGF patients. A 4-h cumulative urine output <350 mL presented the highest accuracy to predict DGF with an AUC of 0.94. The FST was the only significant predictor of DGF in multivariate logistic regression analysis. Moreover, FST was the most accurate predictor of DGF when compared to urinary NGAL, resistive index of renal arteries measured by ultrasonography or effective renal plasma flow measured by 99mTc-MAG3 renography.

These two single-center studies show that FST could improve risk stratification in the early post-transplant period, promptly detecting patients with higher risk of DGF who could benefit from an early initiation of therapeutic interventions. FST was a more accurate predictor of DGF than oliguria (defined as a daily urinary production <400 mL) [55], ultrasonography, 99mTc-MAG3 renography or novel biomarkers such as urinary NGAL. The test was also safe and well tolerated, in line with published results in critically ill patients.

However, although these studies provide an interesting starting point for the application of FST as a predictive tool after kidney transplantation they also suffer significant limitations: both were small sized, single-center studies, limiting external validity of results. The analysis by McMahon et al., was a retrospective review, which means exposure or outcome assessment could not be controlled. Furthermore, furosemide dosage had different timing and dosage in both studies. The possibility of volume depletion after transplant surgery and/or obstructive uropathy due to urinary elimination of blood clots, complications which are commonly associated to active bleeding, were not adequately addressed in these studies. Therefore, additional prospective multi-center studies should be planned to analyze if FST could improve risk stratification and patient management after kidney transplantation.

6. Other Clinical Settings (CKD)

As previously stated, most research regarding the use of FST is centered in the AKI setting. However, Rivero et al. [57] have recently published a prospective study regarding the usefulness of FST as a tool to assess interstitial fibrosis in a sample of CKD patients. To that end, the authors included adult subjects admitted for a kidney biopsy, including transplant recipients. Hypovolemic or subjects with hemodynamic instability were excluded from the study. A standardized dose of 1 mg/kg furosemide, or 1.5 mg/kg furosemide if exposed to loop diuretics during the seven days prior to FST was administered. Fluid therapy was dispensed according to post-FST urine output to avoid furosemide-induced volume depletion. A nephropathologist assessed kidney interstitial fibrosis percentage using morphometry and classified patients in one of three categories: <25%, 26–50% and >50%. Subjects with >50% interstitial fibrosis had a significantly lower urine output after FST, with an inverse correlation between FST response and degree of fibrosis. FST could thus be a potential tool to non-invasively assess interstitial fibrosis, offering a complementary instrument to eGFR and proteinuria to evaluate prognosis and disease progression in CKD patients.

7. Current Limitations and Future Challenges

The FST is a safe, non-invasive, easy to perform, low-cost tool to evaluate the severity of tubular injury which has shown promising initial results in different clinical contexts. Its capacity as a predictive tool could facilitate risk stratification and clinical decision-making in areas as disparate as AKI, kidney transplantation, or CKD. However, there is still a long way to go before the FST can be included in diagnostic and treatment algorithms. Most published clinical research to date is based on small-sized, single center pilot or feasibility studies. Several studies are based on retrospective analysis of patients who received a furosemide bolus, which makes the task of controlling possible sources of bias extremely difficult. Moreover, doses and timing of furosemide administration are highly variable, even in studies framed within the same clinical setting. Standardization of dosage, such as that proposed by Chawla et al. [47] should help to homogenize the FST in order to facilitate comparison of results between studies.

Additionally, some of the published studies solely rely on AUC values to define the predictive capacity of the test. It has been pointed that such statistic may not be the most adequate choice to assess models that predict risk or stratify individuals into risk categories, a setting in which calibration may play a significant role [58]. In these instances, actual or absolute predicted risk, which is not captured by the AUC, could be of outmost interest. Therefore, when comparing models for risk prediction, a combined analysis including global model fit and analysis of calibration and discrimination would be recommended.

8. Conclusions

In summary, tubular stress test assessment using the FST is a rediscovered and promising new tool to stratify risk in different kidney diseases. Multi-center, prospective studies with large enough sample sizes, applying standardized furosemide dosage and timing and comparing the FST to other novel plasma and urinary biomarkers are necessary to adequately validate results and define the possible clinical applications of the test.

Supplementary Materials: Supplementary materials can be found at http://www.mdpi.com/1422-0067/21/9/3086/s1.

Author Contributions: Development of the idea: A.C. and J.B.-M. Writing—Review and Editing: C.A., J.R.S. and A.L.V. Supervision: A.C., E.B.-M. and J.B.-M. All authors have read and agreed to the published version of the manuscript.

Funding: This research received no external funding.

Conflicts of Interest: The authors declare no conflict of interest.

Abbreviations

AKI	acute kidney injury
AKIN	acute kidney injury network
AUC	area under the curve
CKD	chronic kidney disease
CRRT	continuous renal replacement therapy
DGF	delayed graft function
FEM	furosemide excreted mass
FR	furosemide response
FST	furosemide stress test
IL-18	interleukin 18
KIM-1	kidney injury molecule 1
L-FABP	L-type fatty acid binding protein
MC	multi-center
NA	not applicable
NGAL	neutrophil gelatinase-associated lipocalin
P	prospective
R	retrospective
RRT	renal replacement therapy
SC	single-center
TIMP-2	tissue inhibitor of metalloproteinases 2
UO	urine output

References

1. Hoste, E.; Kellum, J.A.; Selby, N.M.; Zarbock, A.; Palevsky, P.M.; Bagshaw, S.M.; Goldstein, S.L.; Cerdá, J.; Chawla, L.S. Global epidemiology and outcomes of acute kidney injury. *Nat. Rev. Nephrol.* **2018**, *14*, 607–625. [CrossRef] [PubMed]

2. Jorge-Monjas, P.; Bustamante-Munguira, J.; Lorenzo, M.; Heredia-Rodríguez, M.; Fierro, I.; Gómez-Sánchez, E.; Hernandez, A.; Álvarez, F.J.; Bermejo-Martin, J.F.; Gómez-Pesquera, E.; et al. Predicting cardiac surgery–associated acute kidney injury: The CRATE score. *J. Crit. Care* **2016**, *31*, 130–138. [CrossRef] [PubMed]
3. Gameiro, J.; Agapito, F.J.; Jorge, S.; Lopes, J.A. Acute kidney injury definition and diagnosis: A narrative review. *J. Clin. Med.* **2018**, *7*, 307. [CrossRef]
4. Bellomo, R.; Ronco, C.; Kellum, J.A.; Mehta, R.L.; Palevsky, P.; Acute Dialysis Quality Initiative Workgroup. Acute renal failure—Definition, outcome measures, animal models, fluid therapy and information technology needs: The Second International Consensus Conference of the Acute Dialysis Quality Initiative (ADQI) Group. *Crit. Care* **2004**, *8*, R204–R212. [CrossRef] [PubMed]
5. Mehta, R.L.; Kellum, J.A.; Shah, S.V.; Molitoris, B.A.; Ronco, C.; Warnock, D.G.; Levin, A. Acute kidney injury network: Report of an initiative to improve outcomes in acute kidney injury. *Crit. Care* **2007**, *11*, R31. [CrossRef]
6. Kellum, J.A.; Lameire, N.; Aspelin, P.; Barsoum, R.S.; Burdmann, E.A.; Goldstein, S.L.; Herzog, C.A.; Joannidis, M.; Kribben, A.; Levey, A.S.; et al. Kidney disease: Improving global outcomes (KDIGO) acute kidney injury work group. KDIGO clinical practice guideline for acute kidney injury. *Kidney Int. Suppl.* **2012**, *2*, 1–138.
7. Thongprayoon, C.; Cheungpasitporn, W.; Kashani, K.B. Serum creatinine level, a surrogate of muscle mass, predicts mortality in critically ill patients. *J. Thorac. Dis.* **2016**, *8*, E305–E311. [CrossRef]
8. Delanaye, P.; Cavalier, E.; Pottel, H. Serum creatinine: Not so simple! *Nephron* **2017**, *136*, 302–308. [CrossRef]
9. Baxmann, A.C.; Ahmed, M.S.; Marques, N.C.; Menon, V.B.; Pereira, A.B.; Kirsztajn, G.M.; Heilberg, I.P. Influence of muscle mass and physical activity on serum and urinary creatinine and serum cystatin C. *Clin. J. Am. Soc. Nephrol.* **2008**, *3*, 348–354. [CrossRef]
10. Delanaye, P.; Mariat, C.; Cavalier, E.; Maillard, N.; Krzesinski, J.-M.; White, C.A. Trimethoprim, creatinine and creatinine-based equations. *Nephron* **2011**, *119*, 187–194. [CrossRef]
11. Van Acker, B.; Koopman, M.; Arisz, L.; Koomen, G.; de Waart, D. Creatinine clearance during cimetidine administration for measurement of glomerular filtration rate. *Lancet* **1992**, *340*, 1326–1329. [CrossRef]
12. Parikh, C.R.; Mishra, J.; Thiessen-Philbrook, H.; Dursun, B.; Ma, Q.; Kelly, C.; Dent, C.; Devarajan, P.; Edelstein, C. Urinary IL-18 is an early predictive biomarker of acute kidney injury after cardiac surgery. *Kidney Int.* **2006**, *70*, 199–203. [CrossRef] [PubMed]
13. Levey, A.S.; Bosch, J.P.; Lewis, J.B.; Rogers, N.; Greene, T.; Roth, D. A more accurate method to estimate glomerular filtration rate from serum creatinine: A new prediction equation. *Ann. Intern. Med.* **1999**, *130*, 461–470. [CrossRef] [PubMed]
14. Levey, A.S.; Stevens, L.A.; Schmid, C.H.; Zhang, Y.L.; Castro, A.F., III; Feldman, H.I.; Kusek, J.W.; Eggers, P.; Van Lente, F.; Greene, T.; et al. A new equation to estimate glomerular filtration rate. *Ann. Intern. Med.* **2009**, *150*, 604–612. [CrossRef] [PubMed]
15. Bragadottir, G.; Redfors, B.; Ricksten, S.-E. Assessing glomerular filtration rate (GFR) in critically ill patients with acute kidney injury - true GFR versus urinary creatinine clearance and estimating equations. *Crit. Care* **2013**, *17*, R108. [CrossRef]
16. Chawla, L.S.; Ronco, C. Renal stress testing in the assessment of kidney disease. *Kidney Int. Rep.* **2016**, *1*, 57–63. [CrossRef]
17. Siew, E.D.; Ware, L.B.; Ikizler, T.A. Biological markers of acute kidney injury. *J. Am. Soc. Nephrol.* **2011**, *22*, 810–820. [CrossRef]
18. Ichimura, T.; Bonventre, J.V.; Bailly, V.; Wei, H.; Hession, C.A.; Cate, R.L.; Sanicola, M. Kidney Injury Molecule-1 (KIM-1), a putative epithelial cell adhesion molecule containing a novel immunoglobulin domain, is up-regulated in renal cells after injury. *J. Biol. Chem.* **1998**, *273*, 4135–4142. [CrossRef]
19. Tanase, D.M.; Gosav, E.M.; Radu, S.; Costea, C.; Ciocoiu, M.; Carauleanu, A.; Lacatusu, C.; Maranduca, M.; Floria, M.; Rezus, C. The predictive role of the biomarker Kidney Molecule-1 (KIM-1) in Acute Kidney Injury (AKI) cisplatin-induced nephrotoxicity. *Int. J. Mol. Sci.* **2019**, *20*, 5238. [CrossRef]
20. Fan, H.; Zhao, Y.; Sun, M.; Zhu, J.H. Urinary neutrophil gelatinase-associated lipocalin, kidney injury molecule-1, N-acetyl-beta-D-glucosaminidase levels and mortality risk in septic patients with acute kidney injury. *Arch. Med. Sci.* **2018**, *14*, 1381–1386. [CrossRef]

21. Murray, P.T.; Wettersten, N.; Van Veldhuisen, D.J.; Mueller, C.; Filippatos, G.; Nowak, R.; Hogan, C.; Kontos, M.C.; Cannon, C.M.; Müeller, G.A.; et al. Utility of urine neutrophil gelatinase-associated lipocalin for worsening renal function during hospitalization for acute heart failure: Primary findings of the urine N-gal acute kidney injury N-gal evaluation of symptomatic heart failure study (AKINESIS). *J. Card. Fail.* **2019**, *25*, 654–665. [CrossRef]
22. Park, M.Y.; Lee, Y.W.; Choi, S.J.; Kim, J.K.; Hwang, S. Urinary cystatin C levels as a diagnostic and prognostic biomarker in patients with acute kidney injury. *Nephrology* **2013**, *18*, 256–262. [CrossRef] [PubMed]
23. Westhuyzen, J.; Endre, Z.H.; Reece, G.; Reith, D.M.; Saltissi, D.; Morgan, T.J. Measurement of tubular enzymuria facilitates early detection of acute renal impairment in the intensive care unit. *Nephrol. Dial. Transplant.* **2003**, *18*, 543–551. [CrossRef] [PubMed]
24. Heise, D.; Rentsch, K.; Braeuer, A.; Friedrich, M.; Quintel, M. Comparison of urinary neutrophil glucosaminidase-associated lipocalin, cystatin C, and ?1-microglobulin for early detection of acute renal injury after cardiac surgery. *Eur. J. Cardio-Thorac. Surg.* **2011**, *39*, 38–43. [CrossRef] [PubMed]
25. Yanishi, M.; Kinoshita, H.; Mishima, T.; Taniguchi, H.; Yoshida, K.; Komai, Y.; Yasuda, K.; Watanabe, M.; Sugi, M.; Matsuda, T. Urinary l-type fatty acid-binding protein is a predictor of early renal function after partial nephrectomy. *Ren. Fail.* **2016**, *39*, 7–12. [CrossRef] [PubMed]
26. Doi, K.; Noiri, E.; Sugaya, T. Urinary L-type fatty acid-binding protein as a new renal biomarker in critical care. *Curr. Opin. Crit. Care* **2010**, *16*, 545–549. [CrossRef]
27. Tang, K.W.A.; Toh, Q.C.; Teo, B.W. Normalisation of urinary biomarkers to creatinine for clinical practice and research—When and why. *Singap. Med. J.* **2015**, *56*, 7–10. [CrossRef]
28. Parikh, C.R.; Mansour, S.G. Perspective on clinical application of biomarkers in AKI. *J. Am. Soc. Nephrol.* **2017**, *28*, 1677–1685. [CrossRef]
29. McMahon, B.A.; Koyner, J.L. Risk stratification for acute kidney injury: Are biomarkers enough? *Adv. Chronic Kidney Dis.* **2016**, *23*, 167–178. [CrossRef]
30. Liu, B.-C.; Tang, T.-T.; Lv, L.-L.; Lan, H.-Y. Renal tubule injury: A driving force toward chronic kidney disease. *Kidney Int.* **2018**, *93*, 568–579. [CrossRef]
31. Yard, B.A.; Daha, M.R.; Kooymans-Couthino, M.; Bruijn, J.A.; Paape, M.E.; Schrama, E.; Van Es, L.A.; Van Der Woude, F.J. IL-1α stimulated TNFα production by cultured human proximal tubular epithelial cells. *Kidney Int.* **1992**, *42*, 383–389. [CrossRef] [PubMed]
32. Baek, J.-H.; Zeng, R.; Weinmann-Menke, J.; Valerius, M.T.; Wada, Y.; Ajay, A.K.; Colonna, M.; Kelley, V.R. IL-34 mediates acute kidney injury and worsens subsequent chronic kidney disease. *J. Clin. Investig.* **2015**, *125*, 3198–3214. [CrossRef] [PubMed]
33. Disteldorf, E.M.; Krebs, C.; Paust, H.-J.; Turner, J.-E.; Nouailles, G.; Tittel, A.; Meyer-Schwesinger, C.; Stege, G.; Brix, S.R.; Velden, J.; et al. CXCL5 Drives neutrophil recruitment in TH17-Mediated GN. *J. Am. Soc. Nephrol.* **2014**, *26*, 55–66. [CrossRef] [PubMed]
34. Geng, H.; Lan, R.; Singha, P.K.; Gilchrist, A.; Weinreb, P.H.; Violette, S.M.; Weinberg, J.M.; Saikumar, P.; Venkatachalam, M.A. Lysophosphatidic acid increases proximal tubule cell secretion of profibrotic cytokines PDGF-B and CTGF through LPA2- and Galphaq-mediated Rho and alphavbeta6 integrin-dependent activation of TGF-beta. *Am. J. Pathol.* **2012**, *181*, 1236–1249. [CrossRef]
35. Meng, X.M.; Tang, P.M.; Li, J.; Lan, H.Y. TGF-beta/Smad signaling in renal fibrosis. *Front. Physiol.* **2015**, *6*, 82. [CrossRef]
36. Zhou, Y.; Xiong, M.; Fang, L.; Jiang, L.; Wen, P.; Dai, C.; Zhang, C.Y.; Yang, J. miR-21–containing microvesicles from injured tubular epithelial cells promote tubular phenotype transition by targeting PTEN protein. *Am. J. Pathol.* **2013**, *183*, 1183–1196. [CrossRef]
37. Strutz, F. EMT and proteinuria as progression factors. *Kidney Int.* **2009**, *75*, 475–481. [CrossRef]
38. Cosentino, C.C.; Skrypnyk, N.I.; Brilli, L.L.; Chiba, T.; Novitskaya, T.; Woods, C.; West, J.; Korotchenko, V.N.; McDermott, L.; Day, B.W.; et al. Histone deacetylase inhibitor enhances recovery after AKI. *J. Am. Soc. Nephrol.* **2013**, *24*, 943–953. [CrossRef]
39. Liu, S.; Soong, Y.; Seshan, S.V.; Szeto, H.H. Novel cardiolipin therapeutic protects endothelial mitochondria during renal ischemia and mitigates microvascular rarefaction, inflammation, and fibrosis. *Am. J. Physiol. Physiol.* **2014**, *306*, F970–F980. [CrossRef]

40. Kang, H.M.; Ahn, S.H.; Choi, P.; Ko, Y.A.; Han, S.H.; Chinga, F.; Park, A.S.; Tao, J.; Sharma, K.; Pullman, J.; et al. Defective fatty acid oxidation in renal tubular epithelial cells has a key role in kidney fibrosis development. *Nat. Med.* **2015**, *21*, 37–46. [CrossRef]
41. Ponto, L.L.; Schoenwald, R.D. Furosemide (frusemide). A pharmacokinetic/pharmacodynamic review (Part II). *Clin. Pharmacokinet.* **1990**, *18*, 460–471. [PubMed]
42. Mariano, F.; Mella, A.; Vincenti, M.; Biancone, L. Furosemide as a functional marker of acute kidney injury in ICU patients: A new role for an old drug. *J. Nephrol.* **2019**, *32*, 883–893. [CrossRef] [PubMed]
43. Brown, C.B.; Ogg, C.S.; Cameron, J.S. High dose frusemide in acute renal failure: A controlled trial. *Clin. Nephrol.* **1981**, *15*, 90–96.
44. Schmidt, C.; Hocherl, K.; Schweda, F.; Kurtz, A.; Bucher, M. Regulation of renal sodium transporters during severe inflammation. *J. Am. Soc. Nephrol.* **2007**, *18*, 1072–1083. [CrossRef] [PubMed]
45. Kunin, M.; Holtzman, E.J.; Melnikov, S.; Dinour, D. Urinary organic anion transporter protein profiles in AKI. *Nephrol. Dial. Transplant.* **2011**, *27*, 1387–1395. [CrossRef] [PubMed]
46. Baek, S.M.; Brown, R.S.; Shoemaker, W.C. Early prediction of acute renal failure and recovery. *Crit. Care Med.* **1973**, *1*, 179. [CrossRef]
47. Chawla, L.S.; Davison, D.; Brasha-Mitchell, E.; Koyner, J.L.; Arthur, J.; Shaw, A.; Tumlin, J.; Trevino, S.A.; Kimmel, P.L.; Seneff, M.G. Development and standardization of a furosemide stress test to predict the severity of acute kidney injury. *Crit. Care* **2013**, *17*, R207. [CrossRef]
48. Koyner, J.L.; Davison, D.L.; Brasha-Mitchell, E.; Chalikonda, D.M.; Arthur, J.; Shaw, A.; Tumlin, J.A.; Trevino, S.A.; Bennett, M.R.; Kimmel, P.L.; et al. Furosemide stress test and biomarkers for the prediction of aki severity. *J. Am. Soc. Nephrol.* **2015**, *26*, 2023–2031. [CrossRef]
49. Van der Voort, P.H.J.; Boerma, E.C.; Pickkers, P. The furosemide stress test to predict renal function after continuous renal replacement therapy. *Crit. Care* **2014**, *18*, 429. [CrossRef]
50. Matsuura, R.; Komaru, Y.; Miyamoto, Y.; Yoshida, T.; Yoshimoto, K.; Isshiki, R.; Mayumi, K.; Yamashita, T.; Hamasaki, Y.; Nangaku, M.; et al. Response to different furosemide doses predicts AKI progression in ICU patients with elevated plasma NGAL levels. *Ann. Intensiv. Care* **2018**, *8*, 8. [CrossRef]
51. Lumlertgul, N.; Peerapornratana, S.; Trakarnvanich, T.; Pongsittisak, W.; Surasit, K.; Chuasuwan, A.; Tankee, P.; Tiranathanagul, K.; Praditpornsilpa, K.; Tungsanga, K.; et al. Early versus standard initiation of renal replacement therapy in furosemide stress test non-responsive acute kidney injury patients (the FST trial). *Crit. Care* **2018**, *22*, 101. [CrossRef] [PubMed]
52. Rewa, O.G.; Bagshaw, S.; Wang, X.; Wald, R.; Smith, O.; Shapiro, J.; McMahon, B.; Liu, K.; Trevino, S.; Chawla, L.; et al. The furosemide stress test for prediction of worsening acute kidney injury in critically ill patients: A multicenter, prospective, observational study. *J. Crit. Care* **2019**, *52*, 109–114. [CrossRef] [PubMed]
53. Sakhuja, A.; Bandak, G.; Barreto, E.F.; Vallabhajosyula, S.; Jentzer, J.; Albright, R.; Kashani, K.B. Role of loop diuretic challenge in stage 3 acute kidney injury. *Mayo Clin. Proc.* **2019**, *94*, 1509–1515. [CrossRef] [PubMed]
54. Borasino, S.; Wall, K.M.; Crawford, J.H.; Hock, K.M.; Cleveland, D.C.; Rahman, F.; Martin, K.D.; Alten, J.A. Furosemide response predicts acute kidney injury after cardiac surgery in infants and neonates. *Pediatr. Crit. Care Med.* **2018**, *19*, 310–317. [CrossRef]
55. McMahon, B.A.; Koyner, J.L.; Novick, T.; Menez, S.; Moran, R.A.; Lonze, B.E.; Desai, N.; Alasfar, S.; Borja, M.; Merritt, W.T.; et al. The prognostic value of the furosemide stress test in predicting delayed graft function following deceased donor kidney transplantation. *Biomarkers* **2017**, *23*, 61–69. [CrossRef]
56. Udomkarnjananun, S.; Townamchai, N.; Iampenkhae, K.; Petchlorlian, A.; Srisawat, N.; Katavetin, P.; Sutherasan, M.; Santingamkun, A.; Praditpornsilpa, K.; Eiam-Ong, S.; et al. Furosemide stress test as a predicting biomarker for delayed graft function in kidney transplantation. *Nephron* **2019**, *141*, 236–248. [CrossRef]
57. Rivero, J.; Rodríguez, F.; Soto, V.; Macedo, E.; Chawla, L.S.; Mehta, R.L.; Vaingankar, S.; Garimella, P.S.; Garza, C.; Madero, M. Furosemide stress test and interstitial fibrosis in kidney biopsies in chronic kidney disease. *BMC Nephrol.* **2020**, *21*, 1–9. [CrossRef]
58. Cook, N.R. Use and misuse of the receiver operating characteristic curve in risk prediction. *Circulation* **2007**, *115*, 928–935. [CrossRef]

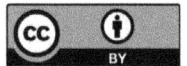 © 2020 by the authors. Licensee MDPI, Basel, Switzerland. This article is an open access article distributed under the terms and conditions of the Creative Commons Attribution (CC BY) license (http://creativecommons.org/licenses/by/4.0/).

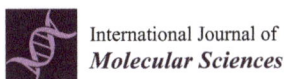

Review

Glomerular Deposition of Nephritis-Associated Plasmin Receptor (NAPlr) and Related Plasmin Activity: Key Diagnostic Biomarkers of Bacterial Infection-related Glomerulonephritis

Takahiro Uchida * and Takashi Oda

Kidney Disease Center, Department of Nephrology and Blood Purification, Tokyo Medical University Hachioji Medical Center, Hachioji, Tokyo 193-0998, Japan; takashio@tokyo-med.ac.jp
* Correspondence: tu05090224@gmail.com; Tel.: +81-42-665-5611; Fax: +81-42-665-1796

Received: 25 March 2020; Accepted: 8 April 2020; Published: 8 April 2020

Abstract: It is widely known that glomerulonephritis (GN) often develops after the curing of an infection, a typical example of which is GN in children following streptococcal infections (poststreptococcal acute glomerulonephritis; PSAGN). On the other hand, the term "infection-related glomerulonephritis (IRGN)" has recently been proposed, because infections are usually ongoing at the time of GN onset in adult patients, particularly in older patients with comorbidities. However, there has been no specific diagnostic biomarker for IRGN, and diagnosis is based on the collection of several clinical and pathological findings and the exclusion of differential diagnoses. Nephritis-associated plasmin receptor (NAPlr) was originally isolated from the cytoplasmic fraction of group A streptococcus as a candidate nephritogenic protein for PSAGN and was found to be the same molecule as streptococcal glyceraldehyde-3-phosphate dehydrogenase and plasmin receptor. NAPlr deposition and related plasmin activity were observed with a similar distribution pattern in the glomeruli of patients with PSAGN. However, glomerular NAPlr deposition and plasmin activity could be observed not only in patients with PSAGN but also in patients with other glomerular diseases, in whom a preceding streptococcal infection was suggested. Furthermore, such glomerular staining patterns have been demonstrated in patients with IRGN induced by bacteria other than streptococci. This review discusses the recent advances in our understanding of the pathogenesis of bacterial IRGN, which is characterized by NAPlr and plasmin as key biomarkers.

Keywords: poststreptococcal acute glomerulonephritis; infection-related glomerulonephritis; nephritis-associated plasmin receptor; plasmin

---

1. Introduction

A wide variety of bacterial infection-related renal diseases are known, among which the most common is acute kidney injury (AKI) [1], which occurs as part of multiple organ failure. Changes in hemodynamics and cytokine expression are thought to be involved in the pathogenesis of AKI.

Bacterial infections also cause renal injury, partly through immune mechanisms. For example, glomerulonephritis (GN) can develop following streptococcal upper respiratory tract or skin infections with a latent period of approximately 10 days. As streptococcal infections are usually cured when GN is diagnosed and there is a distinct infection-free latent period, the GN has been referred to as poststreptococcal acute glomerulonephritis (PSAGN) [2–4].

In previous years, most cases of AGN were PSAGN in children; however, probably owing to the improvement of living environments and the adequate usage of antibiotics, the incidence of PSAGN has been decreasing, particularly in developed countries [4]. Whereas PSAGN is still the most common cause of pediatric AGN, adult AGN cases have been increasing, and those associated with non-streptococcal infections, particularly infections by *Staphylococcus aureus*, are now as common as PSAGN [5]. Thus, a major shift in the epidemiology of AGN has occurred. In Japan, cases of PSAGN, which accounted for more than two-thirds of AGN cases in the 1970s, decreased to about 30% after the 1980s, whereas AGN cases associated with *S. aureus* infections reached 30% in the 1990s [6].

Furthermore, in adult AGN patients, the infection is usually still present at the time when GN is diagnosed. Based on these backgrounds, instead of "postinfectious AGN", the disease concept of infection-related glomerulonephritis (IRGN) has recently been proposed [5]. Notably, whereas in most patients, PSAGN resolves without any specific therapy, the prognosis of patients with IRGN is poor, and older patients, particularly those with an immunocompromised background, such as diabetes mellitus, malignancies, or alcoholism, are reported to be at high risk [7]. Controlling the underlying infection and managing complications are essential for the treatment of IRGN, and immunosuppressive therapy is generally not recommended. However, the prompt diagnosis of IRGN is often difficult because specific diagnostic biomarkers have not yet been identified.

We herein present an overview of our recent understanding of the pathogenesis of bacterial IRGN. Accumulated data suggest that the disease concept of bacterial IRGN can be further expanded, and glomerular deposition of nephritis-associated plasmin receptor (NAPlr), originally considered to be a candidate nephritogenic protein for PSAGN [8] and related plasmin activity [9], can be used as general diagnostic biomarkers of bacterial IRGN. Although infections of various viruses, mycobacteria, fungi, or protozoa are also known to cause IRGN [1], they are not within the scope of this article.

2. NAPlr and Plasmin Activity in Glomeruli as Biomarkers of PSAGN

NAPlr is a 43-kDa protein that was originally isolated from the cytoplasmic fraction of group A streptococcus as a candidate nephritogenic protein for PSAGN [8]. Glomerular NAPlr deposition is detected by immunostaining, and is frequently observed in the early phase of PSAGN; all patients within 2 weeks of disease onset have been reported to show NAPlr deposition [2].

NAPlr was also found to be the same molecule as streptococcal glyceraldehyde-3-phosphate dehydrogenase (GAPDH) [8]. Although GAPDH is a well-known housekeeping gene, it also has pleiotropic functions, such as energy production (glycolysis), regulation of gene expression, and autophagy [10]. In addition, GAPDH from some bacteria, including streptococci, has been shown to have plasmin-binding activity [11,12].

NAPlr binds plasmin and maintains plasmin activity by protecting it from its physiological inhibitors. Plasmin activity can be detected by *in situ* zymography using a plasmin-sensitive synthetic substrate, which is resistant to the addition of α_2-antiplasmin but is completely abrogated by aprotinin, a serine protease inhibitor [9]. Plasmin is considered to cause glomerular damage directly by degrading extracellular matrix proteins and indirectly by activating pro–matrix metalloproteases. Additionally, plasmin can exert proinflammatory function by activating and accumulating inflammatory cells.

NAPlr is also known to convert complement component C3 to C3b, indicating its involvement in the activation of the alternative complement pathway [8]. However, it should be noted that NAPlr deposition is observed mainly in glomerular neutrophils, mesangial cells, and endothelial cells, and its distribution in glomeruli is different from that of C3 and IgG, which are considered to localize within the subepithelial hump [13]. In this regard, NAPlr, which also contains a urokinase-type plasminogen activator receptor (uPAR)-binding site [11], may bind with uPAR expressed on neutrophils, thereby inducing prominent endocapillary inflammation in early phase PSAGN, or NAPlr may be phagocytosed by neutrophils as exogenous material. Thus, glomerular damage from the disease may initially occur in the inner side of the glomerular capillary walls by NAPlr deposition, rather than subepithelial immune complexes.

Streptococcal pyrogenic exotoxin B (SPEB), which is another potential nephritogenic protein of PSAGN with cationic character, has been considered to pass through the glomerular basement membrane and be deposited in the subepithelial area [14]. However, a subsequent study showed that the glomerular distribution of NAPlr and SPEB were essentially similar and that NAPlr staining was dominant [13]. Importantly, as with NAPlr, SPEB has plasmin-binding activity [5]. Thus, it is possible that these 2 (or more) proteins are cooperatively involved in the disease pathogenesis of PSAGN. Figure 1 shows a scheme of the mechanisms involved in the development of PSAGN.

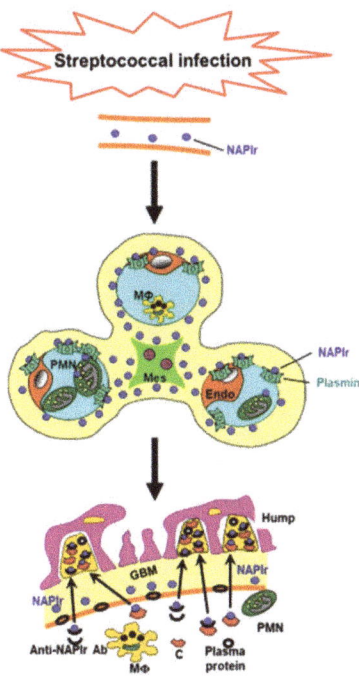

Figure 1. Putative mechanism for the development of poststreptococcal acute glomerulonephritis. Streptococcal infection induces the release of nephritogenic proteins, such as nephritis-associated plasmin receptor (NAPlr), into the circulation. Circulating NAPlr accumulates on the inner side of the glomerular capillary walls, and then traps and maintains the activity of plasmin, which induces glomerular damage by the degradation of extracellular matrix proteins or by activating and accumulating inflammatory cells. Thereafter, immune complexes, formed either *in situ* or in the circulation, pass through the altered glomerular basement membrane (GBM). Accumulation of immune complexes, complements, and plasma proteins forms "humps" on the outer side of the glomerular capillary walls. This scheme is based on the figure from Oda et al. [2]. Ab: antibody; C: complement; Endo: endothelial cell; Mes: mesangial cell; MΦ: macrophage; PMN: polymorphonuclear cell.

Some streptococcal strains have been isolated from PSAGN patients, and such strains have been considered to be "nephritogenic". However, NAPlr, as well as SPEB, have been found in virtually all streptococcal strains [14]. In addition, gene sequences of NAPlr were highly conserved and its protein expression levels were similar between various streptococcal strains [15]. Therefore, it is reasonable to think that any strains expressing NAPlr can be nephritogenic. Another possibility also remains that although NAPlr (and SPEB) are essential molecules, other factors, from both bacteria and the hosts, play important roles in the onset/progression of PSAGN.

There have been several reports showing the occurrence of IRGN in renal transplant recipients, suggesting that IRGN may be a cause of renal allograft injury [16,17]. We have recently encountered a renal transplant recipient who developed PSAGN; notably, NAPlr deposition and plasmin activity were observed in the glomeruli of the patient's transplanted kidney (manuscript in preparation).

3. Streptococcal Infection-related Nephritis (SIRN): Glomerular Diseases with NAPlr Deposition and Related Plasmin Activity Induced by Streptococcal Infection

The unique glomerular staining patterns of NAPlr and plasmin activity were found not only in patients with PSAGN but also in some patients with other glomerular diseases, such as C3 glomerulopathy [18,19], membranoproliferative glomerulonephritis (MPGN) type I [20,21], antineutrophil cytoplasmic antibody (ANCA)-associated vasculitis (both ANCA positive [22] and negative [23]), and IgA vasculitis [24], in which a preceding streptococcal infection is suggested by serological markers, and these cases are referred to as SIRN [2,25]. Although prominent endocapillary proliferation is a common histological feature, the differences in immune responses of the affected hosts may affect the specific histology. In addition, there have been some cases in which patients had a preceding streptococcal infection that initially occurred as PSAGN but later developed into C3 glomerulopathy [26]. It has also been reported that C3 nephritic factor activity is transiently observed in some PSAGN patients during the acute phase of the disease [27]. Thus, the disease concept of SIRN remains to be established, and there are no specific criteria differentiating patients with SIRN from those with the above glomerular diseases. However, it should be noted that streptococcal infections are associated with several forms of GN and that NAPlr and plasmin activity may be biomarkers of these diseases.

4. Glomerular NAPlr Deposition and Plasmin Activity as Candidates of General Biomarkers of Bacterial IRGN

The diagnosis of IRGN is made based on a combination of clinical and pathological findings. Nasr et al. [5] proposed the diagnostic criteria for IRGN as follows, in which at least 3 of the 5 items are required for a positive diagnosis: (1) clinical or laboratory evidence of infection preceding or at the onset of GN, (2) decrease in serum complement levels, (3) endocapillary proliferative and exudative glomerulonephritis, (4) C3-dominant or codominant glomerular immunofluorescence staining, and (5) hump-shaped subepithelial deposits on electron microscopy. The most common pathogen causing bacterial IRGN is staphylococcus, followed by streptococcus and Gram-negative bacteria. Infection sites are diverse, including the upper respiratory tract, skin, lung, and urinary tract, and the identification of foci is sometimes difficult. In addition, disease-specific diagnostic biomarkers have not been identified to date, and there are usually several differential diagnoses that show confounding clinical or pathological characteristics. Therefore, the prompt and accurate diagnosis of IRGN is often difficult.

Interestingly, glomerular NAPlr deposition and plasmin activity have recently been demonstrated in patients with IRGN induced by some bacterial strains, such as *Streptococcus pneumoniae* [28], *Aggregatibacter actinomycetemcomitans* (a Gram-negative coccobacillus that sometimes causes periodontal disease and infectious endocarditis) [29], *Mycoplasma pneumoniae* [30], or *S. aureus* (both methicillin-sensitive and -resistant strains; unpublished observations). The sequences of *S. pneumoniae* GAPDH share high identity with NAPlr, and the C-terminal sequences of *S. pneumoniae* GAPDH, which are most likely to be associated with the plasmin-binding activity, are completely identical to those of streptococcal GAPDH [28]. *M. pneumoniae* GAPDH has been shown to not only have cross-immunoreactivity to the anti-NAPlr antibody but also to have a plasmin-binding function. In addition, *M. pneumoniae* GAPDH has been reported to bind to plasminogen and convert it to plasmin [31]. As shown in Table 1, sequences of GAPDH from *A. actinomycetemcomitans* and *S. aureus* also show high similarity to that of NAPlr at the amino acid level, and *S. aureus* GAPDH has been reported to bind to enzymatically active plasmin [32]. As stated above, GAPDH sequences are highly preserved between streptococcal species [15], and it is, therefore, reasonable that GAPDH from these bacteria have plasmin-binding ability and that its deposition in glomeruli is detected by the anti-NAPlr antibody. However, it should be noted that although the glomerular staining pattern of NAPlr is essentially the same among patients with IRGN, the staining intensity in patients with non-streptococcal IRGN is generally weaker than in those with PSAGN. In this regard, the timing of when a renal biopsy is performed might affect the staining intensity; it could be possible that, in patients with non-streptococcal IRGN, performing renal biopsy during the acute phase is often avoided because of comorbidities or ongoing infection. Another possibility is that positive immunostaining of NAPlr in patients with non-streptococcal IRGN is caused by cross-immunoreactivity to the anti-NAPlr antibody, and is, therefore, weaker than that in patients with PSAGN.

Table 1. Identity and similarity of bacterial GAPDH and streptococcal GAPDH (nephritis-associated plasmin receptor; NAPlr).

Pathogen	Nucleotide		Amino acid	
	Identity	Similarity	Identity	Similarity
Aggregatibacter actinomycetemcomitans	59	59	50	85
Mycoplasma pneumonia	60	60	54	87
Staphylococcal aureus	54	54	67	92

Data are presented as percentages. Nucleotide and amino acid sequences of bacterial GAPDH registered with Kyoto Encyclopedia of Genes and Genomes (http://www.genome.jp/kegg/kegg_ja.html) were used, and identities and similarities were evaluated by Dr. Masayuki Fujino (the AIDS Research Center, National Institute of Infectious Diseases) using genetic information processing software (GENETYX-MAC ver. 18, GENETYX Corporation, Tokyo, Japan).

On the other hand, even if the overall amino acid sequence similarity is not very high, it is possible that some types of bacterial GAPDH, which have a similar steric structure at the antibody-binding site, show cross-immunoreactivity to the anti-NAPlr antibody. Indeed, positive staining for NAPlr and plasmin activity has been used as a marker of IGRN in patients with various forms of glomerulonephritis, such as proliferative glomerulonephritis with monoclonal immunoglobulin G deposits [33] and eosinophilic proliferative glomerulonephritis [34], even if neither the pathogens nor the infection sites could be identified. As the binding site of the anti-NAPlr antibody and that of plasmin in the GAPDH sequence would be different, the GAPDH of some bacteria are expected to bind with plasmin but not react with the anti-NAPlr antibody. In this regard, whether there are IRGN cases in which glomerular plasmin activity is observed without immunoreactivity to the anti-NAPlr antibody needs to be investigated in the future.

Collectively, GAPDH from various bacteria appear to react with the anti-NAPlr antibody and to have plasmin-binding ability, and positivity of the anti-NAPlr antibody and plasmin activity in glomeruli may act as both diagnostic and pathogenetic biomarkers of bacterial IRGN in general. Putative pathogenic mechanisms of IRGN, focusing on NAPlr and plasmin activity as biomarkers, are depicted in Figure 2.

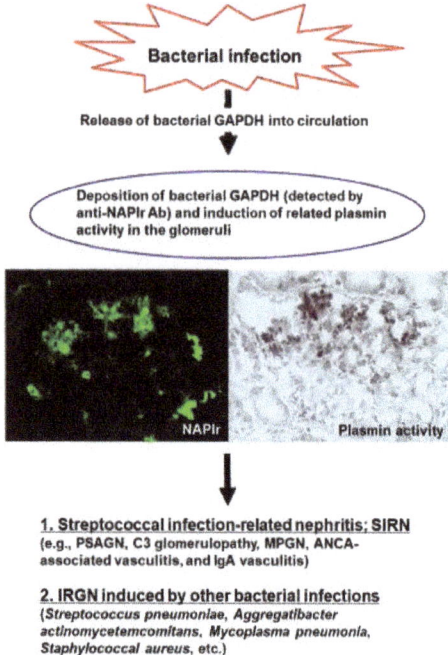

Figure 2. Possible scheme for the pathogenic mechanisms of bacterial infection-related glomerulonephritis (IRGN), focusing on the glomerular deposition of nephritis-associated plasmin receptor (NAPlr) and related plasmin activity. Ab: antibody; ANCA: antineutrophil cytoplasmic antibody; GAPDH: glyceraldehyde-3-phosphate dehydrogenase; MPGN: membranoproliferative glomerulonephritis; PSAGN: poststreptococcal acute glomerulonephritis.

5. NAPlr and Plasmin Activity in Extraglomerular Regions

In the previous study, NAPlr deposition has been observed almost exclusively in the glomeruli of IRGN patients, and the question hence arises as to whether NAPlr deposition is truly limited to the glomeruli. Interestingly, a case of PSAGN complicated by acute interstitial nephritis, in which positive SPEB immunostaining was observed in the interstitium as well as in the glomeruli, has been reported [35]. Although acute tubulointerstitial nephritis after streptococcal infection without obvious GN is rare, such a case has indeed been reported, in which SPEB immunostaining was positive in the affected area [36]. In the former case report [35], the authors also performed immunofluorescence staining of NAPlr using a commercially available antibody but failed to detect its deposition. In this regard, however, it should be noted that immunostaining results can vary depending on the antibodies used and the staining conditions [2]. Thus, whether NAPlr deposition occurs in the tubulointerstitial area or not should be examined more carefully using different antibodies and staining conditions. NAPlr immunofluorescence staining using an original antibody (and *in situ* zymography for plasmin activity) can be performed at the laboratory of Dr. Takashi Oda (Kidney Disease Center, Department of Nephrology and Blood Purification, Tokyo Medical University Hachioji Medical Center; takashio@tokyo-med.ac.jp).

Tubulointerstitial plasmin activity could be found in patients with various renal diseases unrelated to bacterial infection [9,37]. However, NAPlr deposition could not be observed, and plasmin activity was almost exclusively limited to the tubulointerstitial area in the renal tissues of these patients. Although definitive causative roles remain to be solved, this plasmin activity in the tubulointerstitial area may be involved in renal tubulointerstitial inflammation and fibrosis, because plasmin is supposed to induce the infiltration and activation of inflammatory cells and to induce fibrogenesis. Indeed, tubulointerstitial plasmin activity was associated with the degree of tubulointerstitial change, global glomerulosclerosis rate, and estimated glomerular filtration rate [37]. Data regarding tubulointerstitial plasmin activity in patients with IRGN are scarce, and, hence, further accumulation of cases is needed to investigate this matter in more detail.

PSAGN patients rarely show alveolar hemorrhage, and immune complex deposition is suggested in the pathogenesis of alveolar hemorrhage [38]. Therefore, another important issue that remains to be investigated is whether or not NAPlr deposition and related plasmin activity are observed in the lung tissue of patients with PSAGN complicated by alveolar hemorrhage. In this regard, an interesting case of IRGN, in which the causative pathogen was not detected but NAPlr deposition and plasmin activity were observed not only in the glomeruli but also in the renal tubulointerstitial area and pulmonary arteries, has recently been reported [34].

6. Concluding Remarks

NAPlr, isolated from the cytoplasmic fraction of group A streptococcus, has been shown to trap plasmin and maintain its activity and was originally considered as a nephritogenic protein for PSAGN. Indeed, NAPlr deposition and related plasmin activity have been observed to have an almost identical distribution in the glomeruli of early phase PSAGN patients at a high frequency. The interactions among NAPlr, plasmin activity, and SPEB and the association between these elements and complements or immune complexes, both *in vitro* and *in vivo*, should be investigated in future studies.

Some patients with other glomerular diseases, in whom a preceding streptococcal infection is clinically suggested, were found to also show glomerular NAPlr deposition and plasmin activity, and hence, these cases can be referred to as SIRN. Furthermore, such glomerular-staining patterns of NAPlr and plasmin activity are found in some patients with IRGN induced by other bacteria. The amino acid sequence of GAPDH from some types of bacteria show high similarity to the sequence of NAPlr and these bacterial GAPDH molecules appear to have a plasmin-binding ability. Even if the overall similarity is not so high, it is possible that some bacterial GAPDH molecules, which have a similar steric structure at the antibody-binding site, show cross-immunoreactivity to the anti-NAPlr antibody.

It has become evident that bacterial infections are more deeply involved in various renal diseases, including IRGN, than we previously considered. Although the development of noninvasive techniques to detect infections with high sensitivity and high specificity is undoubtedly crucial, the identification of bacterial proteins associated with the pathogenesis of IRGN is also an important ongoing effort. Thus, future studies evaluating the possibility of NAPlr and plasmin activity as common diagnostic biomarkers of bacterial IRGN are anticipated.

Author Contributions: Writing the manuscript draft: T.U.; manuscript revision: T.O. All authors have read and agreed to the published version of the manuscript.

Acknowledgments: We are grateful to Masayuki Fujino at the AIDS Research Center, National Institute of Infectious Diseases, for performing the database searches regarding amino acids and nucleotide sequences of bacterial GAPDH, and to Nobuyuki Yoshizawa at the Hemodialysis Unit, Showanomori Hospital, for his valuable advice and discussions.

Conflicts of Interest: The authors declare no conflict of interest.

References

1. Prasad, N.; Patel, M.R. Infection-Induced Kidney Diseases. *Front. Med.* **2018**, *5*, 327. [CrossRef] [PubMed]
2. Oda, T.; Yoshizawa, N.; Yamakami, K.; Sakurai, Y.; Takechi, H.; Yamamoto, K.; Oshima, N.; Kumagai, H. The role of nephritis-associated plasmin receptor (NAPlr) in glomerulonephritis associated with streptococcal infection. *J. Biomed. Biotechnol.* **2012**, *2012*, 417675. [CrossRef] [PubMed]
3. Soderholm, A.T.; Barnett, T.C.; Sweet, M.J.; Walker, M.J. Group A streptococcal pharyngitis: Immune responses involved in bacterial clearance and GAS-associated immunopathologies. *J. Leukoc. Biol.* **2018**, *103*, 193–213. [CrossRef] [PubMed]

4. Satoskar, A.A.; Parikh, S.V.; Nadasdy, T. Epidemiology, pathogenesis, treatment and outcomes of infection-associated glomerulonephritis. *Nat. Rev. Nephrol.* **2020**, *16*, 32–50. [CrossRef]
5. Nasr, S.H.; Radhakrishnan, J.; D'Agati, V.D. Bacterial infection-related glomerulonephritis in adults. *Kidney Int.* **2013**, *83*, 792–803. [CrossRef]
6. Usui, J.; Tawara-Iida, T.; Takada, K.; Ebihara, I.; Ueda, A.; Iwabuchi, S.; Ishizu, T.; Iitsuka, T.; Takemura, K.; Kawamura, T.; et al. Temporal Changes in Post-Infectious Glomerulonephritis in Japan (1976–2009). *PLoS ONE* **2016**, *11*, e0157356. [CrossRef]
7. Nasr, S.H.; Fidler, M.E.; Valeri, A.M.; Cornell, L.D.; Sethi, S.; Zoller, A.; Stokes, M.B.; Markowitz, G.S.; D'Agati, V.D. Postinfectious glomerulonephritis in the elderly. *J. Am. Soc. Nephrol.* **2011**, *22*, 187–195. [CrossRef]
8. Yoshizawa, N.; Yamakami, K.; Fujino, M.; Oda, T.; Tamura, K.; Matsumoto, K.; Sugisaki, T.; Boyle, M.D. Nephritis-associated plasmin receptor and acute poststreptococcal glomerulonephritis: Characterization of the antigen and associated immune response. *J. Am. Soc. Nephrol.* **2004**, *15*, 1785–1793. [CrossRef]
9. Oda, T.; Yamakami, K.; Omasu, F.; Suzuki, S.; Miura, S.; Sugisaki, T.; Yoshizawa, N. Glomerular plasmin-like activity in relation to nephritis-associated plasmin receptor in acute poststreptococcal glomerulonephritis. *J. Am. Soc. Nephrol.* **2005**, *16*, 247–254. [CrossRef]
10. Butera, G.; Mullappilly, N.; Masetto, F.; Palmieri, M.; Scupoli, M.T.; Pacchiana, R.; Donadelli, M. Regulation of Autophagy by Nuclear GAPDH and Its Aggregates in Cancer and Neurodegenerative Disorders. *Int. J. Mol. Sci.* **2019**, *20*, 2062. [CrossRef]
11. Terao, Y.; Yamaguchi, M.; Hamada, S.; Kawabata, S. Multifunctional glyceraldehyde-3-phosphate dehydrogenase of Streptococcus pyogenes is essential for evasion from neutrophils. *J. Biol. Chem.* **2006**, *281*, 14215–14223. [CrossRef] [PubMed]
12. Bergmann, S.; Rohde, M.; Hammerschmidt, S. Glyceraldehyde-3-phosphate dehydrogenase of Streptococcus pneumoniae is a surface-displayed plasminogen-binding protein. *Infect. Immun.* **2004**, *72*, 2416–2419. [CrossRef] [PubMed]
13. Oda, T.; Yoshizawa, N.; Yamakami, K.; Tamura, K.; Kuroki, A.; Sugisaki, T.; Sawanobori, E.; Higashida, K.; Ohtomo, Y.; Hotta, O.; et al. Localization of nephritis-associated plasmin receptor in acute poststreptococcal glomerulonephritis. *Hum. Pathol.* **2010**, *41*, 1276–1285. [CrossRef]
14. Rodriguez-Iturbe, B.; Batsford, S. Pathogenesis of poststreptococcal glomerulonephritis a century after Clemens von Pirquet. *Kidney Int.* **2007**, *71*, 1094–1104. [CrossRef]
15. Fujino, M.; Yamakami, K.; Oda, T.; Omasu, F.; Murai, T.; Yoshizawa, N. Sequence and expression of NAPlr is conserved among group A streptococci isolated from patients with acute poststreptococcal glomerulonephritis (APSGN) and non-APSGN. *J. Nephrol.* **2007**, *20*, 364–369. [PubMed]
16. Gopalakrishnan, N.; Jeyachandran, D.; Abeesh, P.; Dineshkumar, T.; Kurien, A.A.; Sakthirajan, R.; Balasubramaniyan, T. Infection-related glomerulonephritis in a renal allograft. *Saudi J. Kidney Dis. Transplant.* **2017**, *28*, 1421–1426.
17. Bullen, A.; Shah, M.M. De Novo Postinfectious Glomerulonephritis Secondary to Nephritogenic Streptococci as the Cause of Transplant Acute Kidney Injury: A Case Report and Review of the Literature. *Case Rep. Transplant.* **2018**, *2018*, 2695178. [CrossRef]
18. Sawanobori, E.; Umino, A.; Kanai, H.; Matsushita, K.; Iwasa, S.; Kitamura, H.; Oda, T.; Yoshizawa, N.; Sugita, K.; Higashida, K. A prolonged course of Group A streptococcus-associated nephritis: A mild case of dense deposit disease (DDD)? *Clin. Nephrol.* **2009**, *71*, 703–707. [CrossRef]
19. Suga, K.; Kondo, S.; Matsuura, S.; Kinoshita, Y.; Kitano, E.; Hatanaka, M.; Kitamura, H.; Hidaka, Y.; Oda, T.; Kagami, S. A case of dense deposit disease associated with a group A streptococcal infection without the involvement of C3NeF or complement factor H deficiency. *Pediatric Nephrol.* **2010**, *25*, 1547–1550. [CrossRef]
20. Yamakami, K.; Yoshizawa, N.; Wakabayashi, K.; Takeuchi, A.; Tadakuma, T.; Boyle, M.D. The potential role for nephritis-associated plasmin receptor in acute poststreptococcal glomerulonephritis. *Methods* **2000**, *21*, 185–197. [CrossRef]
21. Okabe, M.; Tsuboi, N.; Yokoo, T.; Miyazaki, Y.; Utsunomiya, Y.; Hosoya, T. A case of idiopathic membranoproliferative glomerulonephritis with a transient glomerular deposition of nephritis-associated plasmin receptor antigen. *Clin. Exp. Nephrol.* **2012**, *16*, 337–341. [CrossRef] [PubMed]
22. Kohatsu, K.; Suzuki, T.; Yazawa, M.; Yahagi, K.; Ichikawa, D.; Koike, J.; Oda, T.; Shibagaki, Y. Granulomatosis With Polyangiitis Induced by Infection. *Kidney Int. Rep.* **2019**, *4*, 341–345. [CrossRef] [PubMed]

23. Yano, K.; Suzuki, H.; Oda, T.; Ueda, Y.; Tsukamoto, T.; Muso, E. Crescentic poststreptococcal acute glomerulonephritis accompanied by small vessel vasculitis: Case report of an elderly male. *BMC Nephrol.* **2019**, *20*, 471. [CrossRef] [PubMed]
24. Kikuchi, Y.; Yoshizawa, N.; Oda, T.; Imakiire, T.; Suzuki, S.; Miura, S. Streptococcal origin of a case of Henoch-Schoenlein purpura nephritis. *Clin. Nephrol.* **2006**, *65*, 124–128. [CrossRef] [PubMed]
25. Iseri, K.; Iyoda, M.; Yamamoto, Y.; Kobayashi, N.; Oda, T.; Yamaguchi, Y.; Shibata, T. Streptococcal Infection-related Nephritis (SIRN) Manifesting Membranoproliferative Glomerulonephritis Type I. *Intern. Med.* **2016**, *55*, 647–650. [CrossRef]
26. Prasto, J.; Kaplan, B.S.; Russo, P.; Chan, E.; Smith, R.J.; Meyers, K.E. Streptococcal infection as possible trigger for dense deposit disease (C3 glomerulopathy). *Eur J. Pediatrics* **2014**, *173*, 767–772. [CrossRef]
27. Fremeaux-Bacchi, V.; Weiss, L.; Demouchy, C.; May, A.; Palomera, S.; Kazatchkine, M.D. Hypocomplementaemia of poststreptococcal acute glomerulonephritis is associated with C3 nephritic factor (C3NeF) IgG autoantibody activity. *Nephrol. Dial. Transplant.* **1994**, *9*, 1747–1750.
28. Odaka, J.; Kanai, T.; Ito, T.; Saito, T.; Aoyagi, J.; Betsui, H.; Oda, T.; Ueda, Y.; Yamagata, T. A case of post-pneumococcal acute glomerulonephritis with glomerular depositions of nephritis-associated plasmin receptor. *CEN Case Rep.* **2015**, *4*, 112–116. [CrossRef]
29. Komaru, Y.; Ishioka, K.; Oda, T.; Ohtake, T.; Kobayashi, S. Nephritis-associated plasmin receptor (NAPlr) positive glomerulonephritis caused by Aggregatibacter actinomycetemcomitans bacteremia: A case report. *Clin. Nephrol.* **2018**, *90*, 155–160. [CrossRef]
30. Hirano, D.; Oda, T.; Ito, A.; Yamada, A.; Kakegawa, D.; Miwa, S.; Umeda, C.; Takemasa, Y.; Tokunaga, A.; Wajima, T.; et al. Glyceraldehyde-3-phosphate dehydrogenase of Mycoplasma pneumoniae induces infection-related glomerulonephritis. *Clin. Nephrol.* **2019**, *92*, 263–272. [CrossRef]
31. Grundel, A.; Pfeiffer, M.; Jacobs, E.; Dumke, R. Network of Surface-Displayed Glycolytic Enzymes in Mycoplasma pneumoniae and Their Interactions with Human Plasminogen. *Infect. Immun.* **2015**, *84*, 666–676. [CrossRef] [PubMed]
32. Modun, B.; Williams, P. The staphylococcal transferrin-binding protein is a cell wall glyceraldehyde-3-phosphate dehydrogenase. *Infect. Immun.* **1999**, *67*, 1086–1092. [CrossRef] [PubMed]
33. Takehara, E.; Mandai, S.; Shikuma, S.; Akita, W.; Chiga, M.; Mori, T.; Oda, T.; Kuwahara, M.; Uchida, S. Post-infectious Proliferative Glomerulonephritis with Monoclonal Immunoglobulin G Deposits Associated with Complement Factor H Mutation. *Intern. Med.* **2017**, *56*, 811–817. [CrossRef] [PubMed]
34. Okabe, M.; Takamura, T.; Tajiri, A.; Tsuboi, N.; Ishikawa, M.; Ogura, M.; Ohashi, R.; Oda, T.; Yokoo, T. A case of infection-related glomerulonephritis with massive eosinophilic infiltration. *Clin. Nephrol.* **2018**, *90*, 142–147. [CrossRef] [PubMed]
35. Ando, F.; Sohara, E.; Ito, E.; Okado, T.; Rai, T.; Uchida, S.; Sasaki, S. Acute poststreptococcal glomerulonephritis with acute interstitial nephritis related to streptococcal pyrogenic exotoxin B. *Clin. Kidney J.* **2013**, *6*, 347–348. [CrossRef]
36. Chang, J.F.; Peng, Y.S.; Tsai, C.C.; Hsu, M.S.; Lai, C.F. A possible rare cause of renal failure in streptococcal infection. *Nephrol. Dial. Transplant.* **2011**, *26*, 368–371. [CrossRef]
37. Uchida, T.; Oda, T.; Takechi, H.; Matsubara, H.; Watanabe, A.; Yamamoto, K.; Oshima, N.; Sakurai, Y.; Kono, T.; Shimazaki, H.; et al. Role of tubulointerstitial plasmin in the progression of IgA nephropathy. *J. Nephrol.* **2016**, *29*, 53–62. [CrossRef]
38. Yoshida, M.; Yamakawa, H.; Yabe, M.; Ishikawa, T.; Takagi, M.; Matsumoto, K.; Hamaguchi, A.; Ogura, M.; Kuwano, K. Diffuse alveolar hemorrhage in a patient with acute poststreptococcal glomerulonephritis caused by impetigo. *Intern. Med.* **2015**, *54*, 961–964. [CrossRef]

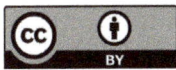 © 2020 by the authors. Licensee MDPI, Basel, Switzerland. This article is an open access article distributed under the terms and conditions of the Creative Commons Attribution (CC BY) license (http://creativecommons.org/licenses/by/4.0/).

MDPI
St. Alban-Anlage 66
4052 Basel
Switzerland
Tel. +41 61 683 77 34
Fax +41 61 302 89 18
www.mdpi.com

International Journal of Molecular Sciences Editorial Office
E-mail: ijms@mdpi.com
www.mdpi.com/journal/ijms

www.ingramcontent.com/pod-product-compliance
Lightning Source LLC
LaVergne TN
LVHW070508100526
838202LV00014B/1816